Breast Imaging Essentials

Niketa Chotai • Supriya Kulkarni

Breast Imaging Essentials

Case Based Review

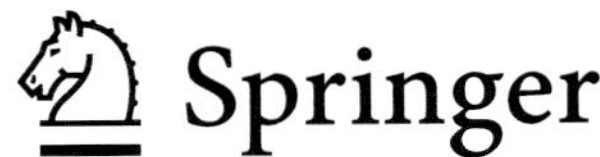

Niketa Chotai
Consultant Breast Radiologist, RadLink
Diagnostic Centre
Visiting Consultant, Tan Tock Seng
Hospital
Singapore

Supriya Kulkarni
Associate Professor
University of Toronto Staff Radiologist
Breast Imaging, Joint Department
of Medical Imaging
University Health Network. Mount Sinai
Hospital. Women's College Hospital
Toronto
ON
Canada

ISBN 978-981-15-1414-2 ISBN 978-981-15-1412-8 (eBook)
https://doi.org/10.1007/978-981-15-1412-8

This Springer imprint is published by the registered company Springer Nature Singapore Pte Ltd.
The registered company address is: 152 Beach Road, #21-01/04 Gateway East, Singapore 189721, Singapore

Preface

Breast imaging has rapidly evolved into a comprehensive multimodality science with increasing impact on interdisciplinary patient management and follow-up. Great strides in technology are enabling the detection of smaller node negative cancers in women. In the era of personalized medicine, the ability to detect smaller cancers allows for better targeting of biologically driven minimally invasive therapies.

The goal of this case review series is to allow a keen student to get an overview of breast imaging and the pertinent aspects of its impact on management. It will also serve as a quick reference guide in the reading room to ensure that the user addresses all points that can guide appropriate workup and thereby impact management.

The book is divided broadly into two parts. Part I provides a broad description of the basic concepts of breast imaging modalities explained in a simple and tangible manner, along with the technical and regulatory aspects. Appropriate illustrations and cases highlight the discussions. Part II brings forth the intricacies arising from the clinical and imaging appearances through a case-based discussion in a question-answer format. This design would help prospective students to prepare for exams/boards. It also prepares the reader for clinical practice by addressing the common differentials and recent advances in breast cancer management. The cases have been categorized based on imaging characteristics or disease groups with an emphasis on specific features, which allows for accurate diagnosis. Each case is followed by notes, highlighting the diagnosis, the possible differentials, and the management principles. Where appropriate, historical information has been included. The goal of the writing style was to avoid onerous discussions and to provide a quick and easy read to the students, young radiologists as well as multidisciplinary practitioners dealing with breast diseases. These are exciting times of rapid technological advancements that are changing the way we manage breast diseases, and we hope to inspire the reader to further pursue the fulfilling field of breast imaging and breast care across the continents.

Writing this book together in different time zones was a unique experience and a testament to how technology has changed the face of communication and education.

We believe that this book will upgrade the reader's understanding of breast care and, in turn, contribute towards our common goal of improving patient care.

Singapore
Toronto, ON, Canada
May 2019

Niketa Chotai
Supriya Kulkarni

Acknowledgments

The material in this book is a summation of my years of learning from various sources. I would like to thank my teachers who have guided me over the years. Deep acknowledgement to my numerous colleagues and students for their invigorating discussions and curiosity that helped me dig deeper and refine my understanding of the subject. I am grateful to my colleague Dr. Ashish Chawla, who inspired me to pen my passion for teaching through this book. I am delighted to acknowledge my publisher, Springer Nature, for making the publication process enjoyable.

My deepest regard and acknowledgment to my co-author Dr. Supriya Kulkarni for enthusiastically accepting the challenging task of co-writing the book with me, despite our 12-h time zone difference.

Needless to say, this work would not have been possible without the constant encouragement and loving support of my family and friends (countless of them). I dedicate this work to you who are the living force behind my very existence.

Niketa Chotai

I would like to dedicate this book to my late mother who was always my inspiration and guiding force. It was her desire that motivated me to document my experience by writing this textbook which hopefully will be one of many. A special thank you to my husband (Shashank) and son (Mukunda) whose incredible selfless support made this possible. To my father, who has always been my pillar of support and care, I offer my gratitude.

Supriya Kulkarni

Special acknowledgement to Dr. Tanvi Jakhi, MD for her excellent and colourful illustrations and artwork depicted in the book.

Contents

About the Authors

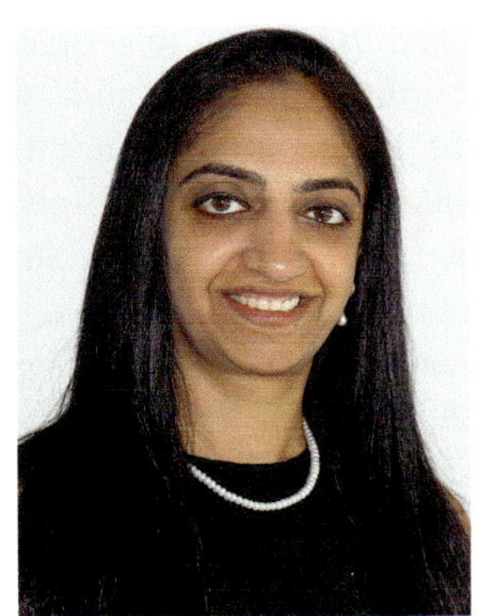

Niketa Chotai, MBBS, MD, DNB, FRCR, FUOT is a consultant radiologist at RadLink Diagnostic Imaging Center and a Visiting Consultant at Tan Tock Seng Hospital, Singapore. Over the past decade, she has been practicing as a breast radiologist. After graduating as an MD (Radiodiagnosis) from King Edward Memorial Hospital, Mumbai University, and as a Diplomate National Board, Delhi, India, she practiced as a consultant radiologist for 5 years in India. She then pursued her FRCR from Royal College of Radiology, UK, and subsequently completed advanced specialist training (AST) from Singapore. Thereafter, she continued her learning journey as a breast imaging fellow at the University of Toronto, Canada.

Dr. Chotai is a registered member of several societies, including the Singapore Medical Council, the Royal College of Radiology, London, and the Maharashtra Medical Council, India. She was in charge of continued medical education activities for the breast subsection of the Singapore Radiology Society from 2015–2017 and is currently acting as the General Secretary for the period 2017–2019. She is actively involved in various research activities and has published in numerous peer-reviewed journals. Dr. Chotai is as passionate about teaching as she is about learning. Over the past few years, she has run courses and workshops on breast imaging and intervention in South Asia. This book is an extension of her passion for sharing her knowledge and growing the breast care community for a healthier world.

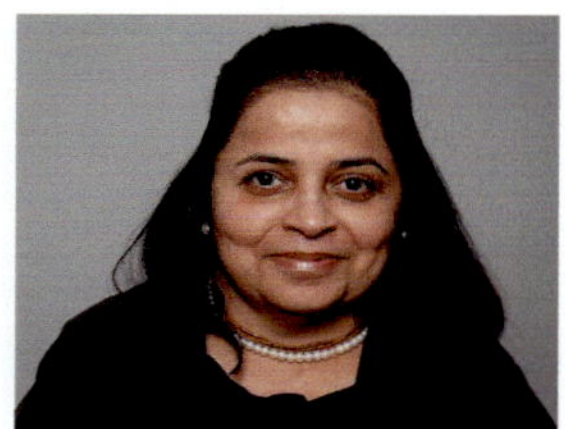

Supriya Kulkarni, MBBS, DMRD, DNB, DABR is a staff radiologist at the Joint Department of Medical Imaging (JDMI) at University Health Network, Mount Sinai Hospital, and the Women's College Hospital, Toronto, Canada. As faculty in the Department of Medical Imaging, University of Toronto, she has over 19 years of experience in the subspecialty practice in breast imaging.

After completing radiology training at the University of Pune and National Board Delhi, India, she pursued fellowship training in pediatric imaging in Melbourne, Australia, and in women's imaging at the University of Toronto following which she was recruited as a subspecialist breast imager at JDMI and as associate professor at the University of Toronto.

Dr. Kulkarni's special focus is on teaching and education internationally and currently manages educational activities for the breast division including CMEs, workshops, and the Women's & Breast Imaging Fellowship Programme (University of Toronto).

She is a recipient of several teaching awards including the prestigious Wightman-Berris Academy individual postgraduate teaching award (2014–2015) and the Outstanding Contribution to Cancer Education Award awarded by the Princess Margaret Cancer Education Program 2017.

She is involved in an advisory capacity for multiple initiatives of the Cancer Care Ontario and the provincial Ontario Breast Screening Program and has served as a Chair of the OBSP Screening of Transgender People Working Group at the Cancer Care Ontario. She is a member of the working group for the breast screening guidelines for the Canadian Association of Radiologists.

Abbreviations

2D	Two dimension
ABUS	Automated breast ultrasound
ACR	American College of Radiology
ADC	Apparent diffusion coefficient
ADH	Atypical ductal hyperplasia
ALH	Atypical lobular hyperplasia
AXLN	Axillary lymph node
BCS	Breast conservation surgery
BCT	Breast conservation treatment
BI-RADS	Breast imaging reporting and data system
CAD	Computer-aided detection
CC	Craniocaudal view
CDR	Cancer detection rate
CESM	Contrast-enhanced spectral mammography
CR	Computerized radiography
DBT	Digital breast tomosynthesis
DCE	Dynamic contrast-enhanced magnetic resonance imaging
DCIS	Ductal carcinoma in situ
DWI	Diffusion weighted Images
EIC	Extensive intraductal component
ER	Estrogen receptor
FCC	Fibrocystic change
FFDM	Full-field digital mammography
HER2	Human epidermal growth receptor
HRT	Hormonal replacement therapy
IDC	Invasive ductal carcinoma
ILC	Invasive lobular carcinoma
IMC	Invasive mammary carcinoma
LABC	Locally advanced breast cancer
LCIS	Lobular carcinoma in situ
LIQ	Lower inner quadrant
LN	Lobular neoplasia
LOQ	Lower outer quadrant
MIP	Maximum intensity projection
MLO	Medio-lateral oblique view
MRI	Magnetic resonance imaging
NAC	Neoadjuvant chemotherapy

PABC	Pregnancy-associated breast cancer
PNL	Posterior nipple line
PR	Progesterone receptor
pCR	Pathological complete response
QC	Quality control
RS	Radial sclerosing lesion
RECIST	Response evaluation criteria in solid tumors
RT	Radiotherapy
TNBC	Triple negative breast cancer
SLNB	Sentinel lymph node biopsy
UIQ	Upper inner quadrant
UOQ	Upper outer quadrant
USG	Ultrasound

Part I

Basics of Breast Imaging

General Considerations in Breast Imaging

1

1.1 Anatomy

The breast is a superficially located structure enveloped between the superficial and the deep layer of fascia overlying the pectoralis muscle. Histologically, the breast consists of 15–20 lobes with lactiferous ducts converging on the nipple and variable amounts of ductal tissue, lobules, adipose tissue, and fibrous stroma. Each lobule consists of about 30 terminal ducts along with acini and surrounding stromal tissue. The extra and intralobular terminal ducts with the acini form the terminal duct lobular units (TDLUs). Thin fibrous bands called Cooper's ligaments anchor the breast within this envelope, posteriorly to the prepectoral facia and anteriorly to the skin. It is supplied by a network of blood vessels and lymphatics (Fig. 1.1).

1.2 Anatomy of Axillary Nodes (Figs. 1.2 and 1.3)

Management of axillary lymph nodes is critical in the locoregional control of breast cancer. The lymph node groups in the axilla are divided based on their position with respect to the pectoralis minor muscle (AJCC classification).

Level I (low axilla): These are the lymph nodes that lie lateral to the lateral border of pectoralis minor muscle.

Level II (mid axilla): These are the lymph nodes that lie between the medial and lateral borders of the pectoralis minor muscle. The interpectoral nodes (Rotter's) lymph nodes are also included in this group.

Level III (apical axilla): These are the lymph nodes that lie medial to the medial margin of the pectoralis minor muscle and inferior to the clavicle. They are also termed as apical or infraclavicular nodes. Metastases to these nodes confers worse prognosis. These nodes are separately identified and evaluated for microscopic evaluation due to their impact on prognosis and treatment.

Internal mammary (ipsilateral): The lymph nodes along the internal mammary vessels, in the intercostal spaces, along the edge of the sternum in the endo-thoracic fascia are termed as internal mammary nodes. Involvement of these nodes in breast cancer may need dedicated mention due to the need for inclusion in treatment planning.

Supraclavicular: These lymph nodes lie in the supraclavicular fossa, a triangle defined by the omohyoid muscle and tendon (lateral and superior border), the internal jugular vein (medial border), and the clavicle and subclavian vein (lower border). Adjacent lymph nodes outside of this triangle are considered to be lower cervical nodes (M1).

Intramammary: The lymph nodes that lie within the breast are termed as intramammary nodes and are considered part of axillary lymph nodes for purposes of categorization and staging.

N. Chotai, S. Kulkarni, *Breast Imaging Essentials*, https://doi.org/10.1007/978-981-15-1412-8_1

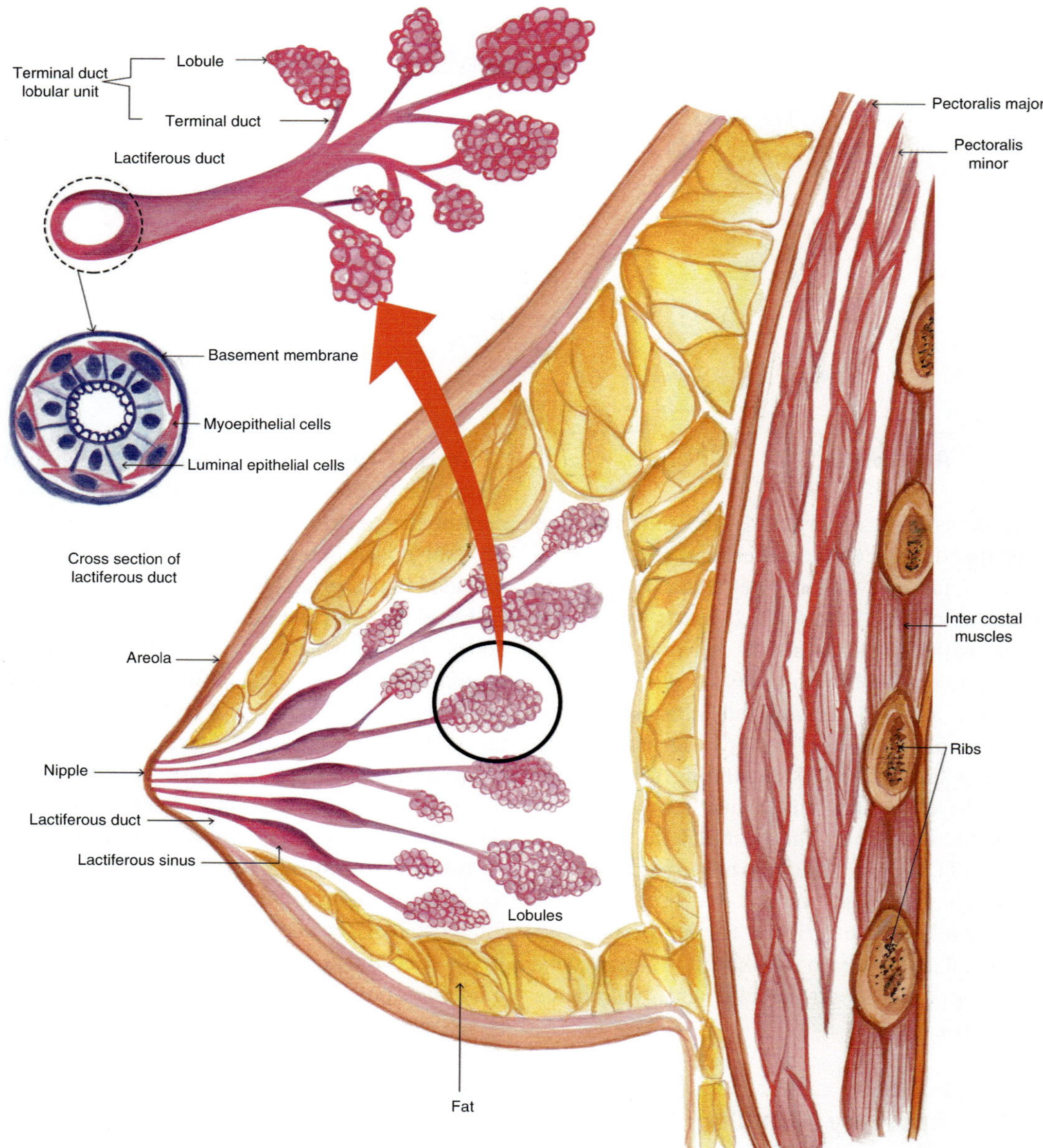

Fig. 1.1 Anatomy of breast showing relationship with chest wall, ribs, and fascia. Inset shows ducts with lobules and histology of duct in cross section

1.3 Scheduling

An individual may be referred to breast imaging for screening (asymptomatic) or diagnostic assessment (symptomatic). Breast assessment consists of a multimodality workup routinely using mammography, ultrasonography, and dynamic contrast-enhanced MRI (DCE). The fibroglandular tissue evolves throughout life in response to the hormonal fluctuations in the body (Estrogen & Progesterone). Monthly cyclical variations with the menstrual cycle can lead to a

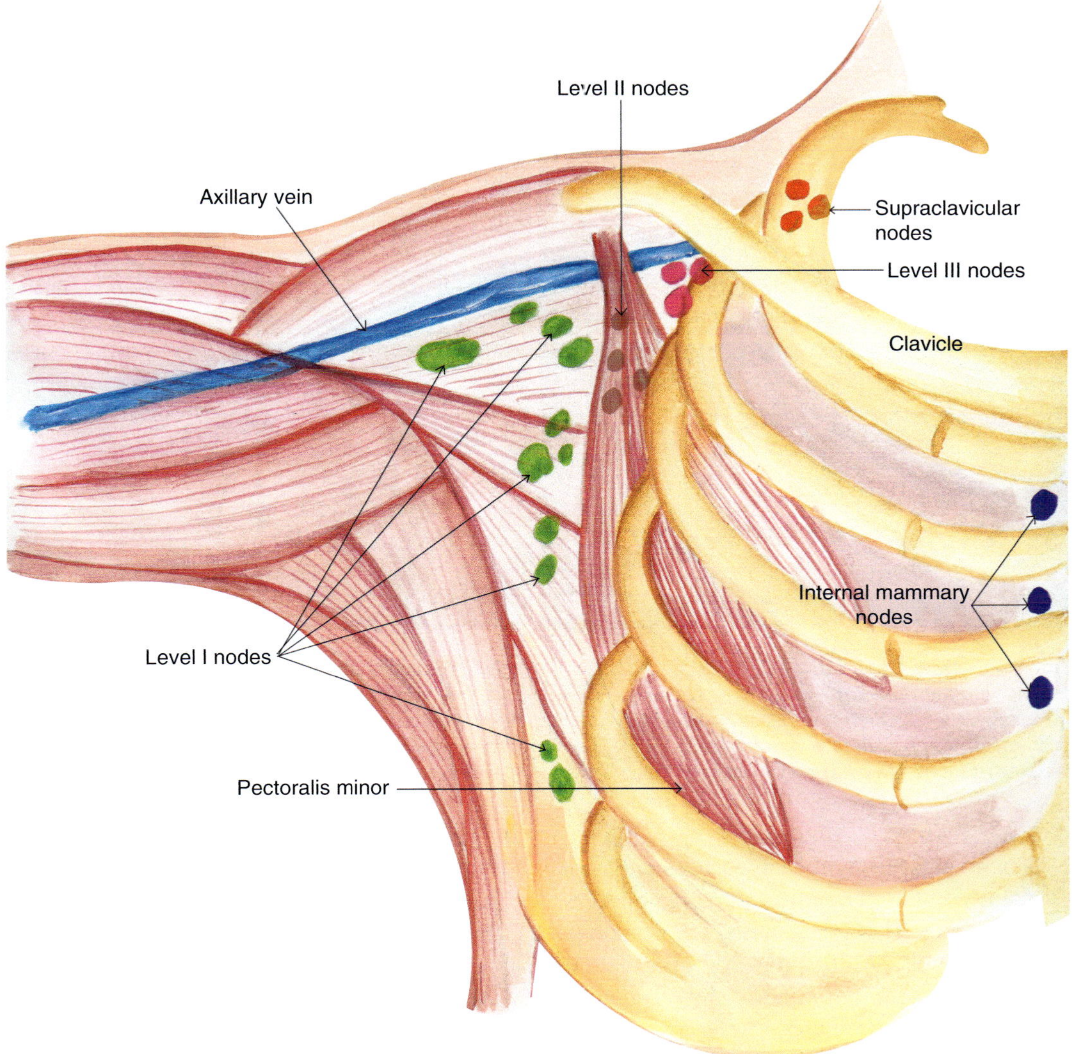

Fig. 1.2 Diagrammatic representation of the axillary lymph node anatomy (Coronal view): Low axillary level I lymph nodes (green) lateral to the pectoralis minor, mid axillary level II lymph nodes (brown) deep to the pectoralis minor, high axillary level III lymph nodes (pink) medial and superior to the pectoralis minor muscle, Internal mammary lymph nodes (purple), supraclavicular nodes (red)

wide variety of changes and water content within the breast; therefore scheduling of tests with respect to the menstrual cycle can be critical.

- **Screening mammogram:** Scheduling of screening mammography is generally not timed with the menstrual cycle, although there is some evidence in literature that it is best performed between the 7th to 16th day (follicular phase) of the menstrual cycle. This allows the breast to be captured in a phase with less interstitial fluid, thus allowing better compression (better quality & less density) and a less painful experience for the patient. Cells are also less susceptible to radiation damage in this phase, thus reducing radiation risk.
- **Diagnostic mammogram:** A diagnostic mammogram is performed at the time the

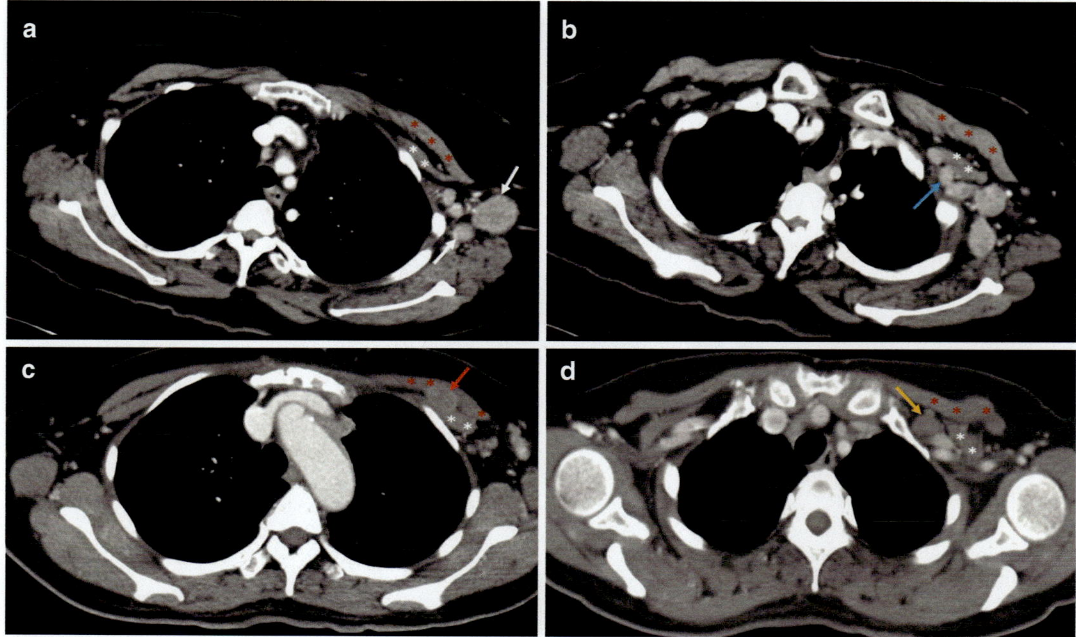

Fig. 1.3 Various level axial images of CT scan in a patient with known breast cancer and metastatic nodes. (**a**) Enlarged left axillary level I nodes (white arrow) are seen lateral to the pectoralis minor muscle (white asterisks). (**b**) Enlarged level II nodes are seen (blue arrow) behind the pectoralis minor muscle. (**c**) Enlarged Rotter's node (red arrow) is seen between the pectoralis major (red asterisks) and pectoralis minor (white asterisks) muscles. (**d**) Enlarged level III node (yellow arrow) is seen medial to the pectoralis minor muscle

patient presents with a breast-related complaint that requires mammographic assessment. This is not timed with the menstrual cycle. Additional work may include digital breast tomosynthesis and/or contrast-enhanced mammography.

- **Breast ultrasound:** Ultrasound is usually used as a diagnostic test and may be performed at any time of the menstrual cycle irrespective of the indication.
- **Dynamic contrast-enhanced magnetic resonance imaging (DCE-MRI):** Cyclical breast changes due to the menstrual cycle impacts background parenchymal enhancement on DCE. It is therefore best to time the DCE with the menstrual cycle to avoid nonspecific parenchymal enhancement, which can lead to false positives and unnecessary intervention. DCE is best performed in the window period between the 7th and the 13th day of the menstrual cycle, particularly in high-risk screening where patient population is younger (Fig. 1.4). Noncontrast breast MRI is only performed for the assessment of implants. For all other indications, intravenous contrast is necessary.

1.4 Patient History and Clinical Details

Breast imaging centers require patients to fill out standard questionnaires (Fig. 1.5 Questionnaire), which address relevant history, risk factors, and clinical symptoms which can affect interpretation of imaging findings and choosing the appropriate tests for the patient. This questionnaire also has a component of

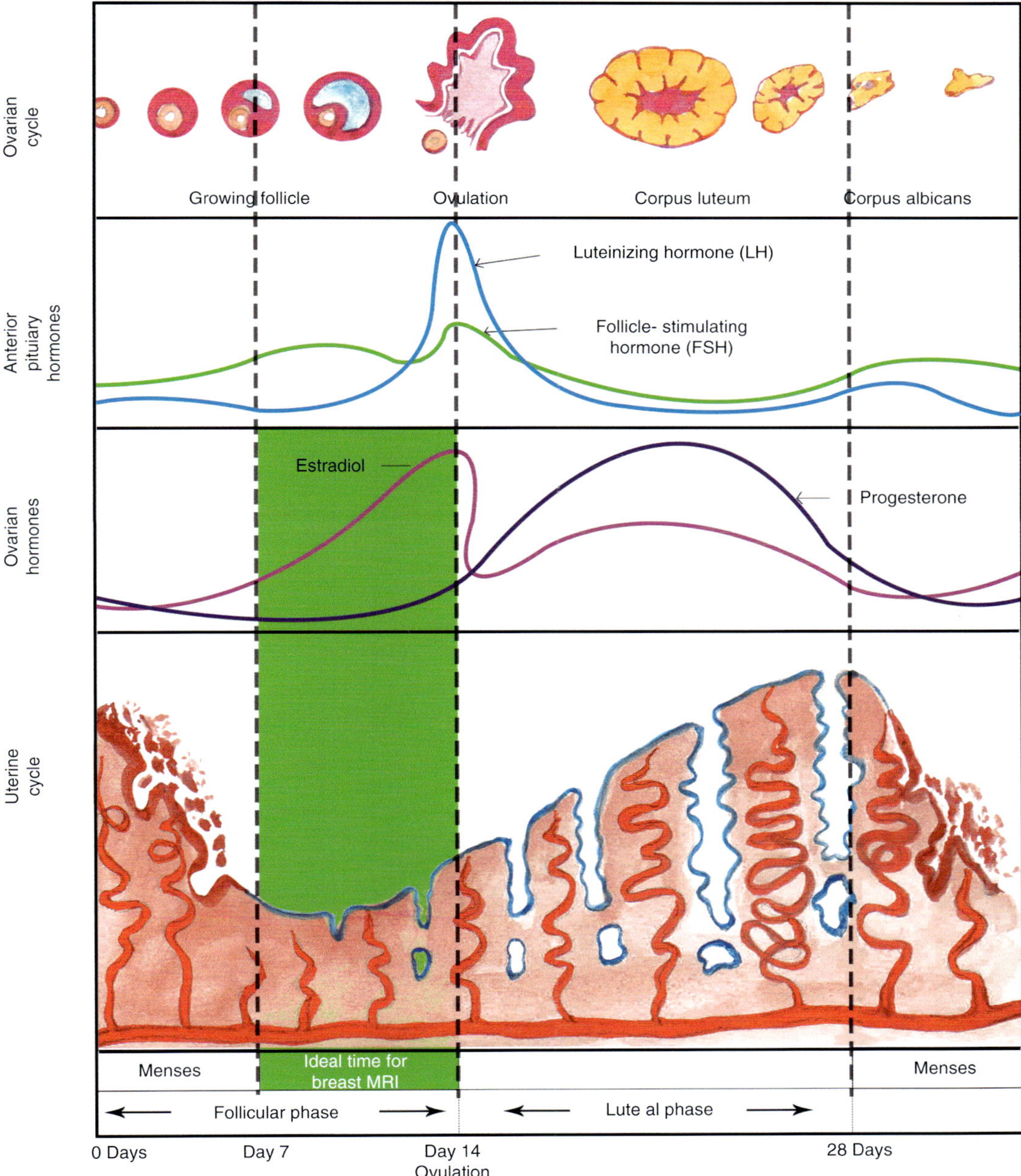

Fig. 1.4 Diagrammatic representation of the menstrual cycle with hormonal changes influencing the ovaries and uterus. The follicular phase (day 7–14) is the best time for breast MRI in premenopausal women (green box)

technical information filled out by the technologist performing the test, which also includes clinical findings noted by the technologists, such as skin discoloration, palpable findings, nipple discharge, nipple retraction, positions of scars, etc., at the time of the mammogram. This information is very useful during reporting of mammograms.

REG. NO : DATE :

NAME : AGE :

***IF YOU ARE PREGNANT OR THINK THAT YOU MAY BE PREGNANT,
PLEASE DISCUSS THIS WITH THE TECHNOLOGIST PRIOR TO THE EXAMINATION****

Previous mammogram : ☐ NO ☐ YES When / Where ________
Previous breast MRI : ☐ NO ☐ YES When / Where ________
Previous breast Ultrasound : ☐ NO ☐ YES When / Where ________

What Is The Reason For Undergoing This Examination?

a. This is a routine examination. I have no breast related complaints.
b. This is a short interval follow-up examination as advised on my previous study.
c. I have some breast related complaint(s)

New lump which can be felt : Right Left Both since
Pain in breast : Right Left Both since
Skin thickening : Right Left Both since
Nipple retraction : Right Left Both since
Nipple discharge : Right Left Both since
Colour of discharge : white/yellow/green/bloodstained
Lumps in the axilla : Right Left Both since

Menstrual Status And History:

When was your last menstrual period?
Are you currently taking Hormone replacement therapy : ☐ No ☐ YES (If yes for how long?)
Are you currently breastfeeding? : ☐ YES since ☐ NO
Have you given birth to children? : ☐ YES ☐ NO
Did you breastfeed? : ☐ YES ☐ NO

Family History

Family history of breast cancer : ☐ YES ☐ NO
☐ Mother at age ☐ Aunt at age ☐ Sister at age ☐ Daughter at age ☐ Grandmother at age
I have had a family member with ovarian cancer : ☐ Yes ☐ No
I have been tested for BRCA genetic mutation

BRCA 1 ☐ Positive ☐ Negative
BRCA 2 ☐ Positive ☐ Negative
I have had breast cancer : ☐ YES ☐ NO ☐ RIGHT ☐ LEFT

I Have Had:

Radiation : ☐ YES When ________ ☐ NO
Chemotherapy : ☐ YES When ________ ☐ NO
Tamoxifen/Arimidex : ☐ YES When ________ ☐ NO
Ovarian cancer : ☐ YES When ________ ☐ NO
Lymphoma : ☐ YES When ________ ☐ NO
Any other type of cancer : ☐ YES When ________ ☐ NO

Surgical History :
Right Breast :

Type of surgery ________ Date ________ Benign ________ Malignant

Left Breast :

Type of surgery ________ Date ________ Benign ________ Malignant
Breast augmentation : Date ________ Type of implant ________
Breast reduction : Date ________
Hysterectomy : ☐ YES ☐ NO When
Oophorectomy : ☐ YES ☐ NO When

Previous breast FNAC/Biopsy:

RIGHT : ☐ Benign ☐ Malignant When
LEFT : ☐ Benign ☐ Malignant When

History of weight loss / weight gain of more than 10 kgs in the past year ☐ YES ☐ NO

Fig. 1.5 Sample patient history questionnaire for a breast clinic

Suggested Readings

AJCC Cancer Staging Manual, Eighth Edition © The American College of Surgeons (ACS), Chicago, Illinois.

Myers ER, Moorman P, Gierisch JM, Havrilesky LJ, Grimm LJ, Ghate S, Davidson B, Montgomery RC, Crowley MJ, McCrory DC, Kendrick A. Benefits and harms of breast cancer screening: a systematic review. JAMA. 2015;314(15):1615–34.

Sardanelli F, Fallenberg EM, Clauser P, Trimboli RM, Camps-Herrero J, Helbich TH, Forrai G. European Society of Breast Imaging (EUSOBI). Mammography: an update of the EUSOBI recommendations on information for women. Insight Imag. 2017;8(1):11–8.

2 Mammography

Mammography may be performed either for screening or for diagnostic (problem-solving) indications. The sensitivity of mammography is approximately 85%, and it rapidly decreases as the breast density increases.

There are two limitations of mammography:

1. False positives: As mammography is a compression technique, there is tissue overlap, which can create artifactual findings leading to "recalls" and additional workup.
2. False negatives: Breast density reduces the sensitivity of mammography by masking (hiding) breast cancer, leading to false negatives. These cancers then may become clinically palpable and present as interval cancers.

These shortcomings, to a certain extent, are addressed by digital breast tomosynthesis (DBT) and adjunctive screening modalities, which will be discussed in the later chapters.

2.1 Mammographicy Technique

Film screen mammography (FSM) has almost been completely replaced by full field digital mammography (FFDM) which is now the standard of care in most countries. FFDM offers better windowing capabilities, contrast, image equalization, and storage.

The multicenter ACRIN DMIST trial in 2005 reported that the overall diagnostic accuracy for breast cancer detection is similar for film screen mammography and digital mammography, but in pre/perimenopausal women and dense breasts, digital mammography is found to be more accurate.

It is also noted that compared to screening with digital mammography, screening with computed radiography (CR) has shown reduced cancer detection (about 10 fewer cancers detected per 10,000 women screened) and its use has been discouraged across some screening programs (e.g., Ontario Breast Screening Program, Canada). CR systems also deliver a higher dose and have poorer image quality as compared to FFDM.

2.2 Quality Assurance in Mammography

Quality of mammography is very critical and entails maintaining quality of mammography equipment, which includes daily, weekly, quarterly, and semiannual quality control (QC) testing procedures and logs, radiation exposure monitoring, and quality of reporting. The responsibility of these lie with the radiologists, technologists, and the medical physicists. Each country has its own organization, which maintains quality assurance in mammography, such as the MQSA administered by the FDA in the United States.

N. Chotai, S. Kulkarni, *Breast Imaging Essentials*, https://doi.org/10.1007/978-981-15-1412-8_2

2.3 Positioning

Two standard views are usually obtained for each breast. These are the cranio-caudal (CC) and medio-lateral oblique (MLO) views. Breast being a skin appendage can be best pulled from the chest wall parallel to the pectoralis major muscle, hence the MLO view allows maximal visualization of the upper breast. Upper inner quadrant is relatively the most fixed region and masses in this area may not be visualized in either view. Nipple is the fixed point of reference.

2.4 Breast Compression

Mammography is a compression technique. Compression spreads out tissue and reduces overlap, reduces scatter, reduces radiation to patient, allows lower kVp, and improves contrast. It also fixes the breast tissue reducing motion blur and improving the image resolution.

2.5 Labeling

Mammograms have to be labeled with a permanent identification label, which includes the patient's demographic information, unique institutional patient identification number, and date of examination. It is mandatory to also record the side and the type of view to be included on the image.

2.6 Breast Composition

Variable proportion of fat and fibroglandular tissue gives four different breast compositions (Fig. 2.1). The ACR suggests the following categories, which should be mentioned in every report.

- Density "A" is entirely fatty breast tissue (Fig. 2.1a).
- Density "B" is scattered areas of fibroglandular density (Fig. 2.1b).

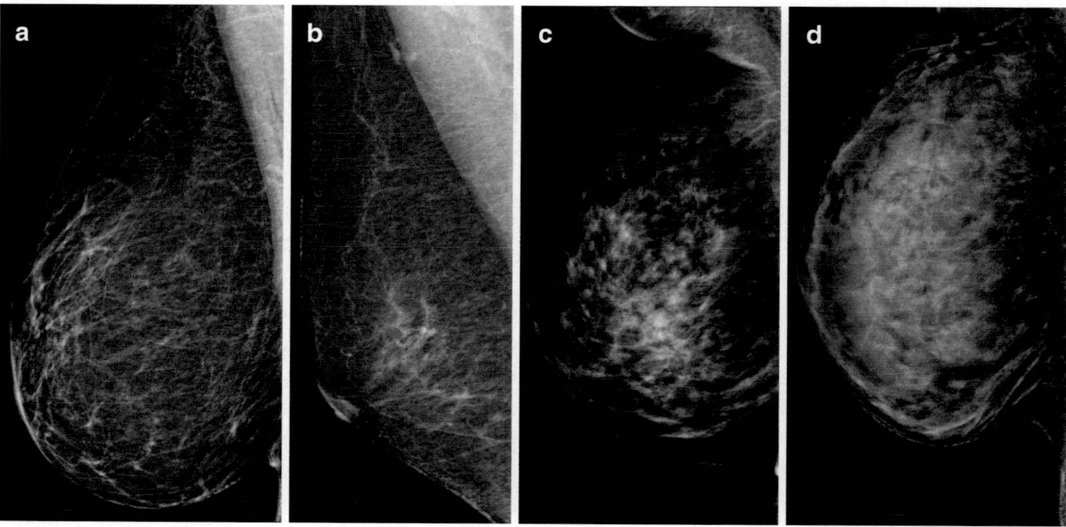

Fig. 2.1 Various breast densities: The mammogram images from left to right show increasing breast density from almost entirely fatty breast (density "A"), scattered fibroglandular parenchyma (density "B"), heterogeneously dense breast parenchyma (density "C"), and extremely dense breast (density "D")

- Density "C" is heterogeneously dense breast tissue that may obscure small masses (Fig. 2.1c).
- Density "D" is extremely dense breast tissue that reduces the sensitivity of the mammogram (Fig. 2.1d).

2.7 Assessing the Adequacy of Mammographic Views

It is important to detect poor positioning in mammographic view to avoid missing breast tissue which may harbor cancer. Things to ensure are:

On MLO view (Fig. 2.2):

- Margin of pectoralis should be convex towards the nipple.
- Inferior extent of the pectoralis muscle should reach at least to posterior nipple line (PNL) or below.
- Nipple should be in profile.
- Inframammary fold should be included.
- Skin folds should be avoided (in axillary region).

On CC view (Fig. 2.3):

- Nipple should be in midline to avoid extended view.
- Nipple should be in profile.
- The length of the PNL should be within 1 cm of length of PNL on the MLO view.
- Retromammary fat should be well included.
- The pectoralis muscle should be seen as far as possible (usually seen in 30% of cases).
- Skin folds should be avoided (laterally).

Lesion description (Lexicon): This is discussed in Chap. 8.

2.8 Approach to Reading a Mammogram

Mammography is about detecting change and hence it is very essential to have multiple prior comparisons before embarking to report. Reviewing the patient questionnaire and technologist documentation is important so that targeted attention can be given to the area of concern.

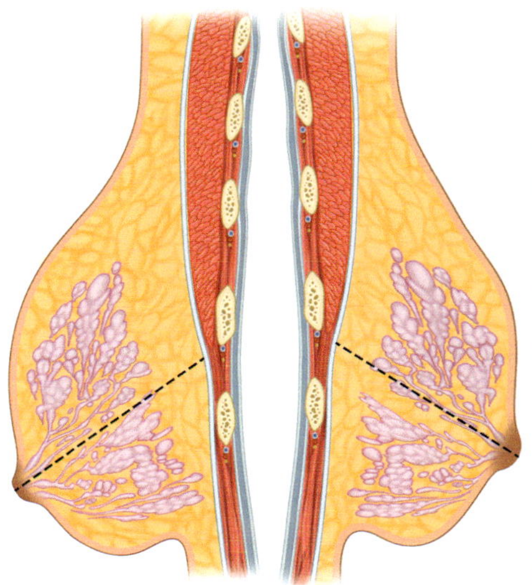

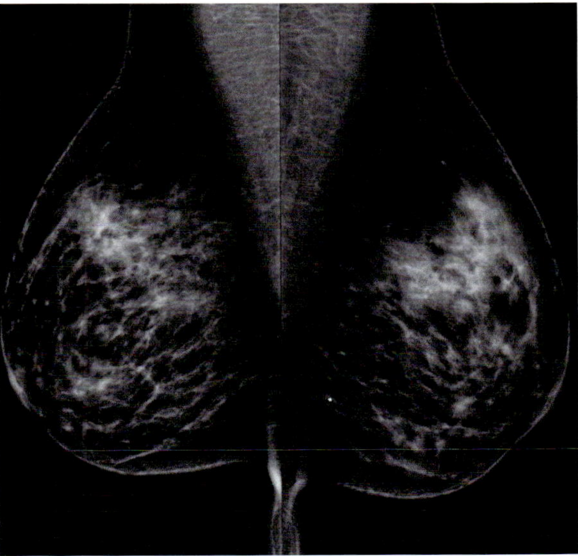

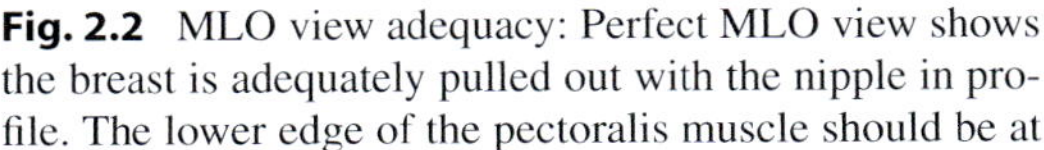

Fig. 2.2 MLO view adequacy: Perfect MLO view shows the breast is adequately pulled out with the nipple in profile. The lower edge of the pectoralis muscle should be at level of the PNL or below and the inframammary fold should be well included. The dotted line represents PNL (Posterior Nipple Line)

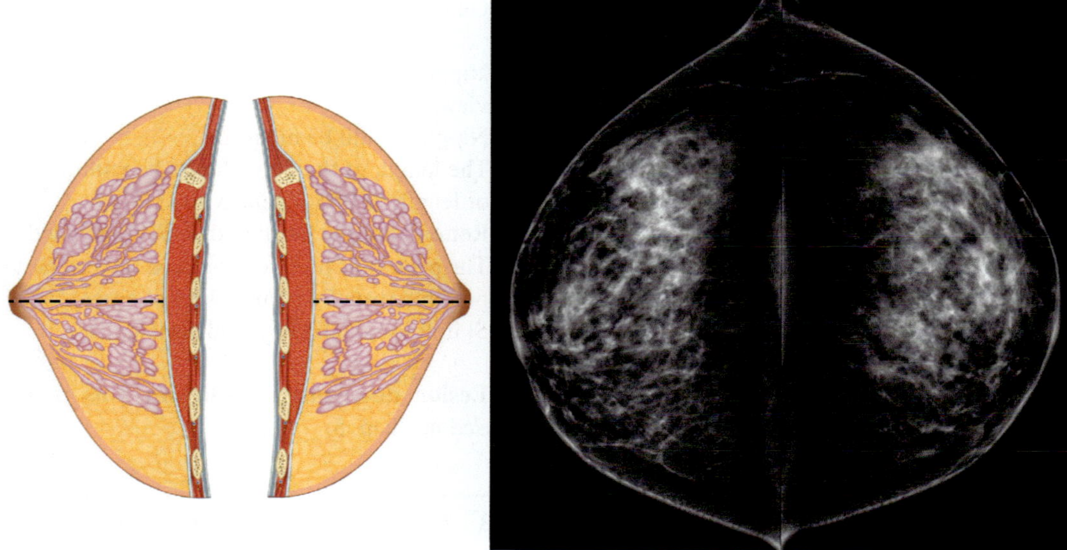

Fig. 2.3 CC view adequacy: Perfect CC view demonstrates maximum breast tissue with retromammary space and some pectoral muscle. Nipple should be in center and in profile. The length of the PNL on CC view must be within 1 cm of the length of the PNL on the MLO view

Reading a mammogram involves mainly detection of abnormality, localization of the abnormality, and sometimes triangulation.

- **Detection of abnormality:** Both breasts should be assessed simultaneously. Each radiologist may have his or her own hanging protocols to review different mammographic views, but the key is to have a side to side comparison and systematically go through each region of the breast. Special regions that may escape attention are the inframammary region, the retroareolar region, and accessory axillary breast tissue, and therefore a systematic approach is very important.
- **Location of abnormality (Figs. 2.4 and 2.5):** The radiologist must provide the location of the abnormality based on the standard mammographic views. On MLO projection, the breast above PNL represents the upper half of breast while the breast below PNL represents the lower half. On CC projection, the breast above PNL represents the outer half (lateral) while the breast below PNL represents the inner half (medial) of the breast. Sometimes additional views, such as a straight lateral view, may be required to determine the exact location of the lesion.
- **Triangulation (Fig. 2.6)**: Triangulation involves lining up the mammographic views from the largest angle (90°) to the lowest angle (0°) from left to right. The lateral view will determine where the lesion lies based on how it moves on the lateral view. "Muffins rise and lead falls" implying medial lesions move up on lateral view (Fig. 2.6a) while lateral lesions fall on lateral views (Fig. 2.6b). With increasing use of DBT, triangulation has become very easy and does not require complex calculations with additional views.

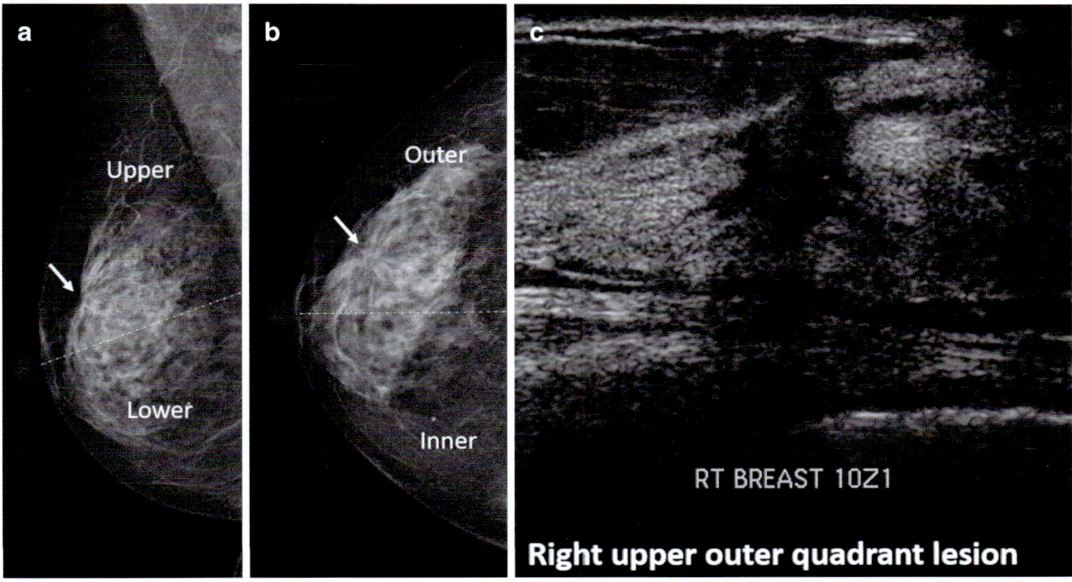

Fig. 2.4 The spiculated mass in upper half on MLO view (**a**) and in outer half on CC view (**b**) suggests that the mass is located in the upper outer quadrant of the right breast, between 9 and 12 o'clock. On ultrasound (**c**) the corresponding mass is seen at 10 o'clock

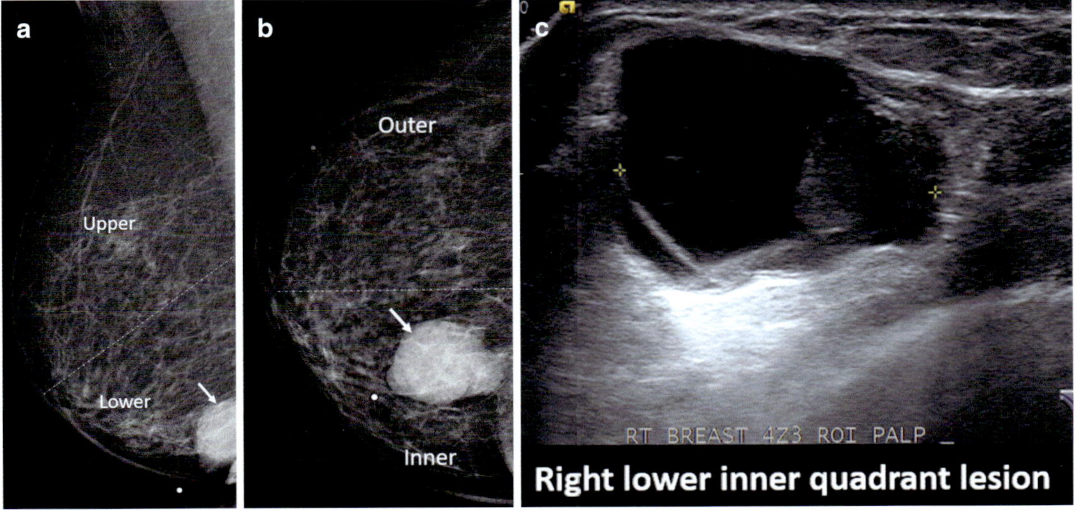

Fig. 2.5 A circumscribed, high-density mass in the lower half on MLO view (**a**) and in the inner half on CC view (**b**) suggests that the mass is located in the lower inner quadrant of the right breast, between 3 and 6 o'clock. On ultrasound (**c**) the corresponding mass is seen at 4 o'clock

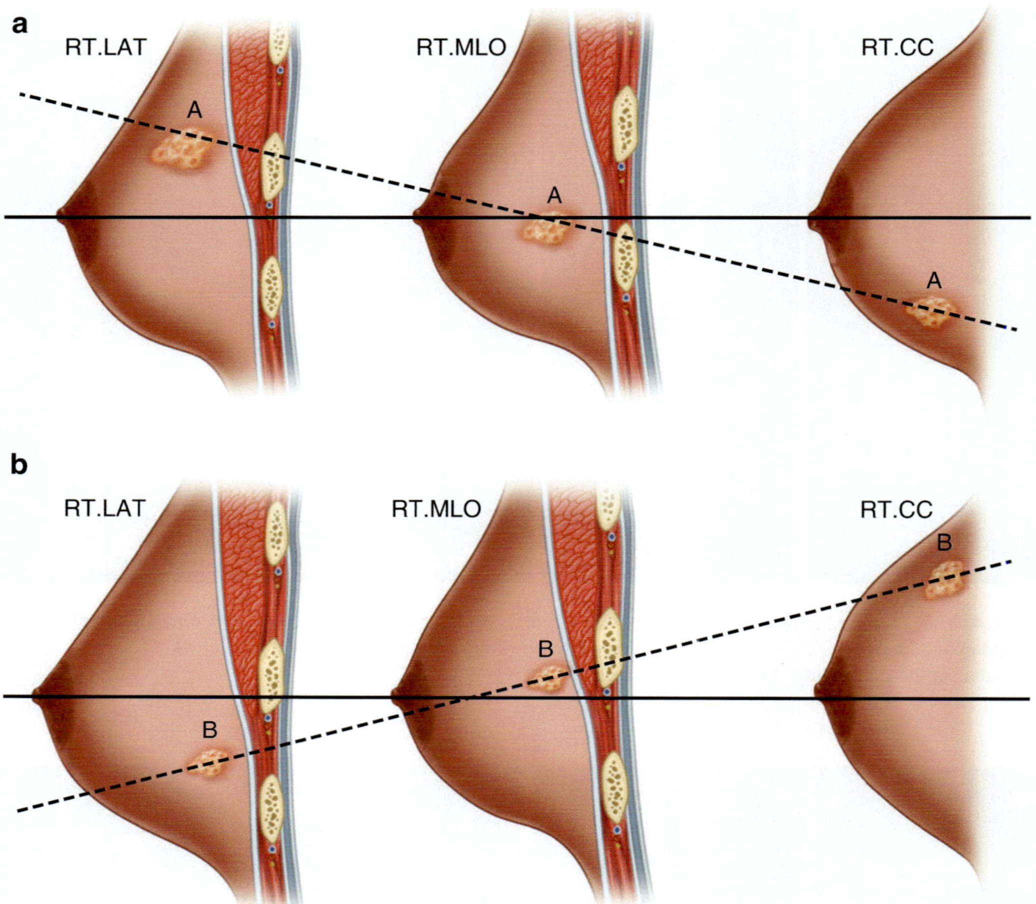

Fig. 2.6 Triangulation is performed by sequentially lining up the mammographic views from the highest degree of tube angulation to lowest, meaning lateral to MLO to CC views. (**a**) The medial lesion will move superiorly on the lateral view compared to the MLO view. (**b**) The lateral lesion will move inferiorly on the lateral view compared to the MLO view. The phrase "muffins rise and lead falls" helps to determine how the lesion moves on the lateral view based on its medial or lateral location

Suggested Readings

Chiarelli AM, Edwards SA, Prummel MV, Muradali D, Majpruz V, Done SJ, Brown P, Shumak RS, Yaffe MJ. Digital compared with screen-film mammography: performance measures in concurrent cohorts within an organized breast screening program. Radiology. 2013;268(3):684–93.

Pisano ED, Gatsonis C, Hendrick E, Yaffe M, Baum JK, Acharyya S, Conant EF, Fajardo LL, Bassett L, D'orsi C, Jong R. Diagnostic performance of digital versus film mammography for breast-cancer screening. N Engl J Med. 2005;353(17):1773–83.

3 Additional Views

Standard MLO and CC views may not be sufficient for confident diagnosis in all cases, and many times additional views are needed before a conclusion is made on mammographic studies (Fig. 3.1). Some common additional views are described below.

Spot compression views (SCV): When focal compression is used over a small area it is called

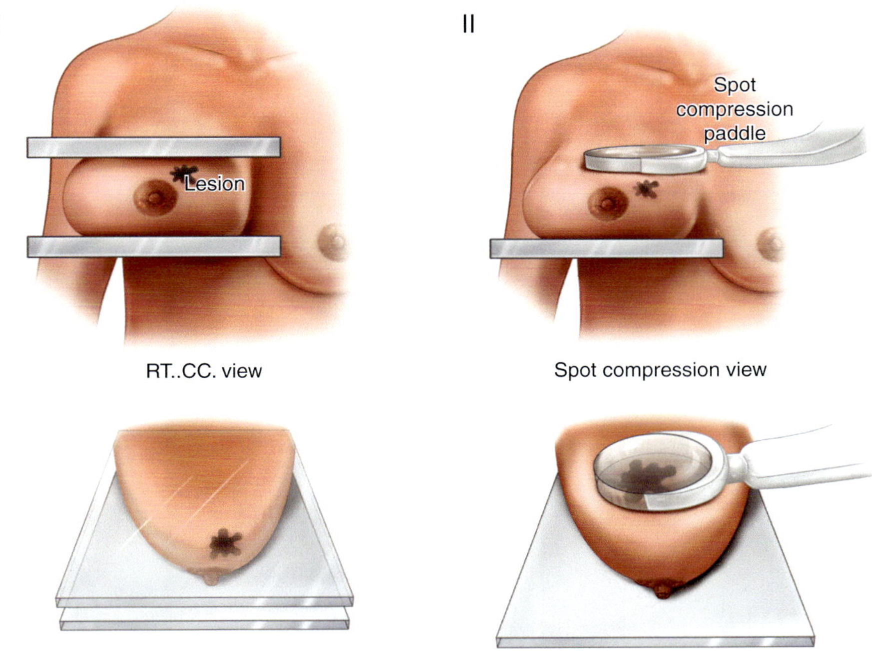

Fig. 3.1 Additional mammographic views: (*i*) Standard cranio-caudal view. Small irregular mass (black) in upper inner quadrant of right breast. (*ii*) Spot compression view: Focal compression to area of interest using compression paddle allows better visualization of the tissue in that area. (*iii*). Spot magnification view: additional view to evaluate and characterize microcalcifications. A magnification platform is used, which brings the breast away from the image receptor and closer to the X-ray source, thereby magnifying the area of interest

N. Chotai, S. Kulkarni, *Breast Imaging Essentials*, https://doi.org/10.1007/978-981-15-1412-8_3

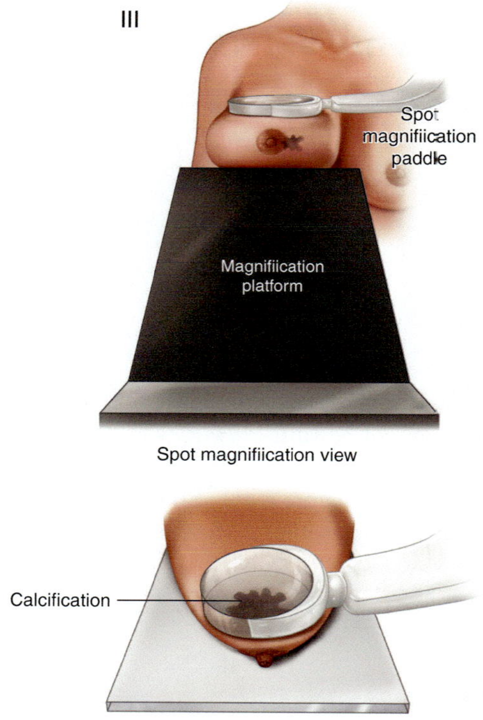

Fig. 3.1 (continued)

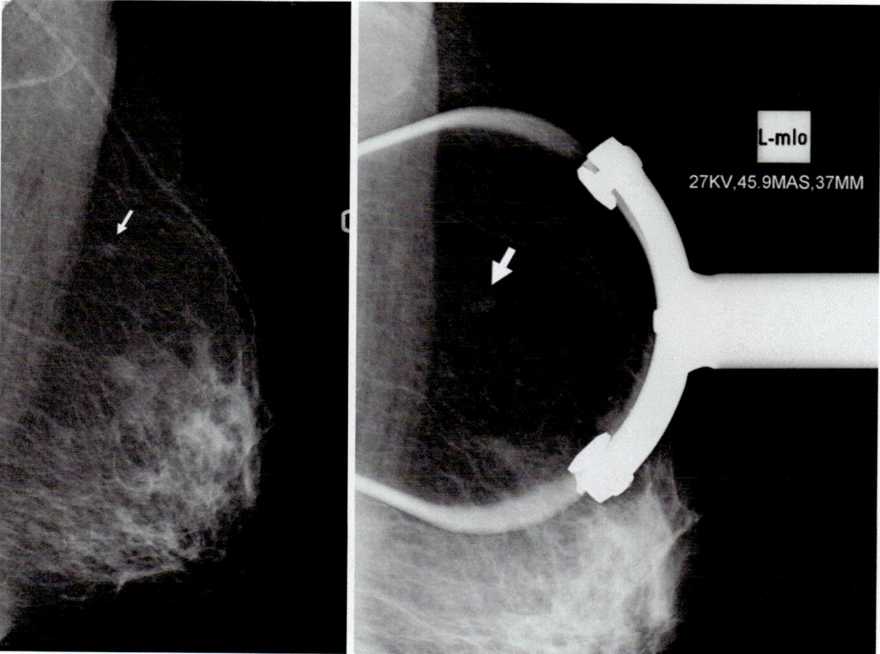

Fig. 3.2 Left MLO view shows a focal isodense asymmetry in the upper half of left breast (white arrow) in prepectoral fat. The asymmetry is persistent (thick white arrow) on spot compression view and likely represents a real lesion. There is no associated microcalcification in this asymmetry. This was later proven to be invasive breast carcinoma

a SCV. A smaller compression paddle is used over small regions of interest, allowing better tissue separation, reducing tissue overlap, and improving resolution. The improved resolution is due to the increased compression which reduces thickness in the examined area and thereby getting the suspicious area closer to the detector surface.

Role of SCV:

- Differentiate true lesion versus tissue overlap (summation) in cases where a focal asymmetry is detected on a mammogram (Fig. 3.2).
- Assessment of margins of a lesion that may have been detected on the mammogram.
- Improve visibility of architectural distortion.

Caveat: Small cancers can get obscured on SCV and may therefore be missed.

It has been shown that DBT negates the need to perform SCV due to its inherent ability to remove tissue overlap, increasing lesion conspicuity and enhancing visualization of architectural distortion.

Magnification (compression) views: Magnification views are used to better evaluate morphology and distribution of microcalcifications (Fig. 3.3). They also help in better lesion margin assessment.

Magnification views allow geometric magnification of small objects within the image. Small focal spot of 0.1–0.15 mm is used with breast compressed over a platform that increases the distance between the breast and the image receptor. This is called the "air gap technique" (Fig. 3.4). Along with narrow collimation, it reduces scatter, thereby allowing acquisition of high contrast magnification images.

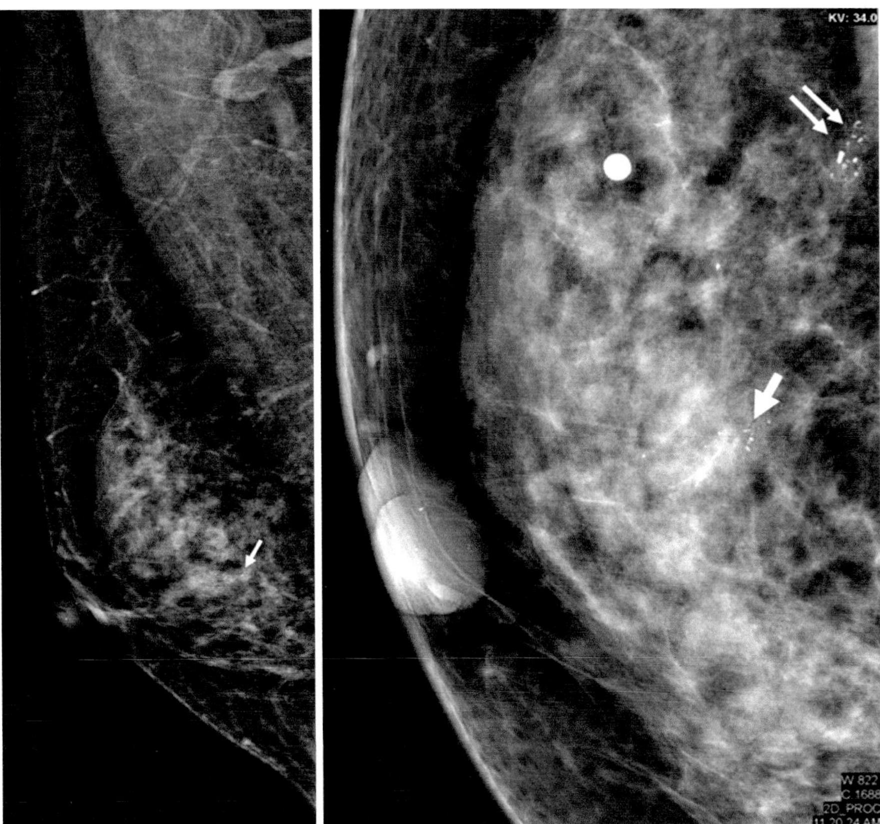

Fig. 3.3 Right MLO view shows a group of microcalcifications in the right central breast (white arrow). Magnified right MLO view shows two groups of coarse heterogeneous microcalcifications (thick white arrow and double white arrows) in the right breast. A few other scattered microcalcifications are also seen in the right breast. Please note that the morphology of microcalcifications is better appreciated on magnification views

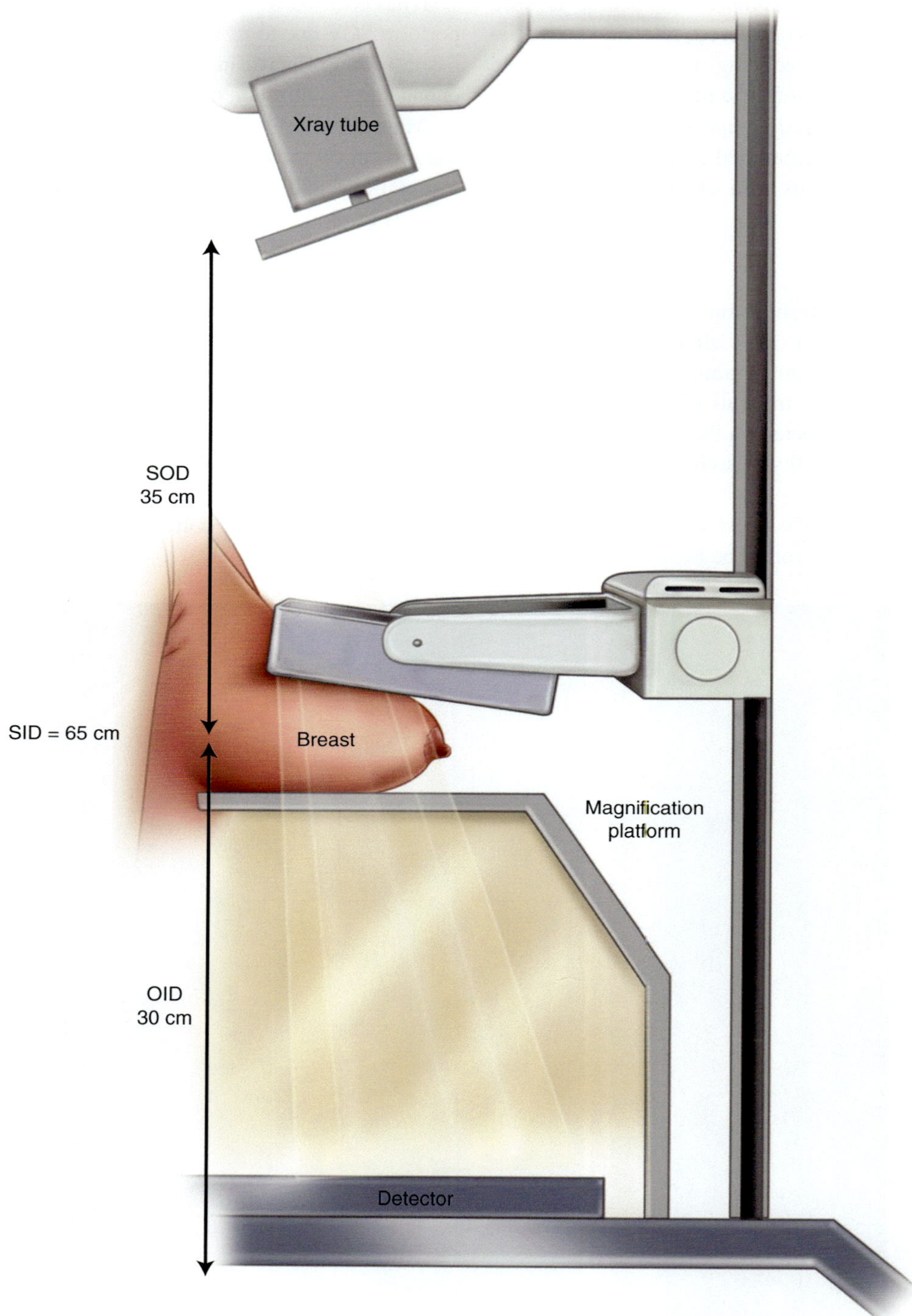

Fig. 3.4 Air gap technique: The addition of an air gap between the breast tissue and the image receptor created by using a magnification platform increases the object-image distance (OID) and reduces the source-object distance (SOD) allowing true geometric magnification of the targeted area. Source-image distance (SID) = OID + SOD

Implant displacement views (Eklund views): Augmented breasts are not completely assessed by two-view mammography. The implants often impede adequate compression, reducing lesion visibility and assessment. Therefore, such breasts are assessed with additional implant displacement views, depending on the mobility and location of the implant. These views are achieved by pushing the implants back and pulling the breast tissue anteriorly into compression (Fig. 3.5). Implant displacement views are easier to perform in retropectoral implants.

Rolled views: In women with uncertain densities/asymmetries, rolled views can unravel overlapping tissue, thus providing additional

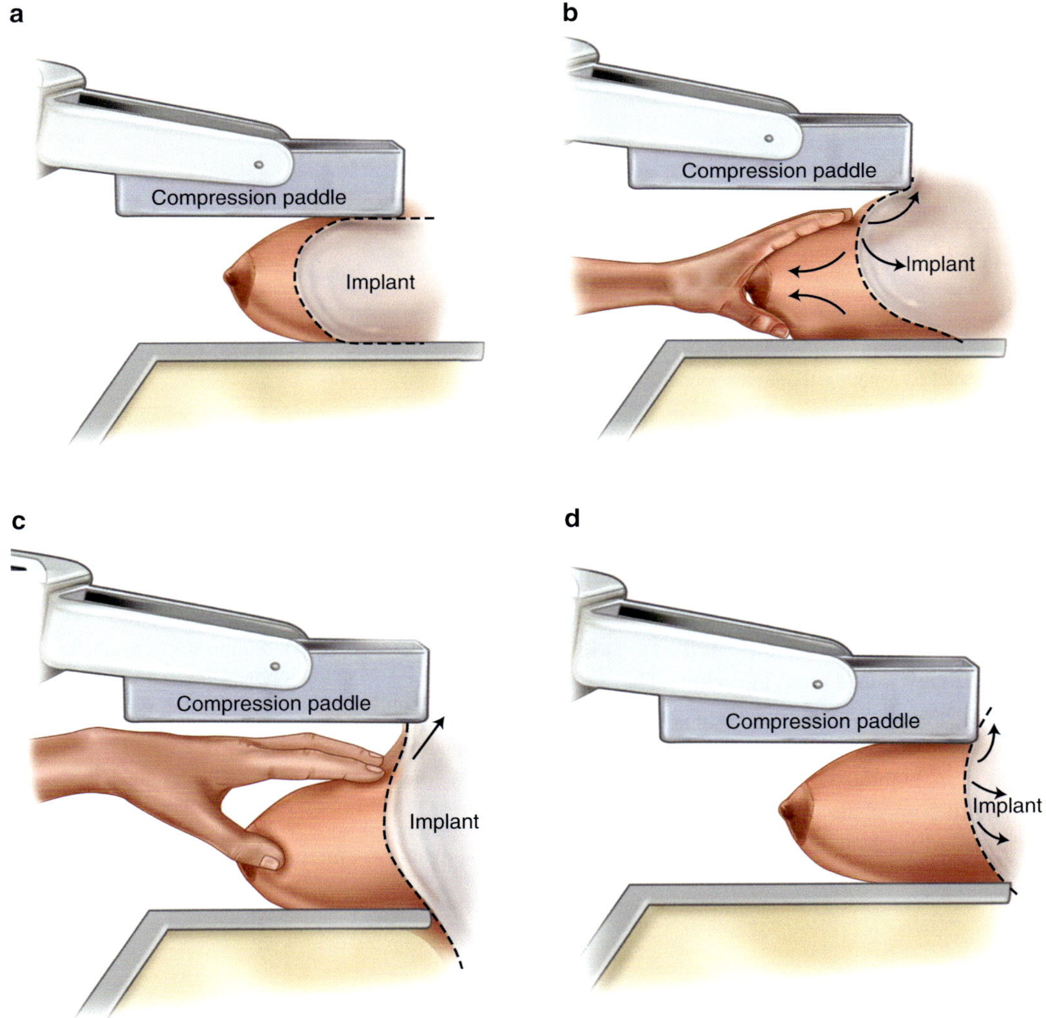

Fig. 3.5 Eklund view: Eklund modified compression technique is used for patients with augmented or reconstructed breasts. (**a**) Standard cranio-caudal compression view with implant obscuring adequate breast tissue visualization. (**b**, **c**) Posterosuperior displacement of the implants with simultaneous traction of the anterior breast. (**d**) Eklund view demonstrating displacement of the implant with greater visualization of the breast tissue

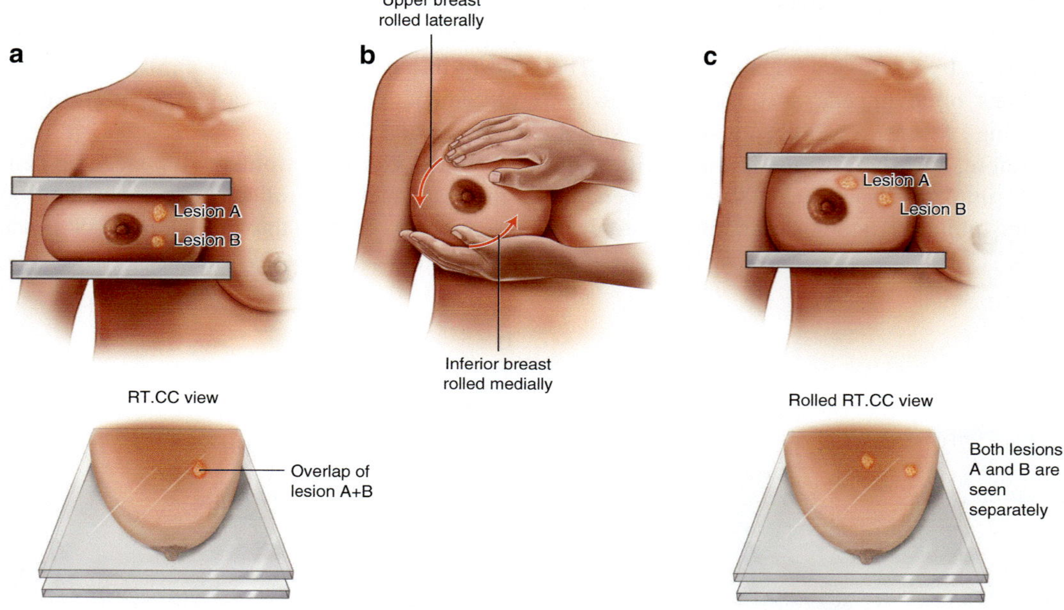

Fig. 3.6 Rolled view: (**a**) Craniocaudal view of right breast showing two superimposing lesions. (**b**) Rolled view performed by rotating the breast medially or laterally around the axis of the nipple. (**c**) The two lesions are now clearly discernible on the rolled CC view

information. These are most effective in the CC projection where the superior or inferior aspect of the breast can be rolled medially or laterally depending on where the lesion is lying in the breast (Fig. 3.6).

Extended lateral/medial, axillary view (Cleopatra view), and cleavage view: These are additional types of views used for assessment of specific areas of the breast, which may not be included on standard mammographic views either due to poor/challenging positioning or due to large size of the breast.

Suggested Readings

Eklund GW. The art of mammographic positioning. In: Radiological diagnosis of breast diseases. Berlin, Heidelberg: Springer; 2000. p. 75–88.

Funke M, Breiter N, Hermann KP, Oestmann JW, Grabbe E. Magnification survey and spot view mammography with a new microfocus X-ray unit: detail resolution and radiation exposure. Eur Radiol. 1998;8(3):386–90.

Hayes R, Michell M, Nunnerley HB. Evaluation of magnification and paddle compression techniques in the assessment of mammographic screening detected abnormalities. Clin Radiol. 1991;44(3):158–60.

4 Breast Ultrasound

Ultrasound is the most commonly used adjunctive modality to mammography. It may be used as the primary imaging modality for women younger than 30 years of age and in lactating/pregnant women. It is independent of breast density. In women more than 30 years of age, ultrasound and/or mammography may be used as the primary modality. Generally, handheld ultrasound with a high-frequency (about 10 MHz), linear array probe is used for breast ultrasound.

Depending on the indication, either a whole breast or targeted ultrasound may be performed.

Indications: There are multiple indications for breast ultrasound. Some of the common indications are enumerated below:

- To evaluate the palpable abnormality or to look for correlation for mammographic abnormality.
- To differentiate from cystic versus solid mass (Fig. 4.1).
- To characterize the features of the lesion like echogenicity, margins, vascularity, and elasticity that help to differentiate benign versus malignant lesions.
- Supplemental screening in dense breasts, especially in high-risk women who are unable to have DCE due to claustrophobia, pregnancy, or lactation.
- To check the extent of disease, e.g., to look for additional foci in breast cancer cases (staging).
- For axillary nodal staging.
- For ultrasound-guided interventions like biopsy, clip placements, and localizations.

Technique: The patient is positioned in an ipsilateral lateral oblique position with the arm raised above the head. Patient should be positioned such that the breast tissue is evenly spread over the chest wall. This allows complete systematic scanning in a clockwise manner from nipple to periphery or vice versa in a radial and antiradial plane (Fig. 4.2). The scanning may also be performed in the transverse and sagittal plane (Fig. 4.3). Depending on the size of the breast, positioning can be adjusted to allow proper scanning. Gentle pressure helps while scanning. Additional software enhancements such as compound imaging and harmonics help in improving image contrast and quality and removing some unnecessary artifacts. Color doppler and elastography can be used to enhance lesion assessment and provide a safe route for biopsy. Unfortunately, ultrasound is an operator-dependent technique, and training of ultrasound personnel can play an important role in the reproducibility and sensitivity of ultrasound. Poor technique reduces the sensitivity to detect lesion.

Labeling: As per the ACR practice guidelines for the performance of breast ultrasound (2011), the following need to be ensured:

- Ultrasound images must be labeled with a permanent identification label, which includes the patient's demographic information, unique

N. Chotai, S. Kulkarni, *Breast Imaging Essentials*, https://doi.org/10.1007/978-981-15-1412-8_4

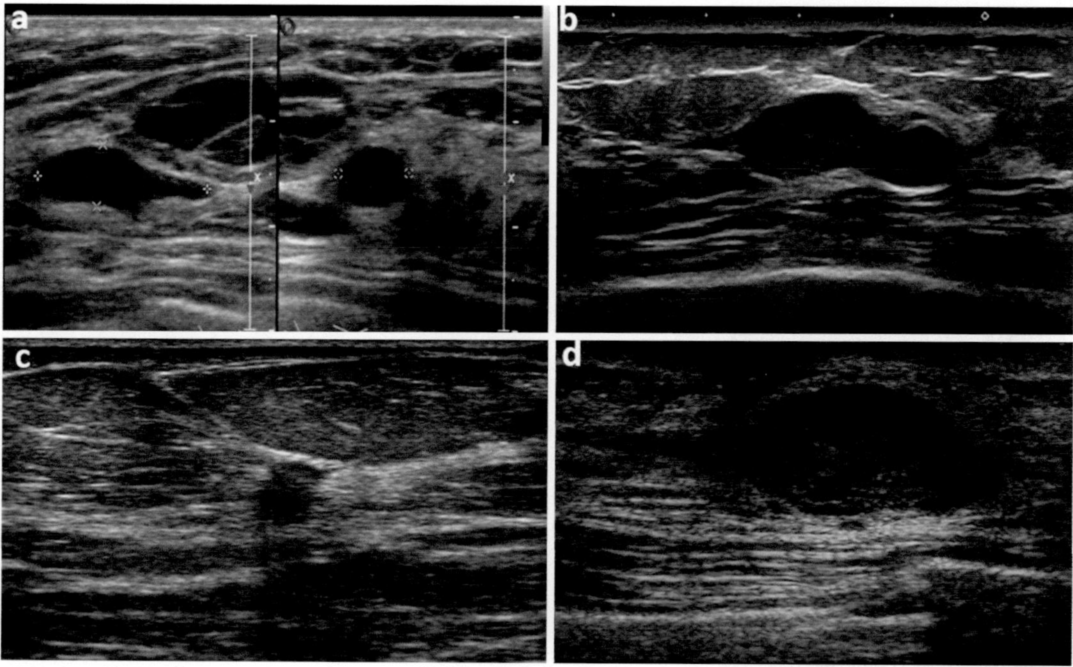

Fig. 4.1 Breast ultrasound: Image (**a**) shows an oval, circumscribed, anechoic lesion with posterior enhancement. This is a simple benign cyst. Image (**b**) shows an oval, circumscribed, hypoechoic lesion in parallel orientation. This lesion has benign imaging features and is a complicated cyst or benign solid breast nodule. Image (**c**) shows an irregular hypoechoic mass with angular margins and antiparallel orientation. Imaging features of this lesion are suspicious for breast cancer. Image (**d**) shows a complex cystic lesion with low-level echoes and mildly thickened posterior wall

institutional patient identification number, and date of examination.

- The breast (left or right) examined should be documented.
- The breast is represented by clock face with the nipple as the center. The anatomic location should be labelled in "o'clock position" and distance from nipple should be documented for each significant (reportable) finding. (Fig. 4.4).
- Position of the transducer (Transverse or Sagittal) should be documented.
- Sonographer or radiologist initials should be included on the image.
- Measurements should be obtained in three planes on a split screen.

Advantages of ultrasound: It is a widely available, easy to use, inexpensive modality that has no ionizing radiation. It is the preferred modality for guiding breast interventions due to easy availability and real-time capabilities.

Limitations:

- Handheld ultrasound is a time-consuming modality.
- It is an operator-dependent modality that requires training and skill.
- Ultrasound has been shown to have a high false positive rate, increasing the need for follow up and false positive biopsies.
- Microcalcifications are difficult to see on ultrasound.
- Posterior chest wall invasion may not be clearly depicted.

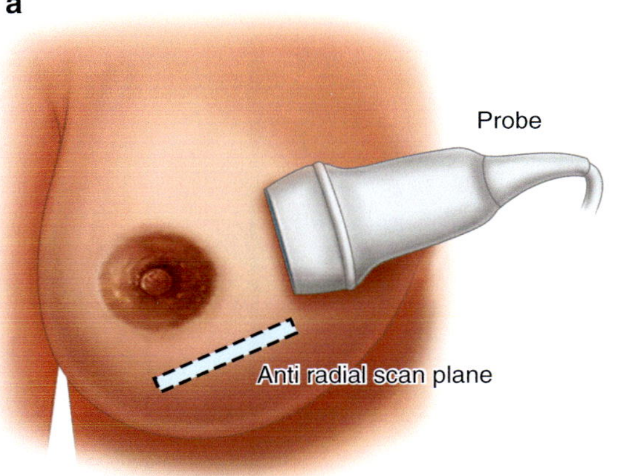

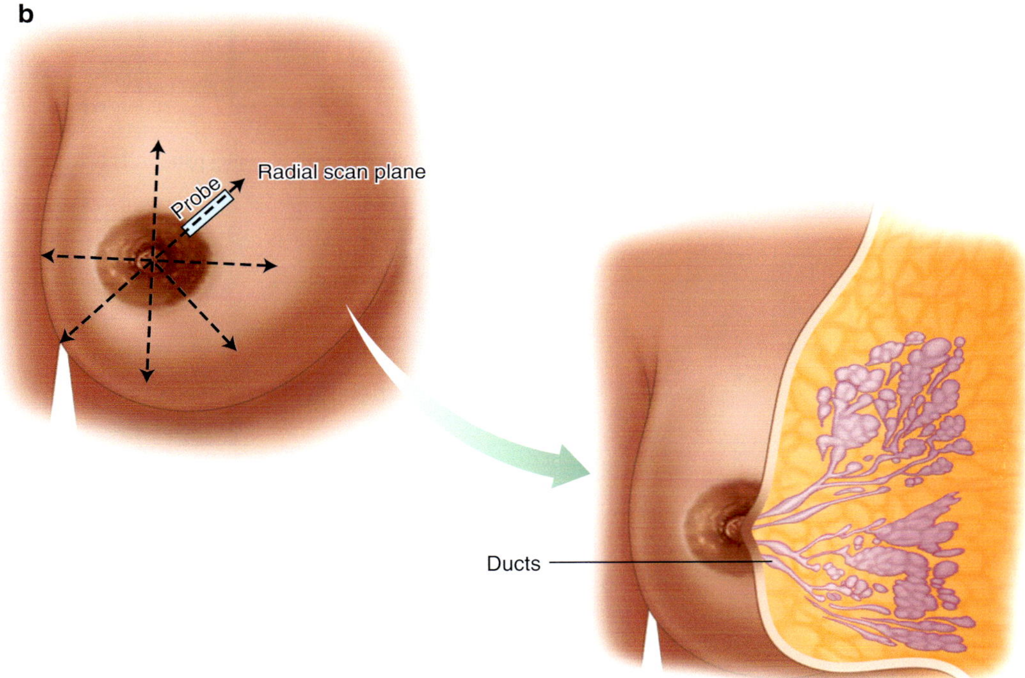

Fig. 4.2 Diagrammatic representation of the different planes of scanning. (**a**) Radial scan with the ultrasound probe parallel to the direction of the ducts (inset). (**b**) Anti-radial scan performed by rotating the probe 90°, i.e., perpendicular to the radial plane

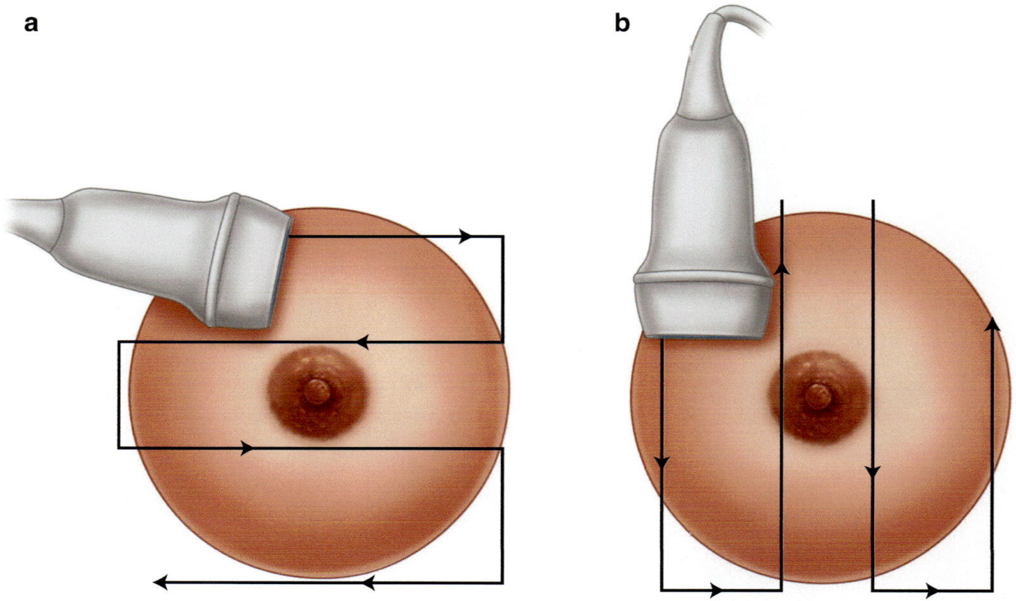

Fig. 4.3 Diagrammatic representation of the techniques of scanning using the grid scanning pattern. Transverse plane: Scan superior to inferior (**b**). Sagittal plane: Scan medial to lateral (**a**)

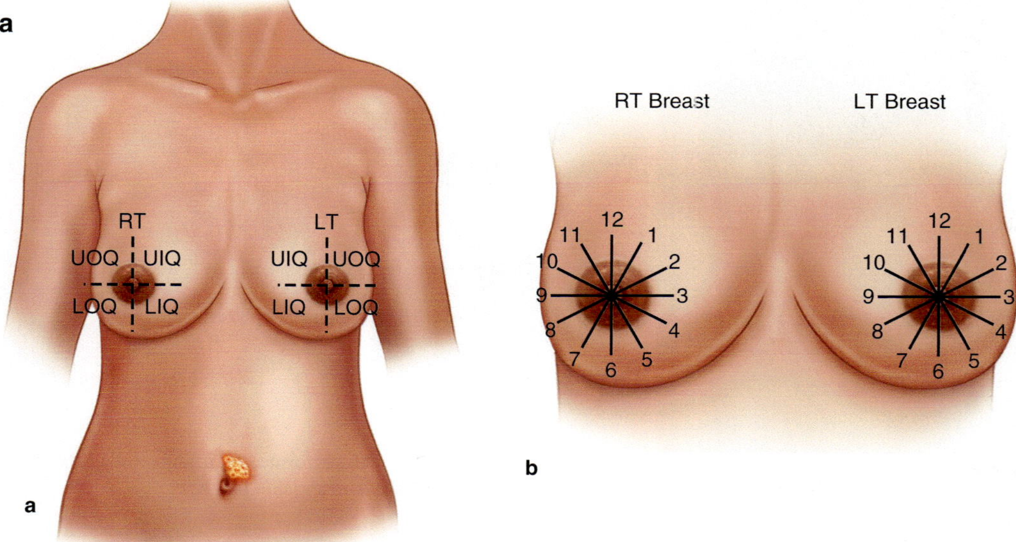

Fig. 4.4 (**a**) Diagrammatic representation of the clock-face position for breast ultrasound. (*a*) Coronal image showing quadrants of both breasts. (*b*) Coronal image of both breasts showing clock-face positions. (*c*) Corresponding locations on the CC view. (**b**) Diagrammatic representation using the ABC and 123 method for lesion location in addition to clock position. (*a*) Lesion A in the right breast at 12 o'clock, about 4 cm superior to the nipple and 1 cm deep is described as RT 12 2 A. (*b*) Lesion B in the right breast at 7 o'clock, about 6 cm from the nipple and 4 cm deep is described as RT 7 3 C

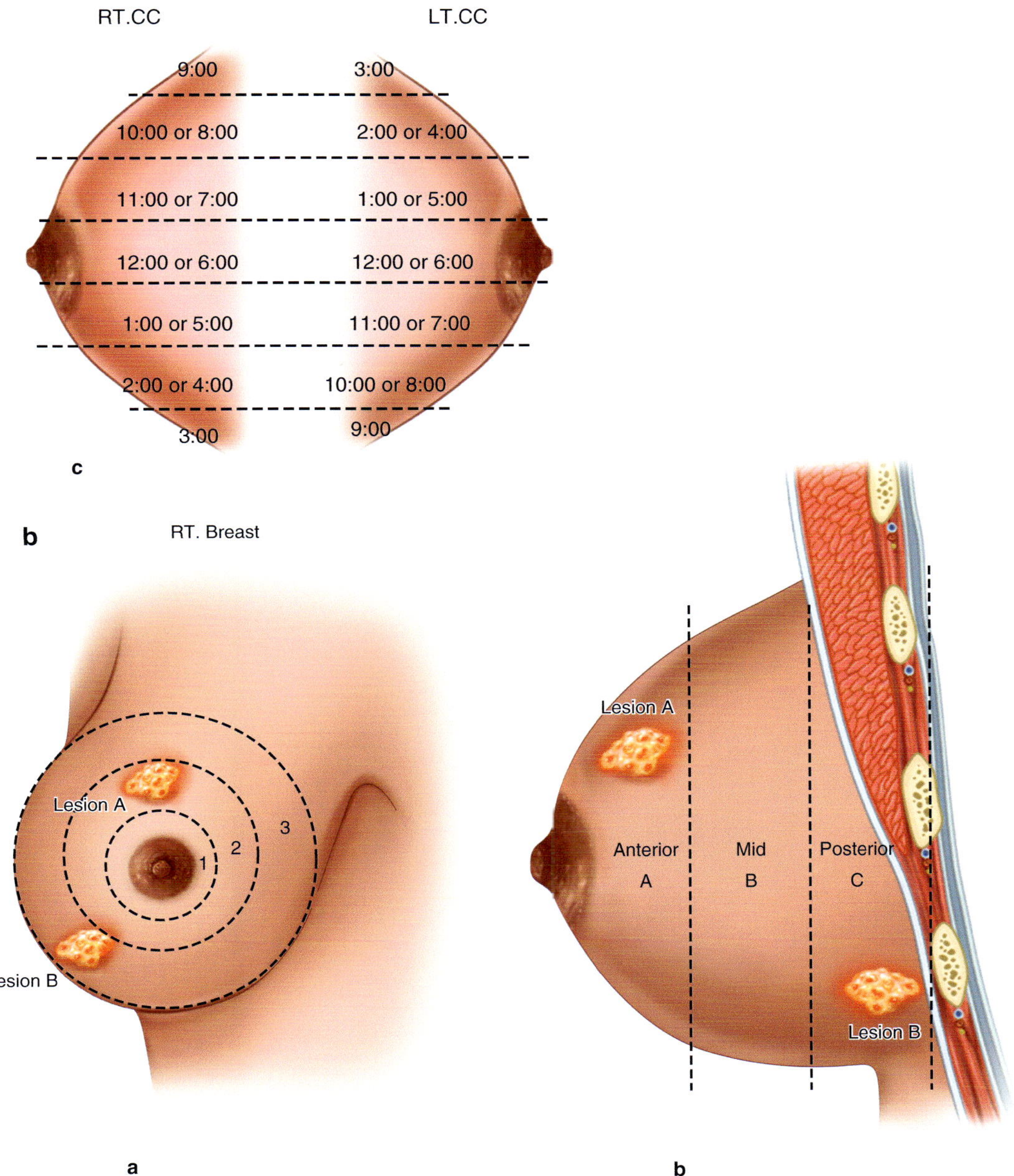

Fig. 4.4 (continued)

Suggested Readings

1. Sehgal CM, Weinstein SP, Arger PH, Conant EF. A review of breast ultrasound. J Mammary Gland Biol Neoplasia. 2006;11(2):113–23.
2. Thigpen D, Kappler A, Brem R. The role of ultrasound in screening dense breasts—a review of the literature and practical solutions for implementation. Diagnostics. 2018;8(1):20.
3. Berg WA. Rationale for a trial of screening breast ultrasound: American College of Radiology Imaging Network (ACRIN) 6666. Am J Roentgenol. 2003;180(5):1225–8.

5 Breast MRI

Breast MRI is the most sensitive test available to detect breast cancer, and its use is rapidly increasing across multiple clinical scenarios.

Indications: The current indications as endorsed by organizations, such as the Society of Breast Imaging, the European Society of Breast Imaging, the American Cancer Society, etc., are as follows.

5.1 Screening

High-Risk Screening

- Known BRCA1 and BRCA2 gene carriers and their untested first-degree relatives.
- Women with lifetime risk more than 25% or greater (using risk assessment models like Tyrer-Cuzick, Gail model, BOADICEA, etc.).
- History of chest irradiation (mantle radiation), e.g., for Hodgkin's lymphoma before the age of 30; starting 8 years after their completed radiation.
- Women with rare genetic syndromes like Cowden syndrome, Le-Fraumeni syndrome, Bannayan-Riley-Ruvalcaba syndrome, and their first-degree relatives.
- Women with diagnosis of LCIS or atypical hyperplasia and dense breast parenchyma (ACR density of C or D).

Foreign Body Injections

Women with free silicone, paraffin, polyacrylamide gel injections in whom mammography and ultrasound is of limited use due to the artifacts created by the injected substance.

Surveillance

Prior personal history of breast cancer at premenopausal age and having dense breast tissue (ACR breast density C or D) at the discretion of the clinician or radiologist, and also in patients who meet the criteria of high-risk screening.

5.2 Diagnostic

- Metastatic axillary adenocarcinoma with occult primary on conventional imaging.
- Silicone implant integrity.
- Newly diagnosed breast invasive breast cancer (Staging) especially if it is an invasive lobular carcinoma (ILC), dense breast parenchyma (ACR breast density C or D), or if the patient is BRCA/High risk patient.
- Locally advanced breast cancer for pre-neoadjuvant treatment (Figs. 5.1 and 5.2).

N. Chotai, S. Kulkarni, *Breast Imaging Essentials*, https://doi.org/10.1007/978-981-15-1412-8_5

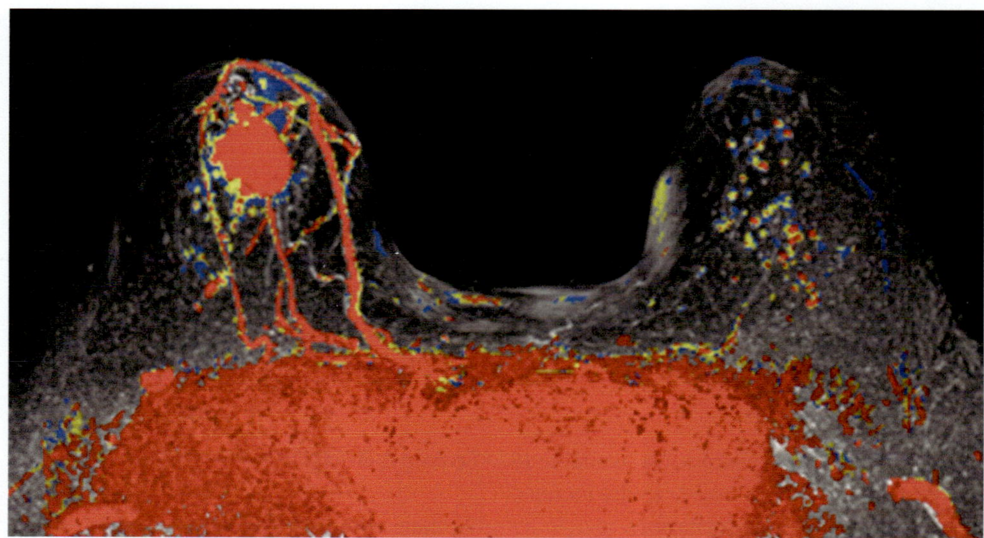

Fig. 5.1 Color angio MIP image of MRI breast shows a large, irregular mass in the right central breast with washout kinetics. Increased vascularity is seen around the mass. The imaging features are highly suspicious for breast malignancy

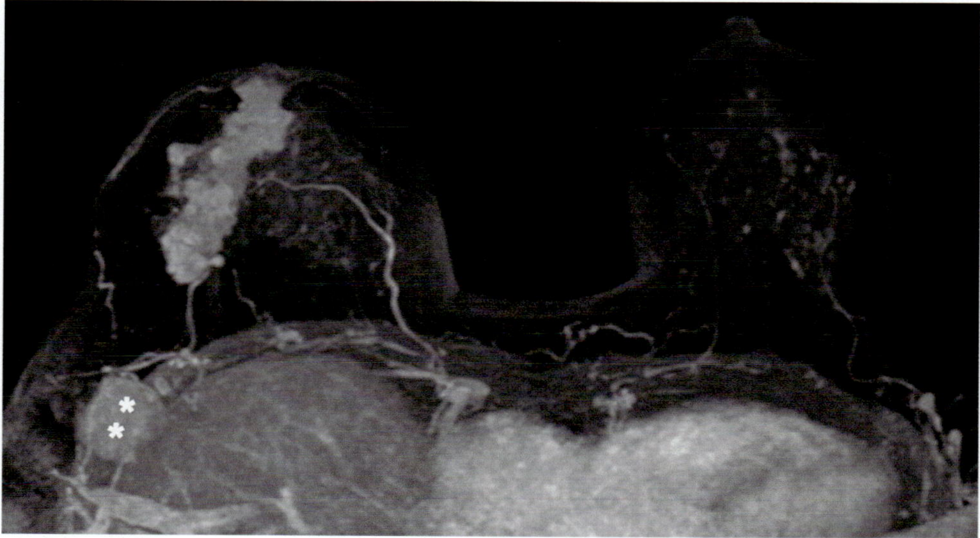

Fig. 5.2 Post-contrast MIP image showing a large irregular mass along the outer half of right breast reaching the retroareolar region. Right nipple retraction is noted. Large level I axillary lymph node is noted (white asterisks)

- Extent of disease (staging) (variable institutional policies): to assess T size, to assess extent of disease burden, lymph node assessment, and involvement of surrounding structures and to look for synchronous contralateral breast cancer (6–9%).
- Assessment prior to re-excision for positive margins.
- Nipple discharge (replacing galactography in many institutions).
- Insufficient conventional imaging/problem solving.

Technique: MRI techniques tend to be vendor specific; however, there are certain basic requirements that have been laid down by the American College of Radiology (ACR). These are as follows:

1. Resolution, contrast, and field strength:
   - In general, 1.5 T magnet strength is considered to be a minimal requirement with a slice thickness of 3 mm or less.
   - In-plane pixel resolution of 1 mm or less (volume averaging).
   - Chemical fat suppression is an absolute must for high-resolution images to optimize contrast between tumor and tissue.
   - Post-contrast subtractions performed as postprocessing. These may produce misregistration for which motion correction algorithm may be applied to reduce misregistration artifacts.
2. Simultaneous bilateral imaging: The breast is a symmetric organ and hence comparison must be available for the same time frame to evaluate true enhancement from spurious background enhancement, thereby reducing false positives.
3. Gadolinium: Bolus of 0.1 mmol/kg gadolinium is utilized with a 10 mL saline flush injected by an automatic injector.
4. Scan time: MRI is a dynamic 3D acquisition and therefore kinetic information is also available, which should be reported. Interval between two sequences should be 4 min or less. Time delay between the injection of contrast and acquisition of the first contrast run is also critical and is vendor specific.
5. Dedicated breast coil: A dedicated breast coil is a must. This has multiple small-diameter coils (elements) arranged to form a larger coil. Signals are therefore received from every single coil. Signals are combined after acquisition, providing increased signal-to-noise ratio with noise reduction.
6. Parallel Imaging: This technique uses phased-array radiofrequency coils which reduce acquisition time while maintaining spatial resolution. This allows production of high-resolution images with simultaneous fat suppression that is essential for breast MRI.
7. Timing of the MRI: As the breast shows cyclical changes with the menstrual cycle, which impacts enhancement on DCE, it is best to time it with the menstrual cycle to avoid nonspecific parenchymal enhancement which can lead to false positives and unnecessary intervention. DCE is best performed in the window period of 7–13 days of the menstrual cycle, particularly in the high-risk screening where patient population is younger.

Risks of gadolinium injection include the following:

- Allergic reactions.
- Nephrogenic systemic fibrosis (safe use in renal disease needs to be evaluated with eGFR).
- Gadolinium retention – reports of retention of gadolinium in the neural tissues has led to restricted use of linear gadolinium contrast agents. The clinical significance of this gadolinium retention is unknown at the current time. Macrocyclic gadolinium agents have been found to be safer.

Standard protocol: A clinical MRI of the breast is about 30-45 min long. Protocols are vendor specific, but these are the sequences that should be part of every protocol:

- Localizer.
- T2W sequence (STIR) with or without fat suppression.
- T1 non-fat sat sequence.
- T1 fat saturated pre-gadolinium sequence.
- T1 3D fat saturated post-gadolinium sequence (minimum 3 runs).
- Diffusion weighted sequence (recommended).
- Post processing:
  1. Subtractions (with motion correction recommended).
  2. Reconstruction sequence (sagittal or axial).
  3. MIP.

Advantages of breast MRI:

1. High sensitivity for detection of breast cancer.
2. High negative predictive value in a screening setting.
3. Allows assessment of both breasts simultaneously.
4. Allows local staging, involvement of surrounding structures and axilla.
5. Reproducible.
6. Breast density does not affect performance.

Limitations of breast MRI:

1. High false positive rates, leading to additional workup, biopsies, patient anxiety, and delays in surgical times.
2. Expensive tests, which may not be available to the population at large.
3. Does not detect microcalcifications.
4. Some patients may not be suitable for the test, such as those with tissue expanders, pacemakers, pregnant women, and those with claustrophobia.

Suggested Readings

Menezes GL, Knuttel FM, Stehouwer BL, Pijnappel RM, van den Bosch MA. Magnetic resonance imaging in breast cancer: a literature review and future perspectives. World J Clin Oncol. 2014;5(2):61.

Millet I, Pages E, Hoa D, Merigeaud S, Curros Doyon F, Prat X, Taourel P. Pearls and pitfalls in breast MRI. Br J Radiol. 2012;85(1011):197–207.

Rahbar H, Partridge SC. Multiparametric MR imaging of breast cancer. Magnet Reson Imag Clin. 2016;24(1):223–38.

6 Screening

Screening is done for apparently *healthy* or *asymptomatic* population (World Health Organization) using simple tests to detect preclinical or early-stage disease. It also helps identify individuals with higher risk than the average population and suggest special tests for early detection of disease in these high-risk individuals.

Breast cancer screening involves periodic bilateral mammography examination performed in asymptomatic average-risk women to detect preclinical asymptomatic breast cancer. Large trials demonstrate a 30% mortality reduction for women over 50 years of age upon receiving systematic population screening with a mammogram and also reduces node-positive cancers. The sensitivity of mammogram to detect breast cancer ranges from 50% to 95% depending on breast density from D to A category. A 15% increase in sensitivity is seen upon switching from screen-film mammography to full-field digital mammogram, particularly in dense breast tissue (DMIST Trial).

Screening mammograms are generally read by trained/accredited radiologist. Batch reading is recommended wherein all screening mammograms are read as a batch in a controlled setting with minimal interruptions or distractions. Double reading (human-CAD or human-human) increases cancer detection by 5–20%.

Supplementary screening: Ultrasonography and MRI are used for supplementary screening. The role of these modalities for supplementary screening has been discussed in the previous chapters.

Digital breast tomosynthesis (DBT): DBT with synthetic views is being used routinely for average-risk screening in several countries in Europe and the USA. Refer to Chap. 7 for more details.

6.1 Average-Risk Population Screening Guidelines

There are minor differences in the screening guidelines by different societies, as summarized below:

1. 40 years +: Once a year [ACR & SBI Guidelines (USA)].
2. 50–70 years: Once every 2 years in the USA, Singapore, the Netherlands, Canada, Australia, New Zealand.
3. 45–55 years: Once a year and subsequently once in 2 years (American College of Surgeons, ACS).
4. 50–70 years: Once every 3 years in the UK (NHS).

6.2 High-Risk Population Screening Guidelines

1. 30–69 years: Annual mammogram and DCE-MRI.
2. >69 years: Standard average risk protocol.

N. Chotai, S. Kulkarni, *Breast Imaging Essentials*, https://doi.org/10.1007/978-981-15-1412-8_6

High-risk screening is offered to the following:

1. Known BRCA1 and BRCA2 carriers and their untested first-degree relatives.
2. Women with lifetime risk more than 25% or greater (Risk assessment models Tyrer-Cuzick, Gail model, BOADICEA, etc.).
3. History of chest irradiation (mantle radiation), e.g., for Hodgkin's lymphoma before the age of 30, starting 8 years after their completed radiation.
4. Women with rare genetic syndromes like Cowden syndrome, Le-Fraumeni syndrome, and Bannayan-Riley-Ruvalcaba syndrome, and their first-degree relatives.
5. Women with diagnosis of LCIS or atypical hyperplasia and ACR C or D breast density.

Suggested Readings

Fuller MS, Lee CI, Elmore JG. Breast cancer screening: an evidence-based update. Med Clin N Am. 2015;99(3):451.

Lee W, Peters G. Mammographic screening for breast cancer: a review. J Med Radiat Sci. 2013;60(1):35–9.

Tabar L, Dean PB. Thirty years of experience with mammography screening: a new approach to the diagnosis and treatment of breast cancer. Breast Cancer Res. 2008;10(4):S3.

7 Digital Breast Tomosynthesis

Mammographic sensitivity drops as the density of the breast tissue increases. As it is a compression technique, it is fraught with two shortcomings:

1. False negatives: Superimposition of tissue, leading to masking of abnormalities especially in dense breast tissue; 15–30% of breast cancers can be missed.
2. False positives: Superimposition of tissue leads to summation artifacts, which lead to recall rates artifactual findings, causing high recall rates of 10–12%. This also leads to additional costs and patient anxiety.

Digital breast tomosynthesis (DBT) is a technique developed to overcome these two shortcomings of mammography. The X-ray tube moves within a fixed arc (15°–50° depending upon the vendor) obtaining multiple low-dose exposures. The data is reconstructed in the form of a stack of thin 1.0 mm slices in the direction of breast compression (Fig. 7.1). This allows slicing of the dense tissues and enhancing an object at a specific depth while blurring out the objects at other levels.

7.1 Performance of DBT for Screening

Several trials and studies have been published evaluating the role of DBT in breast cancer screening (Oslo Trial, STORM Trial, TOMMY trial, etc.). The performance of DBT has been better than 2D. The two most important benefits of DBT are increased cancer detection rate (CDR) for invasive mammary carcinoma and reduced recall rate. Increased cancer detection is achieved because of the tomographic technique which makes the cancers more conspicuous (visible) in the surrounded blurred tissue. DBT is very good at detecting architectural distortion and spiculations, thereby picking up cancers that produce the above-described features (Fig. 7.2). As compared to 2D, DBT can increase CDR by about 40% especially when the breast tissue is dense. DBT has also been shown to increase CDR in fatty breast tissue, indicating that the benefit of DBT is seen across all breast densities. DBT leads to better characterization of masses, distortions, and asymmetries leading to an upgrade in their BI-RADS features. For example, a perceived asymmetry on 2D may be characterized as an irregular mass on DBT.

It is important to remember that tumor growth patterns may not be concentric and may be perceived only on one view and therefore DBT should be performed in two views as opposed to one view, when possible. Studies have shown that adding a single-view DBT does increase cancer detection, but adding two views further increases cancer detection.

Studies (ASTOUND Trials) have shown that supplementary screening with ultrasound shows a higher CDR compared to DBT; however, false

N. Chotai, S. Kulkarni, *Breast Imaging Essentials*, https://doi.org/10.1007/978-981-15-1412-8_7

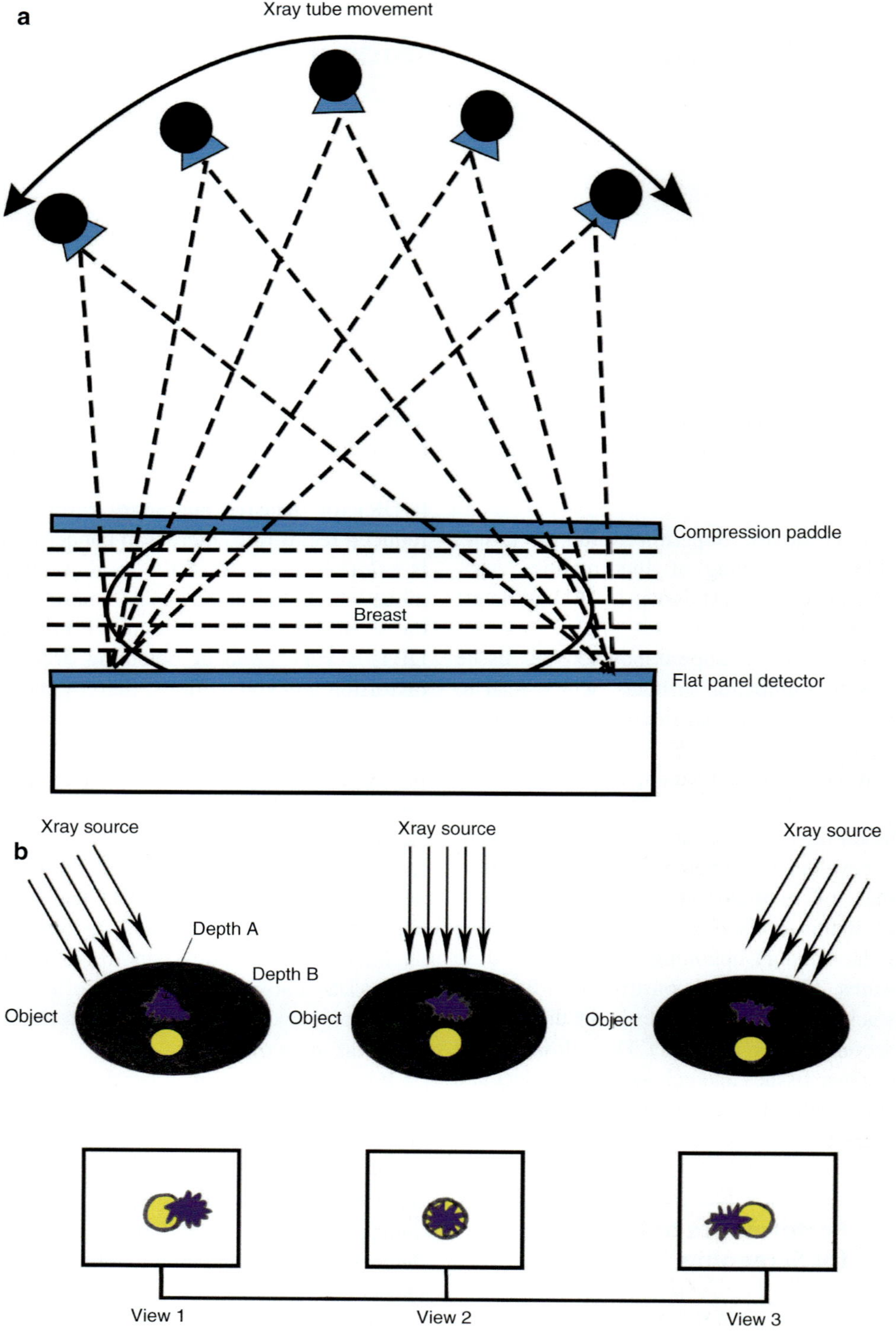

Fig. 7.1 Diagrammatic representation of digital breast tomosynthesis. (**a**) The X-ray source rotates around the breast in an arc in a limited range and projection images are formed on the detector. These are then reconstructed into slices through the breast along the *z*-direction. (**b**) Depending on the position of the X-ray source, the projections help differentiate overlapping lesions enabling depth resolution and reducing superimposition

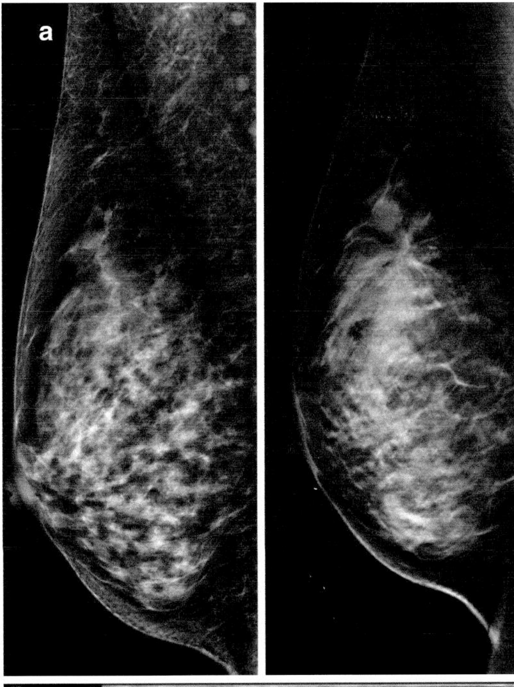

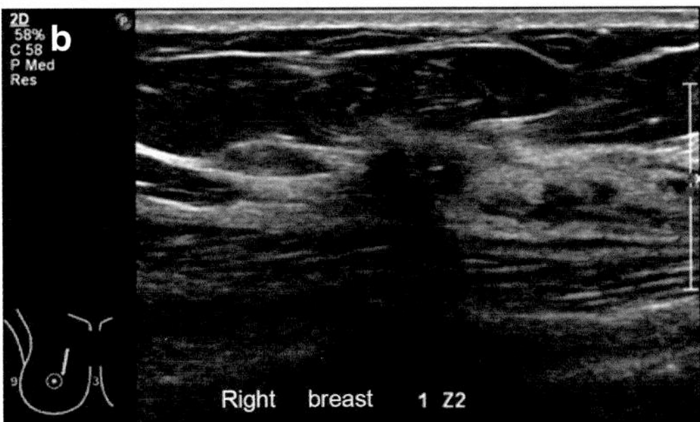

Fig. 7.2 (**a**) Right MLO view shows dense breast parenchyma without any obvious abnormality. Corresponding DBT image shows architectural distortion in the upper half of right breast. (**b**) Ultrasound shows a suspicious mass in the right breast at 1 o'clock in the area of distortion, which on histology revealed invasive ductal carcinoma of the tubular variety

positive rates are much higher with ultrasound compared to DBT.

DBT has shown reduction in recall rates by 20–40% depending on individual practice and has shown to be particularly useful in younger radiologists who are new to the practice as opposed to more experienced breast radiologists. DBT minimizes tissue overlap, thereby preventing spurious densities and symmetries.

7.2 DBT and Calcifications

Individual calcifications may be depicted on multiple slices in the three-dimensional DBT study, and they're sometimes better and more quickly appreciated on the two-dimensional projection image. Obtaining co-registered 2D and DBT simultaneously helps overcome this limitation. Improving technologies allow detection of microcalcifications on DBT and its synthesized view, which is comparable to FFDM in about 92%. Microcalcifications should still be assessed by standard true magnification views.

7.3 DBT and Radiation Dose

Addition of DBT to 2D doubles the radiation dose to the breast. For a thickness of a standard 4.5 cm breast phantom, the average mean dose is around 2.5 mGy (varies from vendor to vendor) per view which is still within the FDA approved dose of 3 mGy per exposure. It is an important consideration especially if DBT is used as a regular screening tool with repeatedly higher exposure annually. It is also important to understand that if the thickness of the breast were to be greater than the standard phantom then the dose would also increase as dose is directly proportional to the thickness of the breast. For example, if you were to compare a dose for a single projection of a breast that is 4.5 cm thick on compression (standard phantom) versus a breast that was 10 cm thick on compression, the dose absorbed by the thicker breast would be much higher than the standard phantom. If DBT were to be performed on its own without 2D views, then the radiation dose would be comparable or even be lower than a standard 2D views. However, we do need the synthetic 2D views for assessment of calcifications and also for comparison with older studies.

7.4 DBT and Synthetic View

Postprocessing algorithms are available, which use the reconstructed stack of image slices to create a synthetic 2D (s2D) image. Studies have shown that s2D images are comparable in all respects with a standard 2D FFDM image and are also FDA approved. This removes the need to perform standard 2D images with DBT thereby addressing the question of increased radiation due to 2D + DBT studies. Several centers in the USA and in Europe have completely replaced standard 2D images with s2D images for screening mammograms.

7.5 DBT and Time

The time required to complete a 2D + DBT is longer, thereby increasing the duration of compression. This can result in increased motion artifacts. When s2D is used instead of a 2D FFDM, the timing is significantly decreased, making it easier for the patient to stay still, thereby reducing patient related motion artifacts.

The time required to read a DBT is also longer than reading a 2D mammogram as there is a large number of slices to review. There is a learning curve effect when a radiologist first starts to read a DBT study and gradually the workflow becomes normalized.

7.6 DBT for Diagnostic Workup

Decrease in recall rates with DBT is mostly seen in densities and asymmetries, thereby reducing the number of spot compression views (SCV) for these findings. DBT performs well for margin assessment of mass lesions and therefore the need for SCV for DBT detected mass lesions is eliminated. Overall, women recalled following DBT screening tend to have abbreviated workup.

Women recalled following a 2D FFDM findings greatly benefit from a full breast DBT versus a SCV as it allows not only assessment of the noted abnormality but also allows the rest of the breast to be screened for other 2D FFDM occult abnormalities. s2D views can also be obtained with no additional radiation burden to the patient. If a very small area needs to be assessed, DBT spot compression views with s2D views can be performed, although it is counterintuitive to deny DBT assessment of the remainder breast.

In the diagnostic workup of mass lesions, DBT shows them more conspicuously, demonstrates the halo sign, margins, surrounding distortion, and spiculations far better than 2D. Intralesional fat densities, oil cysts, are better seen on DBT, helping assessment of postoperative scar abnormalities.

Skin lesions presenting as breast masses are easily seen on the skin on DBT. Tortuous vessels producing spurious masses on 2D FFDM are easily unraveled on DBT. Vascular calcifications which may present as indeterminate new group of calcifications can be demonstrated to be in the vessel wall on DBT thus avoiding unnecessary intervention and biopsy.

In the setting of a known breast cancer, DBT can show additional lesions otherwise undetected on 2D FFDM. Serendipitous detection of synchronous contralateral breast cancer is also seen with DBT, especially in dense breast tissue.

7.7 DBT Biopsy and Contrast-Enhanced DBT

For DBT-only lesions DBT-guided biopsy capability is essential and therefore should be available. DBT with contrast-enhanced mammography is also now available and its use in staging will be of great value, especially in areas where MRI staging is unavailable.

Suggested Readings

Ciatto S, Houssami N, Bernardi D, Caumo F, Pellegrini M, Brunelli S, Tuttobene P, Bricolo P, Fantò C, Valentini M, Montemezzi S. Integration of 3D digital mammography with tomosynthesis for population breast-cancer screening (STORM): a prospective comparison study. Lancet Oncol. 2013;14(7):583–9.

Hooley RJ, Durand MA, Philpotts LE. Advances in digital breast tomosynthesis. Am J Roentgenol. 2017;208(2):256–66.

Skaane P, Sebuødegård S, Bandos AI, Gur D, Østerås BH, Gullien R, Hofvind S. Performance of breast cancer screening using digital breast tomosynthesis: results from the prospective population-based Oslo Tomosynthesis Screening Trial. Breast Cancer Res Treat. 2018;169(3):489–96.

8 BI-RADS Lexicon

BI-RADS is an acronym for Breast Imaging-Reporting and Data System, which was designed as a quality assurance tool originally for use with mammography. The system is a collaborative effort of many groups but is published and trademarked by the American College of Radiology (ACR).

The system is designed to standardize reporting to be used by reporting radiologists, and since then has also been expanded and adapted to be used with ultrasonography and MRI.

Breast Imaging-Reporting and Data System (BI-RADS) was first released by the American College of Radiology in 1993. Since then various editions have been published over time, the last (fifth) edition was released in 2013.

BI-RADS suggests use of standardized numerical codes to be assigned by the reporting radiologist after interpreting a mammogram, ultrasound, or MRI. The main purpose of this is to allow concise and unambiguous understanding of patient records between various medical facilities and multiple doctors.

The BI-RADS codes not only provide standardization of reporting and communication but is also a very robust tool for quality control and audit.

In addition to the BI-RADS categories, the BI-RADS atlas also describes:

1. Standardized terminology along with images of relevant examples that should be used for reporting. These are called BI-RADS descriptors.
2. Standardized reports for each modality (refer to Chapter 9).
3. Auditing tools.

BI-RADS Assessment Categories

Assessment category	Management	Likelihood of cancer
0: Incomplete evaluation	Recall for additional imaging and/or comparison with prior study	NA
1: Negative	Routine screening	Essentially 0%
2: Benign	Routine screening	Essentially 0%
3: Probably benign	Short-term follow-up	0–2%
4: Suspicious 4A: Low suspicion 4B: Moderate suspicion 4C: High suspicion	Tissue diagnosis	2–95% 2–9% likelihood of cancer 10–49% likelihood of cancer 50–94% likelihood of cancer
5: Highly suggestive of cancer	Tissue diagnosis	≥95% likelihood of cancer
6: Known biopsy proven cancer	Appropriate treatment	NA

BI-RADS Hierarchy: 5 > 4 > 0 > 6 > 3 > 2 > 1

N. Chotai, S. Kulkarni, *Breast Imaging Essentials*, https://doi.org/10.1007/978-981-15-1412-8_8

Suggested Reading

D'Orsi CJ, Sickles EA, Mendelson EB, Morris EA, et al. ACR BI-RADS® Atlas, Breast Imaging Reporting and Data System. Reston, VA: American College of Radiology; 2013.

9 Organization of Breast Imaging Reports

Concise and organized breast imaging reports need to be issued, which are compliant with the ACR BI-RADS descriptors. It is a good idea to have the BI-RADS reference card handy at your reporting station.

Report structure.

9.1 Indication for Examination

- Clinical history as provided on the referral note should be recorded within the report. For example, patient referred for routine screening or for diagnostic work following a specific clinical symptom or for a short-term 6-month follow-up (BIRADS 3), etc.
- Pertinent prior history must be recorded, such as prior biopsies, etc.
- Clinical findings, duration, and location should be recorded.
- Hormonal status if applicable should be recorded (MRI).

9.2 Breast Composition Description

It is a subjective assessment; however, as far as possible consistency should be maintained from study to study. Composition should be described in words and not just as letters (A, B, C, and D).

9.3 Clear Description of any Important Findings

Mammograms

- Mass (describe location, size, shape, margin, density, and associated features).
- Calcifications (location, morphology, distribution, and associated features).
- Architectural distortion (location and associated features).
- Asymmetry (location and associated features).
- Skin, nipple, nodes, etc., should also be included in the description, specially if there are any abnormal findings.

Ultrasound

- Mass (location, size, shape, orientation, margins, echo pattern, posterior features).
- Calcifications (in or outside of a mass, intraductal calcifications).
- Associated features (architectural distortion, duct, skin changes edema, vascularity, elasticity).
- Axillary findings.

N. Chotai, S. Kulkarni, *Breast Imaging Essentials*, https://doi.org/10.1007/978-981-15-1412-8_9

MRI

- MRI technique.
- Amount of fibroglandular tissue (FGT).
- Amount of background parenchymal enhancement.
- Presence of implants.
- Unique finding like mass or non-mass enhancement in the breast, axillary and internal mammary node status, and any significant extramammary findings.

9.4 Comparison with Prior Study

Comparison may be helpful in some findings when stability would change the management. If the finding is obviously benign then comparison may not be necessary. If the finding is unequivocally suspicious, then comparison may be irrelevant.

9.5 Assessment Category

Specific BI-RADS assessment 0–6 should be used as final assessment category for clear communication. The BI-RADS assessment categories are generally associated with the likelihood of cancer and management recommendations.

9.6 Management

This refers to the next suggested step depending on the finding of the current study. This is generally linked to the BI-RADS category assessment. For example, BI-RADS 0 means that the study is incomplete and management includes further evaluation or comparison to reach a final decision. BI-RADS 1 and 2 would mean that the patient can continue with routine screening follow-up. BI-RADS 4 and 5 indicate the need for tissue diagnosis as the next step of management.

Suggested Reading

D'Orsi CJ, Sickles EA, Mendelson EB, Morris EA, et al. ACR BI-RADS® Atlas, Breast Imaging Reporting and Data System. Reston, VA: American College of Radiology; 2013.

10 Emerging Technologies

Early detection of breast cancer saves lives and saves the breast. Mammogram has stood the test of time over the last few decades and has proven to reduce mortality from breast cancer around the globe. At the same time, the medical fraternity has realized the limiting effect of breast density on the sensitivity of mammogram to detect early/small breast cancers. New technological developments have helped overcome this limitation.

Digital breast tomosynthesis (DBT) is one such development in mammographic technology that we have discussed in Chapter 7. Here we discuss breifly about other technologies namely contrast-enhanced mammography, automated breast ultrasound (ABUS) and elastography.

10.1 Contrast Enhanced Mammogram (Fig. 10.1)

Contrast enhanced mammography is a technique when a mammogram is performed with intravenous injection of an iodine-based contrast medium. The principle of tumor neo-angiogenesis is used to detect the area of enhancement in the breast. There are two approaches in contrast-enhanced mammogram: temporal enhanced contrast mammogram (TECM) and dual energy contrast-enhanced spectral mammogram (CESM).

In TECM, one breast is compressed in a selected projection and a precontrast mask image is obtained. This is followed by contrast injection and multiple postcontrast acquisitions from 1 to 5 min. Postcontrast images are then subtracted from the mask image to obtain contrast enhancement. This method can provide temporal kinetic enhancement of the lesion similar to MRI. The main limitation of this method is that following a full dose of contrast injection, only a single projection of one breast is obtained. Compression may cause patient discomfort, misregistration artifacts due to patient motion, and occasionally compression may not allow contrast uptake in lesion, leading to false negatives.

In CESM, the contrast is injected while the patient is in a sitting position and the breast is yet to be compressed. Imaging is started 2 min after contrast injection. For each standard projection (CC and MLO), the imaging involves a pair of low- and high-energy exposures. The images are acquired using an anti-scatter grid. Low-energy images are obtained at about 26–31 kVp using molybdenum and rhodium target and molybdenum and rhodium filter. These images are "regular" mammographic images. Though the iodine is already present in the breast, it is not visualized as the exposure is done at an energy level that is below the k-edge of iodine which is 33.2 keV. The high-energy images are obtained using a molybdenum target and an aluminum plus copper filter with peak kilovoltage values of 45–49 kVp. This

N. Chotai, S. Kulkarni, *Breast Imaging Essentials*, https://doi.org/10.1007/978-981-15-1412-8_10

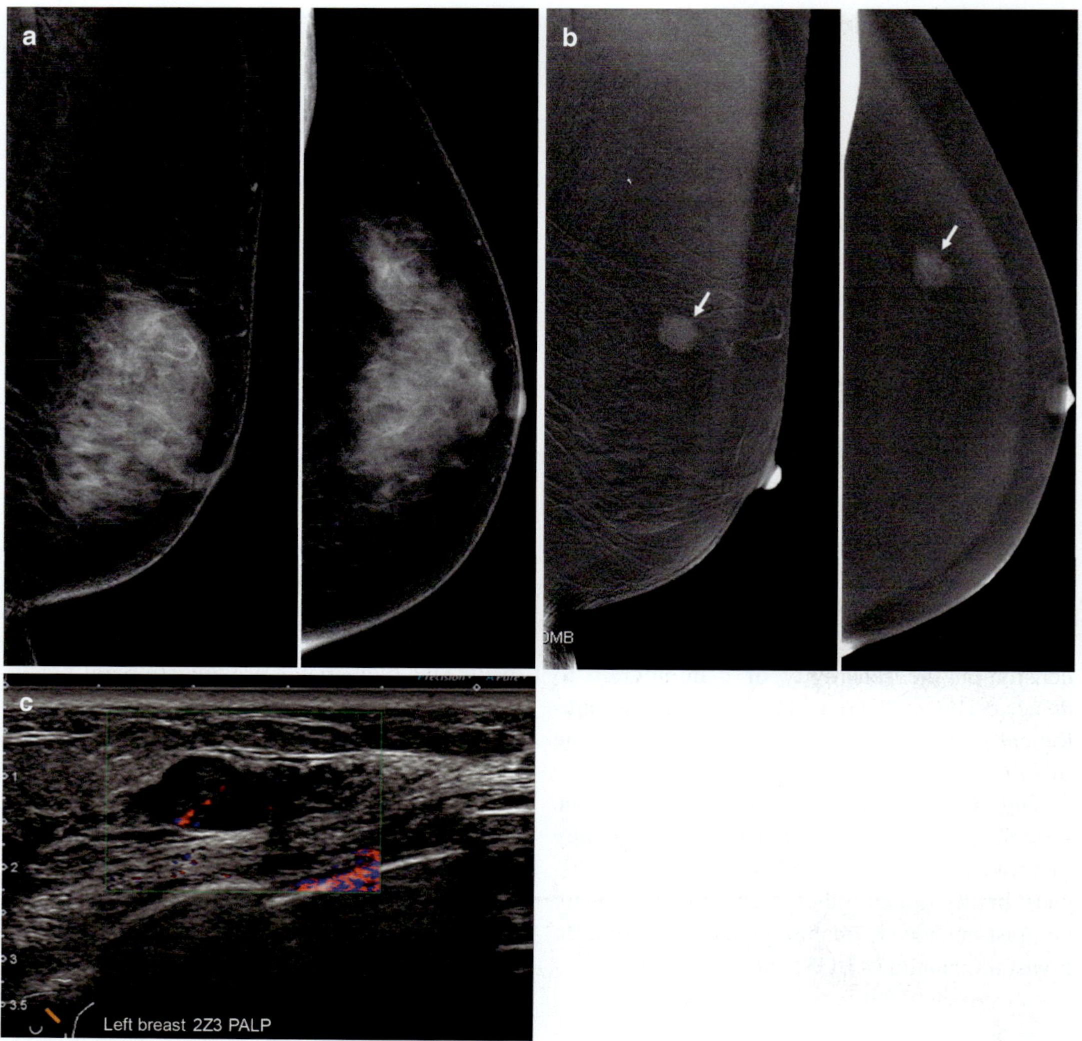

Fig. 10.1 A 60-year asymptomatic female for screening mammogram. (**a**) Left MLO and CC mammogram shows dense breast parenchyma. No suspicious findings. (**b**) Contrast-enhanced mammogram shows an enhancing lesion in the upper outer quadrant of the left breast (white arrow). (**c**) Targeted ultrasound of upper outer quadrant of the left breast shows a 1.3 cm round, mixed echogenic lesion with microlobulated margin. Post-biopsy histology revealed papillary carcinoma

x-ray spectrum is above the k-edge of iodine, and therefore the images obtained contain information on lesion enhancement. The data available from high- as well as low-energy exposures are then processed to obtain a recombined image that provides information on contrast enhancement. In this technology, with single injection of contrast, both the breasts are imaged in two projections providing adequate information. Each breast is compressed for only a few seconds for every exposure, making this a more acceptable procedure by the patient.

By using this technique, functional information is added, which increases the sensitivity of mammogram to detect breast cancer.

Several studies have shown CESM to have a higher sensitivity than mammogram and quite similar to MRI.

10.2 Elastography (Fig. 10.2)

Elasticity by definition is the ability of a body to resist a distorting influence and to return to its original size and shape when that influence or force is removed. In breast lesions, the loss of elasticity leads to tissue stiffness.

Ultrasound elastography allows the evaluation of "stiffness" of the breast lesion in a non-invasive way. Benign breast tissue is more likely softer and more elastic whereas in a malignant mass perilesional tissue more likely loses elasticity making the lesion stiffer. Measurement of this tissue elasticity increases the specificity of

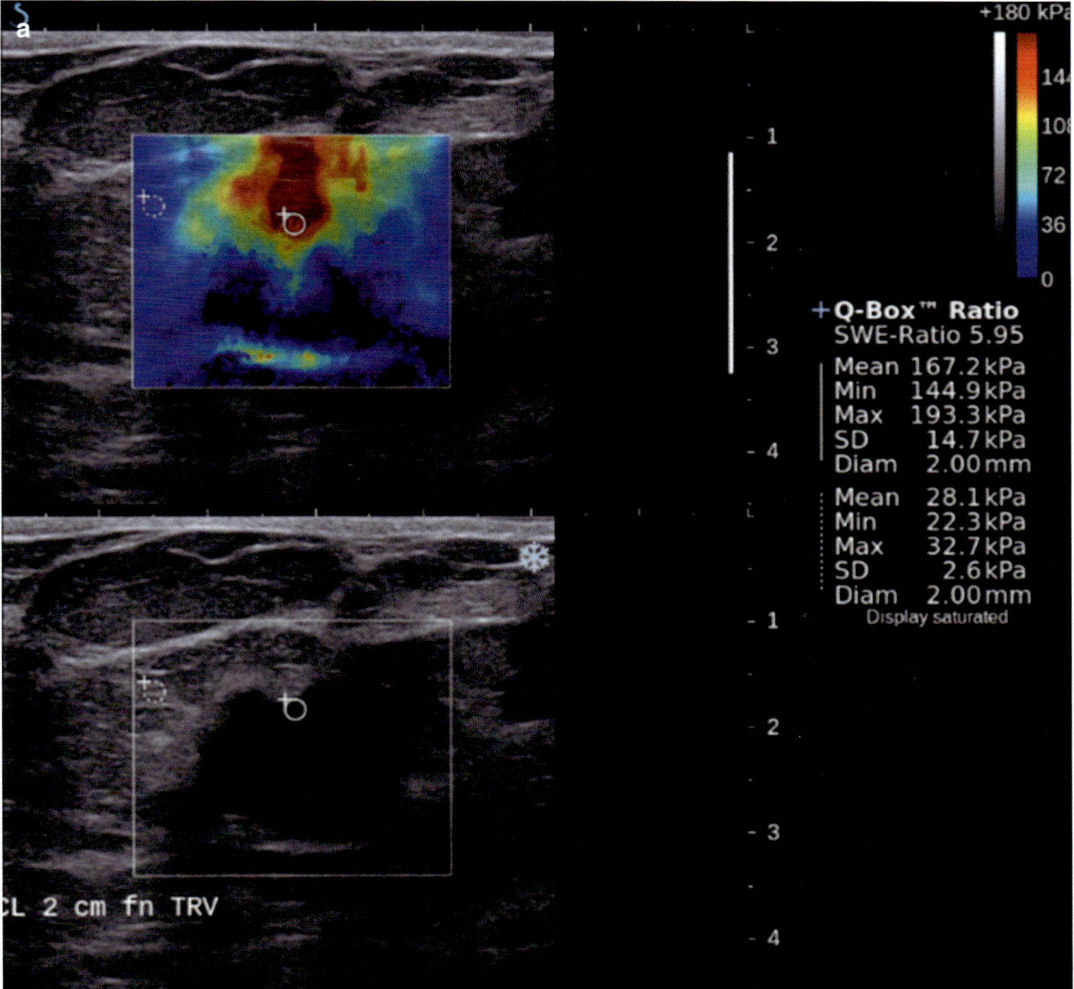

Fig. 10.2 Shear wave elastography: (**a**) 55-year-old woman with mass in left breast. Shear wave elastography superimposed on ultrasound image (top) shows that mass has very stiff peripheral region with light green, yellow, orange, and red colors and high elasticity values (mean elasticity, 167.2 kPa; maximum elasticity, 193.3 kPa; elasticity ratio, 5.95). Ultrasound image (bottom) shows that mass has irregular angular margins, is taller than wide, and was considered to be BI-RADS category 5. Pathologic diagnosis on core biopsy was invasive ductal carcinoma. (**b**) 48-year-old woman with mass in left breast. Shear wave elastography superimposed on ultrasound image (top) shows that the mass has homogeneously blue color and low elasticity values (mean elasticity, 25.0 kPa; maximum elasticity, 29.7 kPa; elasticity ratio, 1.88). Ultrasound image (bottom) shows that mass has mostly smooth margins with one small protuberance along the upper medial edge (white arrow), mass was considered to be BI-RADS category 4. Pathologic diagnosis on core biopsy was a fibroadenoma

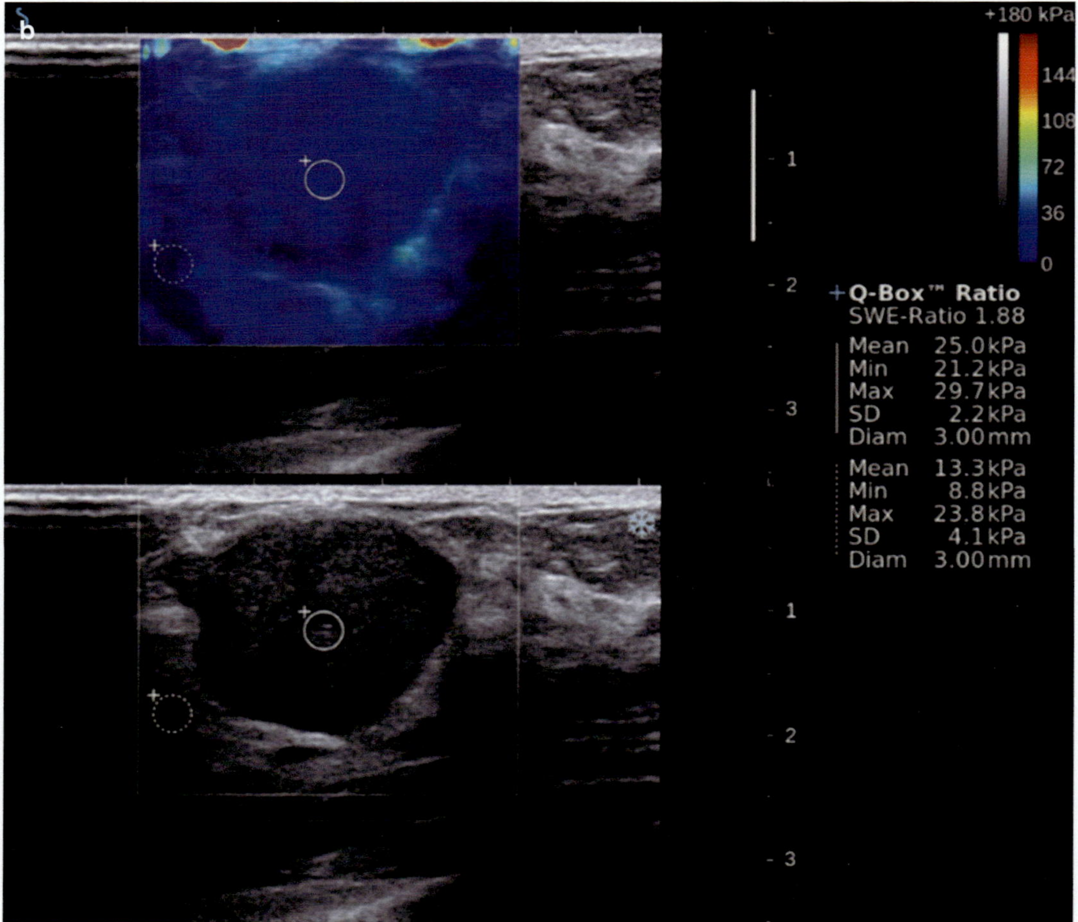

Fig. 10.2 (continued)

the B-mode ultrasound to about 89.8% and accuracy to 88.3% in characterization of breast lesions. This leads to reduction of false-positive results, thereby by avoiding unnecessary breast biopsies.

There are two types of elastography techniques in clinical use:

Static Ultrasound Elastography: Strain Imaging

Strain elastography provides qualitative assessment of tissue deformation and does not require specific software. The main disadvantages are lack of quantitative assessment, operator dependency, and reproducibility.

Dynamic Ultrasound Elastography: Shear Wave Imaging

Shear wave elastography is a quantitative assessment and values of stiffness of tissues are represented in kiloPascals (kPa).

Sensitivity of shear wave elastography is higher (up to 95.8%) compared to strain elastography (up to 81.7%) in differentiating benign from malignant breast lesions. It is also more reproducible. In contrast, strain elastography is found to be more specific (93.7%) compared to shear wave elastography (84.8%).

The latest BI-RADS fifth edition has included elastographic features as an important tool to increase the specificity of breast lesions. Based on elastographic features, lesions can be classified as soft, intermediate, and hard. Elastography can be used to modify the grayscale BI-RADS characterization of breast lesions; e.g., a soft lesion characterized as BI-RADS category 3 on grayscale ultrasound imaging may be downgraded to a BI-RADS 2 avoiding unnecessary short-term follow-up. Similarly, a hard lesion characterized as BI-RADS 3 may be upgraded to BI-RADS 4A and subjected to a biopsy, reducing a false negative.

Caveat: Morphology is considered the most significant criterion in BI-RADS 4B, 4C, and 5 category lesions when malignancy is suspected. Elastographic features alone should not be used to downgrade suspicious looking lesions which need a core biopsy. This may lead to missed cancers.

Automated Breast Ultrasound (ABUS) (Fig. 10.3)

Handheld ultrasound (HHUS) is shown to be a useful adjuvant modality to mammography and increases cancer detection by at least 4–6/1000 screening studies. Handheld ultrasound is however limited as it is operator dependent, time consuming, and requires training and skills.

Automated breast ultrasound (ABUS) addresses some of the important limitations of HHUS, such as operator dependency and long scanning time. ABUS allows fast acquisition, increases reproducibility, and separates the time of image acquisition from image interpretation.

ABUS uses large footprint transducer (about 15 cm long) mounted on a mechanical arm.

To ensure adequate contact of the transducer with the skin, a replaceable membrane cover is used over the transducer. The patient lies in the supine position with the ipsilateral arm extended over the head. Generally, three scans of 1 min each are performed for medial, central, and lateral parts of breast covering the entire breast. The scan is performed from inferior to superior direction. The acquired data is processed and then displayed on dedicated workstations in native axial as well as reconstructed sagittal and coronal planes, with 0.5–1 mm thickness.

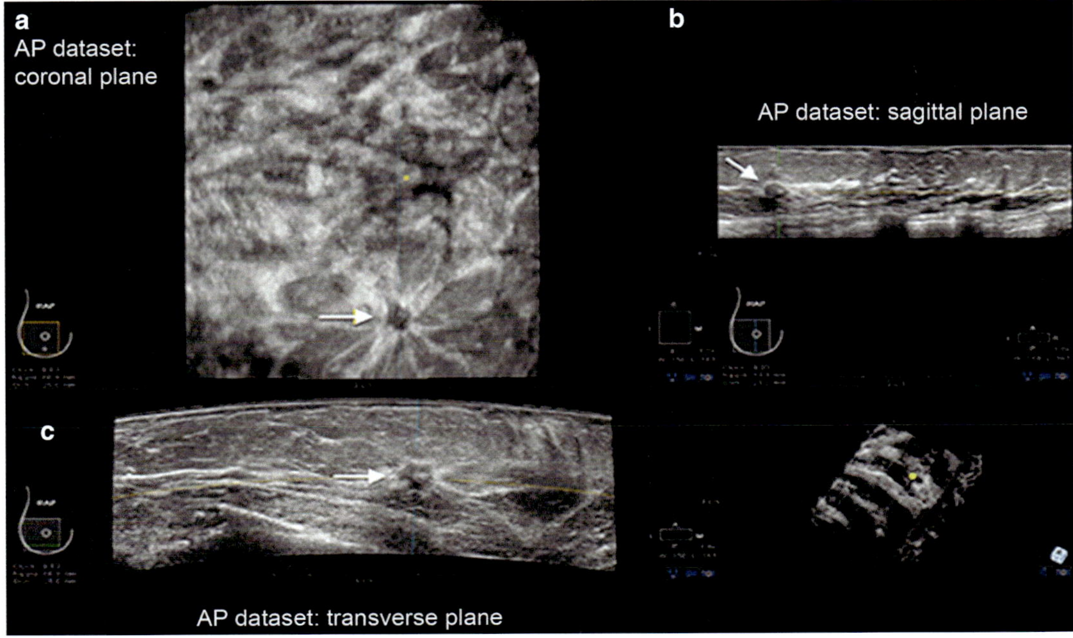

Fig. 10.3 Automated breast ultrasound (ABUS) images in coronal (**a**), sagittal (**b**), and axial (**c**) projections show an irregular mass in the right breast (white arrow). Architectural distortion around the mass is well seen on coronal view radiating from the mass and thus increasing the visibility of this lesion

ABUS is generally performed as a supplementary screening test in addition to mammography. An increase in cancer detection up to 3.6/1000, significant increase of sensitivity, ability to detect small sub centimeter cancers, and increase in recall rates have been reported upon addition of ABUS to routine mammography. Once trained, a lower reading time and reduced recall rate have been reported as compared to HHUS.

Advantages

- Less operator dependent. Easy to train the staff to perform this study.
- Less time required to acquire the images. The workflow can be better streamlined.
- Provides multi-axial images. It is better to identify architectural distortion.
- Higher reproducibility.

Limitations

- Retroareolar, peripheral tissue, and axillary region are not well scanned.
- Inability to allow dynamic evaluation like compression, color doppler imaging, elastography, etc.
- Difficult skin contact producing air artifacts, especially in drooping breasts, post-operative deformed breasts, etc.
- Inability to perform breast interventions.

Suggested Readings

Chang JM, Won JK, Lee KB, Park IA, Yi A, Moon WK. Comparison of shear-wave and strain ultrasound elastography in the differentiation of benign and malignant breast lesions. Am J Roentgenol. 2013;201(2):W347–56.

Fallenberg EM, Dromain C, Diekmann F, Engelken F, Krohn M, Singh JM, Ingold-Heppner B, Winzer KJ, Bick U, Renz AD. Contrast-enhanced spectral mammography versus MRI: initial results in the detection of breast cancer and assessment of tumour size. Eur Radiol. 2014;24(1):256–64.

Itoh A, Ueno E, Tohno E, Kamma H, Takahashi H, Shiina T, Yamakawa M, Matsumura T. Breast disease: clinical application of US elastography for diagnosis. Radiology. 2006;239(2):341–50.

Jochelson MS, Dershaw DD, Sung JS, Heerdt AS, Thornton C, Moskowitz CS, Ferrara J, Morris EA. Bilateral contrast-enhanced dual-energy digital mammography: feasibility and comparison with conventional digital mammography and MR imaging in women with known breast carcinoma. Radiology. 2013;266(3):743–51.

Kelly KM, Richwald GA. Automated whole-breast ultrasound: advancing the performance of breast cancer screening. Semin Ultrasound CT MRI. 2011;32(4):273–80.

Lobbes MB, Smidt ML, Houwers J, Tjan-Heijnen VC, Wildberger JE. Contrast enhanced mammography: techniques, current results, and potential indications. Clin Radiol. 2013;68(9):935–44.

Wing-Fai Au F, Ghai S, Moshonov H, Kahn H, Brennan C, Dua H, Crystal P. Diagnostic performance of quantitative shear wave elastography in the evaluation of solid breast masses: determination of the most discriminatory parameter. Am J Roentgenol. 2014;203:W328–36. https://doi.org/10.2214/AJR.13.11693.

Zanotel M, Bednarova I, Londero V, Linda A, Lorenzon M, Girometti R, Zuiani C. Automated breast ultrasound: basic principles and emerging clinical applications. Radiol Med. 2018;123(1):1–2.

Part II

Case Based Review

11 Calcifications

11.1 Case 11.1

History: 49-year-old woman with history of left lumpectomy for ductal carcinoma in situ 4 years ago presents for routine surveillance mammogram. Family history of breast cancer in mother and two sisters.

Questions

Q1. Describe the findings on mammogram (Fig. 11.1a–c) with appropriate lexicon.
Q2. What would you recommend next? What would be appropriate BI-RADS category?
Q3. Please provide possible differentials for this finding.
Q4. Describe the findings on ultrasound (Fig. 11.1d) and MRI (Fig. 11.1e).
Q5. What would you recommend next?

Answers

A1. Bilateral mediolateral oblique (MLO) (Fig. 11.1a) and craniocaudal (CC) (Fig. 11.1b) views of both breasts show heterogeneously dense breast parenchyma. Two groups of microcalcifications are noted in the right breast: one in right mid central breast (white arrow) and other in the right lower outer quadrant in the posterior third of the breast (double white arrow). No obvious mass or architectural distortion is seen in the right breast. Architectural distortion in the upper outer quadrant of the left breast and the partially retracted nipple is a postoperative change from the prior known lumpectomy. Spot magnification view (Fig. 11.1c) of the right breast shows both the groups of microcalcifications with coarse heterogeneous morphology (white arrows). In addition, they are variable in shape, size, and density, indicating pleomorphic morphology. A few other scattered microcalcifications are seen in the right breast and nipple. No obvious associated mass or architectural distortion is identified with the microcalcifications.

A2. Comparisons with prior mammograms is suggested if available. If the microcalcifications were to be new or showed interval changes, they would be deemed BI-RADS 4 and further stereotactic biopsy would be necessary.

In women presenting with microcalcifications, a breast ultrasound may be performed to look for an associated mass which would suggest an invasive component. If a mass is found, an ultrasound-guided biopsy would be preferred.

A3. Possible differentials for coarse heterogeneous microcalcifications include:
(a) Fibroadenoma.
(b) Stromal fibrosis.

N. Chotai, S. Kulkarni, *Breast Imaging Essentials*, https://doi.org/10.1007/978-981-15-1412-8_11

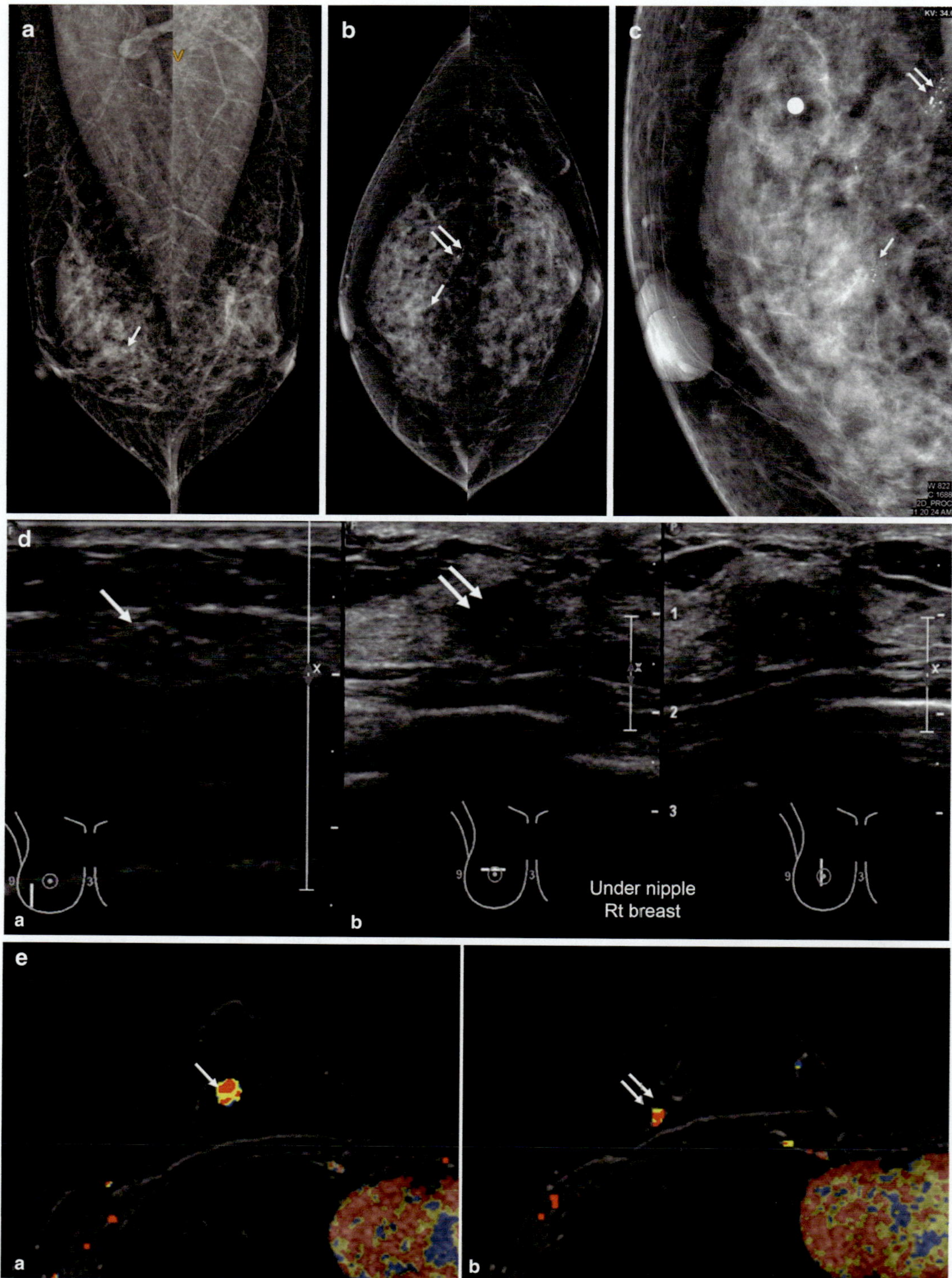

Fig. 11.1 (**a**) Bilateral MLO views. (**b**) Bilateral CC views. (**c**) Right CC magnification view. (**d**) (*a*, *b*) Right breast ultrasound. (**e**) (*a*, *b*) Axial DCE T1WI MRI color angiomaps of the right breast

(c) Post-traumatic from evolving dystrophic calcifications (fat necrosis).
(d) ADH.
(e) DCIS.
(f) IDC.

A4. Figure 11.1d—Right breast ultrasound shows an oval, hypoechoic mass with internal calcifications at 8 o'clock location (white arrow) and another round hypoechoic mass with irregular margin in the deep retroareolar region (double white arrows). These correlate to the previously described grouped microcalcifications on the mammogram.

Figure 11.1e Post contrast axial MRI color angiomaps.

MRI demonstrates a round, heterogeneously enhancing mass with irregular margins in the central right breast with washout kinetic (white arrow).

Small focal non-mass enhancement with washout seen in the lateral aspect of the right breast (double white arrows).

Diagnosis: Two groups of new suspicious microcaclfications correlating with suspicious masses on ultrasound and MRI. BI-RADS 4.

Ultrasound-guided biopsy was performed for both these masses. A post-biopsy specimen was also acquired to confirm retrieval of microcalcifications.

Histopathology: Atypical Ductal Hyperplasia (ADH).

A5. ADH is considered to be a high-risk lesion with a reported upgrade rate to DCIS in up to 20% and up to 35–40% when microcalcifications are associated with a solid mass on ultrasound as in our case.

An ultrasound-guided hook wire surgical excision is suggested.

Surgical Histopathology: On excision, the right central breast mass revealed intermediate grade DCIS and 8 o'clock mass revealed low-grade DCIS.

Patient underwent right mastectomy with reconstruction.

Notes

Breast Calcifications

Breast calcifications are very common, particularly in women older than 50 years of age. Although most calcifications are benign, breast cancer can present as microcalcifications and hence it is important to evaluate them carefully. Microcalcifications need to be assessed for their morphology and distribution, as these features can give an indication about the likelihood of malignancy. Magnification views should be performed for the assessment of microcalcifications.

Morphology

Typically, benign calcifications are likely to show the following morphology:

(a) Coarse calcification (dystrophic, popcorn, etc.)
(b) Large rod-like calcification (secretory calcifications).
(c) Tram track calcification (vascular).
(d) Rim calcifications (calcified cyst wall or oil cyst).
(e) Milk of calcium (layering suggesting microcystic adenosis).
(f) Scattered bilateral punctate calcifications (sclerosing adenosis).
(g) Skin calcifications (lucent polygonal).
(h) Suture calcifications (seen in surgical bed, linear and dense, may show shape of a knot).

Typically, malignant calcifications are likely to show the following morphology:

(a) **Amorphous** (Case 11.2).

These are small, hazy microcalcifications without specific shape or form. Bilateral, symmetrical, multiple groups of amorphous microcalcifications are generally benign and are categorized as BI-RADS 2. A single group of amorphous microcalcifications in grouped/regional/segmental or linear distribution presenting as a unilateral or a new finding is considered suspicious. The PPV of amorphous calcifications is 20% and therefore they are classified as BI-RADS 4B category.

(b) **Coarse heterogeneous** (Case 11.1).

Coarse heterogeneous microcalcifications are irregular, conspicuous calcifications that are generally larger than 0.5 mm and smaller than 1 mm. Multiplicity, bilaterality, and stability favor benign etiology. A single group of coarse heterogeneous microcalcifications, especially associated with some fine pleomorphic calcifications, has a positive predictive value up to 13% for breast cancer and hence is classified as BI-RADS 4B category.

(c) **Fine pleomorphic** (variable in shape, size, and density) (Case 11.5).

Fine pleomorphic (crushed stone) microcalcifications vary in size and shapes and are usually more conspicuous than the amorphous calcifications. There is about 20–45% risk of malignancy. These calcifications are categorized as BI-RADS 4B. Differential diagnosis: Ductal carcinoma in situ (DCIS), ADH, flat epithelial atypia (FEA), papilloma, fibrocystic change, etc.

(d) **Linear/linear branching** (Case 11.6).

Fine linear or linear branching microcalcifications descriptor is used for microcalcifications confirming to ductal pattern. These may be dot-dash or snake skin pattern or casting calcifications. Their morphology indicates an intraductal location. The calcifications may be thin branching, irregular, or curvilinear, <0.5 mm in diameter. They may be discontinuous. The PPV is about 70% and therefore they are categorized as BI-RADS 4C. Differential diagnosis includes DCIS (generally high grade) or IDC, ADH, Papilloma, occasionally early secretory calcifications or ruptured inflamed duct.

Distribution

There are five typical distribution described namely, diffuse, regional, segmental, linear, and grouped. The term **"grouped"** microcalcifications is used to include a minimum of five calcifications within 1 cm of each other or a larger number of calcifications that are grouped within 2 cm of each other.

11.2 Case 11.2

History: 45-year-old average-risk woman presents for regular screening mammogram. She was recalled for additional workup for a new finding.

Questions

Q1. Describe the microcalcifications with appropriate lexicon on mammogram views provided (Fig. 11.2a, b). What would you advise next?

Q2. What is the probability (risk) of cancer associated with these microcalcifications?

Q3. Please provide possible differentials for this finding.

Q4. Given the pathology diagnosis, what further management is suggested?

Answers

A1. Left MLO and CC views (Fig. 11.2a) and left breast magnification views (Fig. 11.2b) are provided. Heterogeneously dense breast parenchyma is noted (ACR breast density C). There is a group of small, indistinct microcalcifications in the 3 o'clock position in the mid third of the left breast (white arrows). Magnification views reveal a loose group with amorphous morphology (white arrows). There is no associated architectural distortion or mass noted. Ultrasound is unlikely to find any corresponding abnormality.

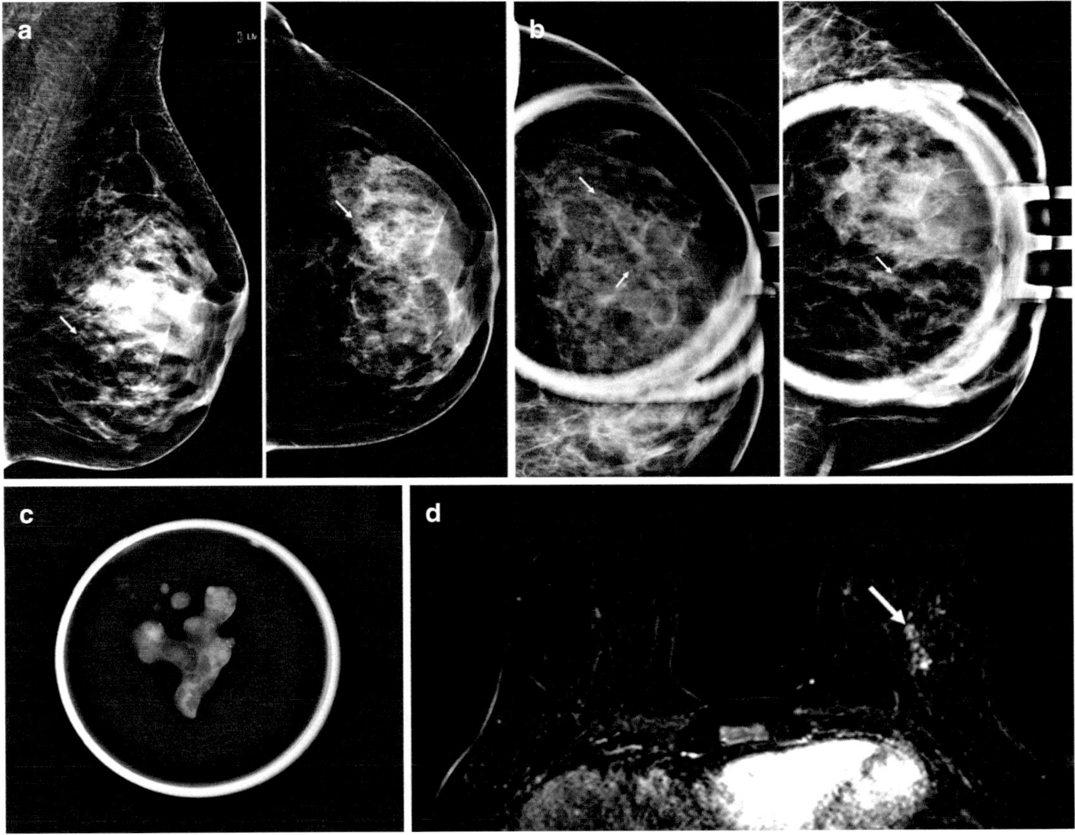

Fig. 11.2 (**a**) Left MLO and CC views. (**b**) Left CC and lateral magnified views. (**c**) Post-stereotactic biopsy specimen. (**d**) Axial DCE T1WI MRI of breasts

Given that these microcalcifications are a new finding with amorphous morphology, they are considered indeterminate and therefore classified as BI-RADS 4B. A stereotactic biopsy is suggested.

A2. Risk of cancer with a new group of amorphous microcalcifications is about 20–25% (most cancers are low-grade DCIS with less than 10% being IDC, especially if they are associated with mass on ultrasound).

A3. Possible differentials for grouped amorphous microcalcifications are:
   (a) Benign etiology like fibrocystic change, papilloma, fibroadenoma (FBA), sclerosing adenosis.
   (b) High-risk lesions like ADH, atypical lobular hyperplasia (ALH), LCIS.
   (c) Malignant lesions like DCIS or IDC.

Diagnosis: Stereotactic biopsy of these microcalcifications was performed. Fig. 11.2c shows a specimen radiograph with microcalcifications.

Histopathology: Lobular carcinoma in situ (LCIS).

A4. LCIS would be considered a concordant pathology. Wire-guided localization and excision biopsy of these microcalcifications is suggested to exclude a more significant pathology, such as invasive mammary carcinoma. DCE MRI (Fig. 11.2d) shows linear non mass enhancement (white arrow) in the left breast correlating with the region of microcalcifications.

Notes

Ductal and Lobular Proliferations

Atypical Ductal Hyperplasia (ADH)

ADH histologically is ductal proliferation with cellular atypia but not enough volume of involved ducts to demonstrate architectural atypia required to call it DCIS. There is a great deal of variability in how pathologists report ADH versus DCIS.

ADH most commonly presents as a mammographic finding of grouped amorphous microcalcifications and occasionally as grouped coarse heterogeneous (Case 11.1) or punctate microcalcifications. Occasionally architectural distortion may be seen. Some ADH can present as a mass on ultrasound and as incidental non-mass enhancement on MRI.

ADH is considered to be a high-risk lesion with an upgrade rate of 20% to DCIS and up to 35–40% when microcalcifications are associated with a solid mass on ultrasound. Risk of upgrade is higher with synchronous carcinoma and in younger women. ADH increases the risk of breast cancer bilaterally by 4–5 times which further increases to 7–13 times if there is additional family history of breast cancer in a first-degree relative.

Lobular Neoplasia (LN)

Lobular Neoplasia (LN) includes atypical lobular hyperplasia (ALH) and lobular carcinoma in situ (LCIS), both originating from the same cell type. LN is a proliferative disease arising in the terminal duct lobular unit and is seen as an incidental finding in about 2% of all breast biopsies, particularly in perimenopausal women. Classification of LN is guided by strict application of pathologic criteria.

ALH and LCIS are considered high-risk lesions. Increased relative risk of breast cancer is about threefold which further increases to eightfold if there is associated history of a first-degree family member with breast cancer. LN does not show any typical imaging findings and is usually detected incidentally during workup of some other findings. Rarely they may be associated with microcalcifications, in which case they should be viewed with caution. LCIS is multicentric in more than 80% of the cases, bilateral in 30–60% of the cases and shows a few varieties; the main being the classic and the pleomorphic types.

Management

Both ADH and lobular neoplasia confer a long-term increased risk of breast cancer and should trigger discussion of risk-reduction and surveillance strategies. Surgical excision is standard of care for ADH identified on core biopsy. Surgical excision is also recommended for "nonclassic" LCIS, such as pleomorphic LCIS and LCIS with comedo-necrosis, and for LCIS found on core biopsy of enhancing lesions on MRI. For classic LCIS, management requires multidisciplinary involvement and assessment of confounding risk factors. For ALH, surgical excision may be deferred when there is no mass lesion, no accompanying ADH, and biopsy was performed by large core vacuum-assisted biopsy with excellent sampling and concordance with the target image.

11.3 Case 11.3

History: 46-year-old average-risk woman presents for a baseline screening mammogram.

Questions

Q1. Describe the abnormality on mammogram and provide possible differentials.
Q2. Describe the findings on ultrasound.
Q3. What are the common presenting symptoms in this condition?

Answers

A1. Bilateral MLO (Fig. 11.3a) and CC (Fig. 11.3b) views show extremely dense breast parenchyma. This reduces the sensitivity of the mammogram. There are several, up to 0.5 mm size, round calcifications seen with nearly symmetrical, diffuse distribution in both breasts. Some of the microcalcifications show "Tea-Cup" appearance on MLO projection (white arrows); suggesting

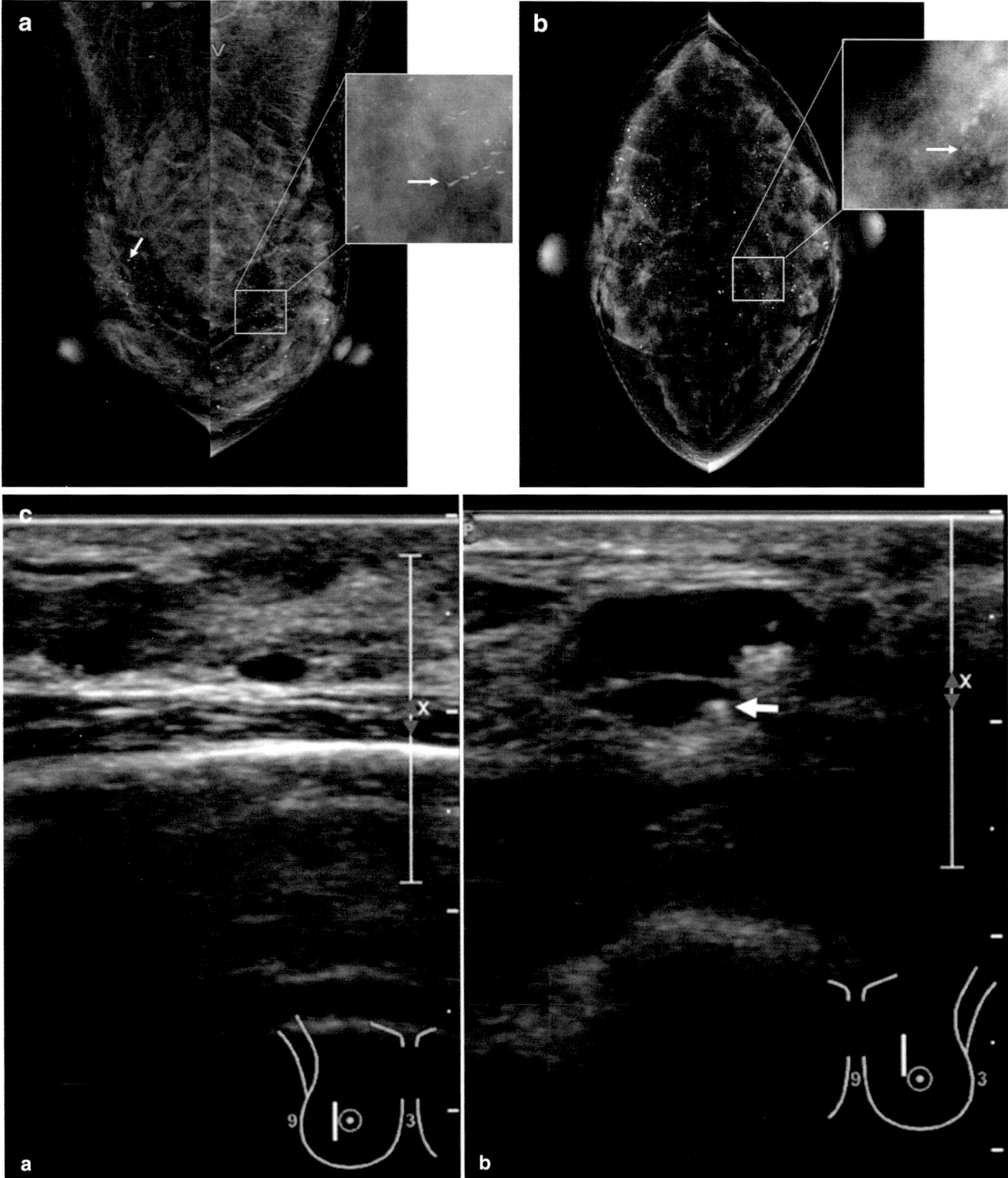

Fig. 11.3 (**a**) Bilateral MLO views with a left lateral magnification view. (**b**) Bilateral CC views with a left CC magnification view. (**c**) (*a*, *b*) Targeted bilateral breast ultrasound

calcium in the microcysts. On CC projection, they appear smudged (white arrow). They do not show suspicious morphology or distribution. There is no obvious associated mass or architectural distortion identified with the microcalcifications. Skin, subcutaneous tissue and nipple appear unremarkable. Findings suggest *microcystic adenosis* which is a spectrum of fibrocystic change. Category: BI-RADS 2.

Differentials for diffusely distributed, round calcifications would include: adenosis (microcystic adenosis, blunt duct adenosis & sclerosing adenosis), fibrocystic change (FCC), columnar cell lesions, ADH, ALH or LCIS, skin calcifications, and rarely extensive low-grade DCIS.

A2. Ultrasound images of both breasts (Fig. 11.3c) show a few subcentimeter cysts in both breasts. Echogenic foci (white arrow) suggesting calcifications are seen in left breast cysts. In conjunction with the mammogram, the ultrasound findings suggest diffuse bilateral breast fibrocystic changes.

Category: BI-RADS 2. Routine follow-up is recommended.

A3. Most common presenting symptoms are mastalgia or palpable lump. Rarely the patient may have nipple discharge (cysts may communicate with ducts).

Notes

Bilateral, nearly symmetrical distribution of round, smooth calcifications are more in favor of benign etiology. No biopsy is required for diffuse calcifications with benign morphology. Any suspicious morphology or distribution or interval change within the area of previously documented diffuse bilateral microcalcifications should prompt a stereotactic biopsy.

Fibrocystic Change (FCC)

FCC is considered in the spectrum of normal variants and hence the term fibrocystic change rather than fibrocystic disease. On histology, there is a combination of micro- and macrocysts, fibrosis, and adenosis. Usual intraductal hyperplasia is commonly present. The calcium is generally seen in adenosis.

There is 1.5–2 times increased risk of breast cancer in these proliferative breast changes without atypia. The risk may be higher if it is associated with cellular atypia.

Mammographic findings include bilateral, multiple, partially circumscribed masses and diffusely scattered bilateral microcalcifications (punctate and/or amorphous and/or coarse heterogeneous). Calcifications occuring in microcysts may show layering on lateral mammographic views (Tea cups—microcystic adenosis).

Ultrasound appearance includes multiple cysts/complicated cysts or microcysts that may show calcifications. Discrete masses due to fibrosis may also be seen in some cases.

MRI Variable sized cysts or clusters of cysts are noted. These may show rim enhancement when inflamed. Associated fibrosis may present as diffuse/regional or focal enhancement which may lead to false-positive findings prompting histological correlation for differentiation from malignant disease.

11.4 Case 11.4

History: 71-year-old woman presents for a screening mammogram.

Questions

Q1. Describe the findings and give the appropriate BI-RADS category.

Q2. Describe the typical appearance of this finding.

Answers

A1. Bilateral MLO (Fig. 11.4a) and CC views (Fig. 11.4b) show heterogeneously dense breast parenchyma. There are several smooth rod-like linear calcifications seen in both breasts (white arrows), radiating from nipple. Most of them are more than 1 mm in diameter and about 4–5 mm long. Some of them show central lucency suggesting calcification in duct wall. There is no associated mass or architectural distortion in either breast. The morphology and distribution of these calcifications suggest benign etiology and are typical for secretory calcifications.

Category: BI-RADS 2. Routine follow-up is recommended.

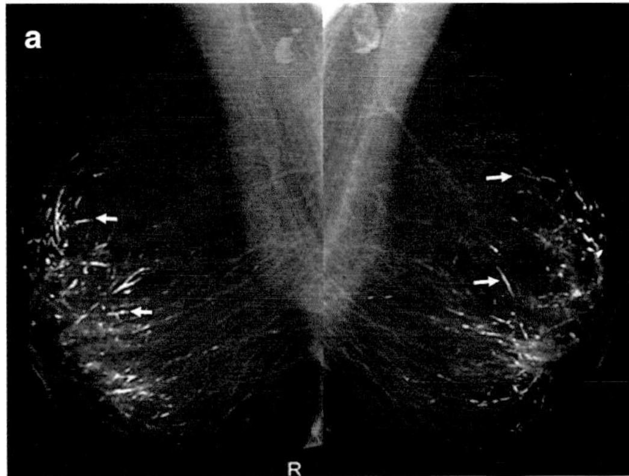

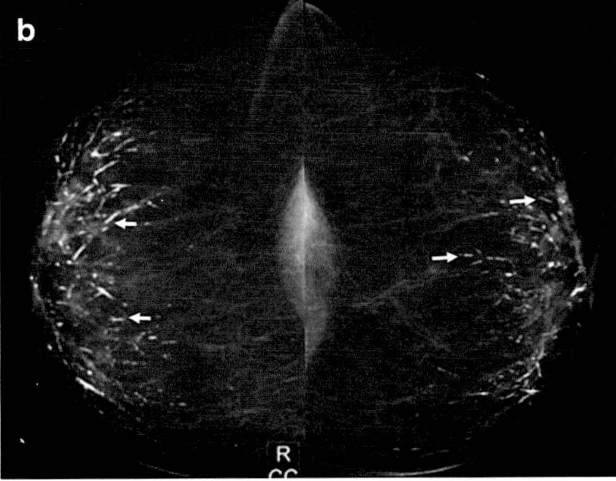

Fig. 11.4 (**a**) Bilateral MLO views. (**b**) Bilateral CC views

A2. Secretory calcifications are smooth, >1 mm in diameter, bilateral, and diffusely distributed with ductal pattern, directed towards nipple. Ultrasound and MRI may identify mammary duct ectasia.

Rarely, in their early phase, the secretory calcifications may be thin, linear/branching, and may simulate calcifications from DCIS, and hence new or developing secretory calcifications need to be carefully assessed.

Notes

Secretory Calcifications (Plasma Cell Mastitis)

These calcifications show rod-like or needle-like configuration and sometimes may be difficult to differentiate from linear calcifications associated with DCIS. Secretory calcifications, however, are thicker measuring >1 mm in diameter, which allows them to be differentiated from the fine linear calcifications that are seen with DCIS. These calcifications are generally occur bilaterally seen incidentaly in asymptomatic, older women and are associated with duct ectasia.

11.5 Case 11.5

History: 49-year-old average-risk woman for screening mammogram.

Questions

Q1. Describe the abnormality on given mammogram (Fig. 11.5a, b). What would you recommend next?

Q2. Patient underwent biopsy of the abnormality at an outside facility. Pathology revealed sclerosing adenosis. What would you recommend next?

Q3. What would you recommend next?

Answers

A1. Magnification views of the right breast in a lateral (Fig. 11.5a) and craniocaudal (CC) (Fig. 11.5b) views show heterogeneously dense breast parenchyma. There is a large group of pleomorphic microcalcifications in the lower inner quadrant of the right breast, in segmental distribution, extending from the retroareolar region (double white arrows) posteriorly to the chest wall (white arrows). There is no obvious associated mass or architectural distortion identified with the microcalcifications. Overlying skin and subcutaneous tissue appear unremarkable. The morphology and distribution of these microcalcifications are suspicious and are categorized BI-RADS 4. An ultrasound may be performed to exclude an underlying mass.

A2. Pathology diagnosis of sclerosing adenosis is discordant with imaging findings and a repeat biopsy is suggested.

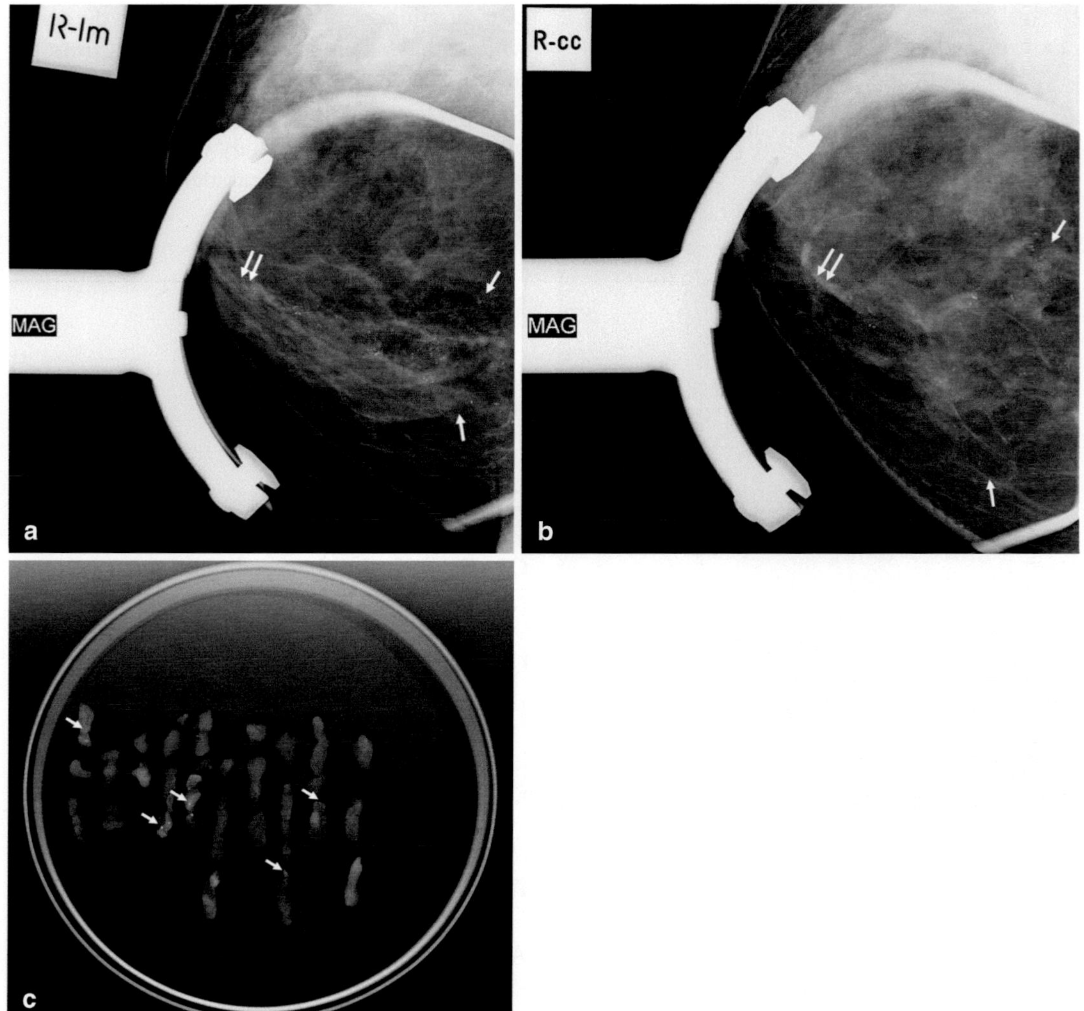

Fig. 11.5 (**a**) Right lateromedial spot magnification view. (**b**) Right CC spot magnification view. (**c**) Post-biopsy specimen radiograph

A repeat biopsy was performed. Figure 11.5c shows biopsy specimen radiography to confirm retrieval of microcalcifications in the sample (with at least 5 cores showing microcalcifications) (white arrows).

Histopathology: High-grade DCIS.

A3. Pathological diagnosis of DCIS is concordant. A surgical consultation is suggested. Given the extent of high-grade DCIS, there is likelihood of underlying occult microinvasive disease, and hence a sentinel lymph node biopsy (SLNB) may be recommended to exclude involvement of axillary lymph nodes.

Similar to invasive mammary carcinoma, hormonal receptor status (estrogen and progesterone receptors) of DCIS may also be tested. Postoperative Tamoxifen therapy may be suggested in hormone-positive DCIS to reduce the risk of recurrence.

Notes

Ductal Carcinoma In Situ (DCIS)

DCIS develops as malignant epithelial cells lining the terminal duct lobular unit (TDLU) remain confined to ducts without invasion of the basement membrane. DCIS is considered a direct precursor of most invasive breast cancers. Till 1980, DCIS constituted about 1–5% of breast cancers. After 1980 due to widespread mammographic screening, DCIS now constitutes about 15–25% of all newly diagnosed breast cancers (about 25–30% of all screen-detected cancers and 5% of all symptomatic cancers).

DCIS is considered to be a precursor of invasive ductal carcinoma (IDC), and if not treated almost half of them are likely to progress to IDC. The time of progression may vary from 1–4 years for high-grade DCIS to almost 10–20 years for low-grade DCIS.

Symptomatic pure DCIS commonly presents with blood-stained nipple discharge, palpable lump, or Paget's disease of nipple. Palpable DCIS is more likely to be associated with biologically aggressive behavior such as high grade or comedonecrosis.

Histologically DCIS is divided as low-, intermediate-, and high-nuclear-grade DCIS. High-grade DCIS is associated with central comedonecrosis. About 70–80% DCIS are ER positive, 30–50% are HER2/neu positive.

On mammography, 70–80% of DCIS may present with microcalcifications. Grouped amorphous microcalcifications are more commonly associated with low-grade DCIS while fine linear branching or casting calcifications are more commonly associated with high-grade DCIS.

About 10% of DCIS presents as a mass without microcalcifications. The presence of mass raises possibility of invasive component. Mammography underestimates the extent of disease in nearly 30% of cases; especially in micropapillary and cribriform types.

Skip lesions are known in DCIS; more so in low-grade DCIS. High-grade DCIS is more likely to be multifocal and contiguous.

On ultrasonography, extensive microcalcifications may be detected along with underlying solid mass. Ultrasound-guided biopsy of the mass should be performed in an effort to exclude underlying invasive disease.

MRI has about 88–95% sensitivity for the detection of DCIS. Non-mass enhancement with clumped internal enhancement, and linear/segmental distribution are common findings on MRI. It has been reported that with increasing nuclear grade of DCIS, the sensitivity of mammogram to detect DCIS reduces. Kuhl et al., in her prospective study, reported that nearly 48% of high-grade DCIS were missed on mammogram.

Management

The common surgical treatment for DCIS is lumpectomy with clear margins or mastectomy for multicentric or extensive DCIS (>5 cm). Sentinel lymph node biopsy (SLNB) may be performed when DCIS is associated with microinvasion on biopsy, large volume of high-grade DCIS, especially comedo-type DCIS, multicentric DCIS, or in women undergoing mastectomy for DCIS.

Axillary nodal metastasis is found in about 2% of pure DCIS suggesting occult invasion. In women undergoing wide local excision for DCIS, adjuvant radiotherapy has been shown to reduce the local recurrence rate by almost 50% without any overall survival benefit. Adjuvant hormonal therapy with Tamoxifen, in ER/PR-positive DCIS, has been shown to reduces local recurrence rate by 32–50% without influence on overall mortality or ipsilateral invasive breast cancer risk.

Opponents of screening mammography argue that DCIS which would not progress to invasive disease or lead to mortality need not be treated. But currently, the factors causing progression of DCIS to IDC are not known. This precludes identification of DCIS which can forgo surgical treatment. This mandates surgical treatment of all screen-detected (asymptomatic) DCIS which potentially leads to overdiagnosis and overtreatment.

11.6 Case 11.6

History: 51-year-old average-risk woman presents for baseline screening mammogram.

Questions

Q1. Describe the abnormality on the provided mammogram (Fig. 11.6a, b). What would you recommend next?

Q2. Describe the abnormality on Fig. 11.6c and give BI-RADS Category on magnification views and ultrasound images (Fig. 11.6d).

Q3. Ultrasound-guided biopsy of the mass was performed. Histology revealed DCIS. What would you recommend next?

Answers

A1. Bilateral MLO (Fig. 11.6a) and CC views (Fig. 11.6b) show extremely dense breast parenchyma. There is a group of suspicious microcalcifications in the upper outer quadrant of the right breast (white arrows). The microcalcifications are seen extending into the nipple (thick white arrow). There is no mass or architectural distortion identified with the microcalcifications.

Next step would be to perform magnification views of the right breast for better assessment of the morphology, distribution, and extent of the microcalcifications. An ultrasound may be performed to exclude underlying mass. If there is a mass on ultrasound, then an ultrasound-guided biopsy is suggested. If not, one should proceed to a stereotactic biopsy preferably with a vacuum-assisted device.

A2. Magnification views of the right breast in two orthogonal projections (Fig. 11.6c) show "segmental" distribution of the microcalcifications with fine linear branching morphology. A few coarse heterogenous and pleomorphic microcalcifications are also noted. The microcalcifications are seen extending into the nipple. There is no mass or architectural distortion identified in this region. This finding is suspicious and categorized BI-RADS 4C.

Ultrasound images (Fig. 11.6d) show a large, irregular mixed solid cystic mass with microlobulated margins between the 12 and 2 o'clock positions in the right breast. The mass shows internal calcifications (white arrows) and vascularity. It shows parallel orientation. No posterior features noted. This mass is felt to correlate with the microcalcifications in the right breast. Biopsy of this lesion under ultrasound guidance is recommended. Specimen radiograph of the biopsy samples should be performed to ensure retrieval of the microcalcifications.

A3. Malignant histology of DCIS is concordant with the morphology of microcalcifications. Further surgical consultation and surgical management is suggested. This woman underwent a right mastectomy.

Notes

Paget's Disease

Paget's disease was first described by Sir James Paget in 1874 as a condition where a woman presents with nipple ulceration, almost always secondary to underlying malignancy. More than 80–90% cases of Paget's disease are secondary to underlying DCIS or invasive breast cancer. It is rare and accounts for about 1–3% of breast cancers. Common presenting symptoms are nipple-areolar complex erythema, eczema, ulceration, and induration with possible nipple retraction and some times blood-stained nipple discharge.

Mammography may be completely normal or may show thickening of nipple-areolar complex, asymmetric density, and nipple retraction. Occasionally, malignant calcifications which may extend into the nipple or a discrete breast

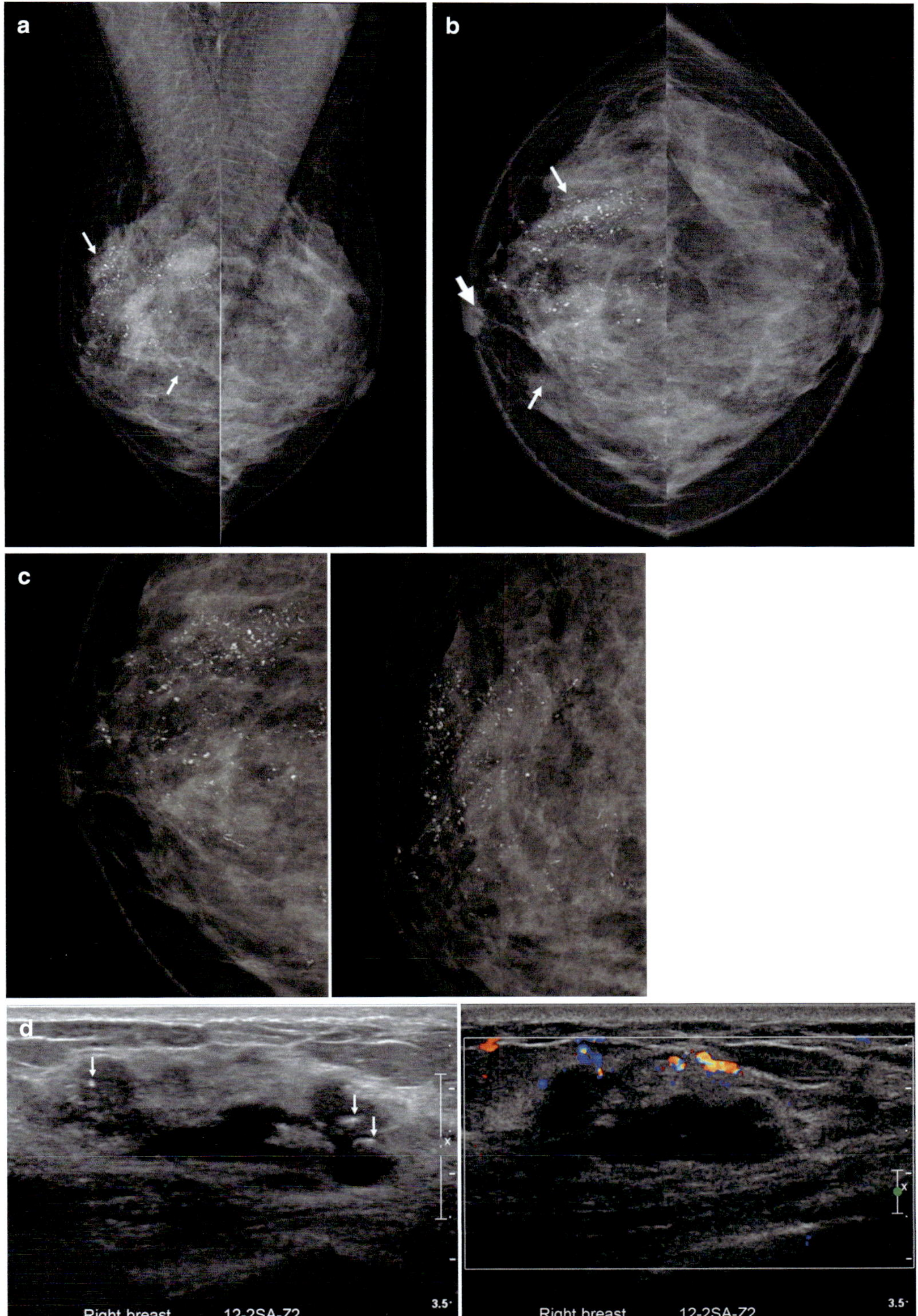

Fig. 11.6 (**a**) Bilateral MLO views. (**b**) Bilateral CC views. (**c**) Right breast spot magnification views in orthogonal projections. (**d**) Targeted right breast ultrasound

mass may be seen. The mass may be retro-areolar or at a distant location. Ultrasound demonstrates solid masses and retroareolar abnormalities. MRI may show thickening and enhancement of nipple-areolar complex, an underlying mass, enhancing DCIS or a combination of these findings.

Infiltration of the epidermis of the nipple by typical malignant cells called Paget cells is the main characteristic of this disease. A Paget cell is a large round or oval cell with clear or pale, abundant cytoplasm with an enlarged pleomorphic and hyperchromatic nucleus. A skin punch biopsy of the nipple-areolar complex is needed to establish the diagnosis. Once confirmed, complete imaging workup is necessary to identify occult disease and subsequent staging.

Management: Paget's disease is treated by mastectomy, with or without axillary dissection. However, in two-thirds of patients the cancer tends to be confined to central quadrant of the breast, and these women can be successfully treated with breast conservation therapy with a central lumpectomy followed by adjuvant radiation therapy.

Case 11.6 shows malignant microcalcifications extending into the nipple. Involvement of the nipple does not imply the diagnosis of Paget's disease unless malignant Paget cells are demonstrated in the epidermis of the nipple and there are characteristic nipple changes clinically. Patient had no clinically visible nipple changes and therefore did not have Paget's disease.

11.7 Case 11.7

History: 55-year-old woman underwent a screening mammogram and was recalled for right magnification views for microcalcifications.

Questions

Q1. Describe the microcalcifications with appropriate lexicon on magnification views provided in Fig. 11.7a.

Q2. Histology showed DCIS for which the patient underwent wide local excision. Her 2-year postoperative surveillance mammogram is available (Fig. 11.7b). Describe the abnormality.

Q3. Describe the abnormality and appropriate BI-RADS on spot magnification views (Fig. 11.7c) and ultrasound images (Fig. 11.7d).

Q4. Ultrasound-guided biopsy of the mass was performed, and histology revealed high-grade DCIS. What would you recommend next?

Answers

A1. Magnification views of right breast in two orthogonal projections (Fig. 11.7a) are provided. There is a group of microcalcifications seen in the inferomedial right retroareolar region. The microcalcifications have round pleomorphic morphology with linear/branching distribution (white arrows). Category: BI-RADS 4B.

A stereotactic biopsy showed DCIS and patient subsequently underwent a lumpectomy followed by radiotherapy.

A2. Right MLO and CC views (Fig. 11.7b) show heterogeneously dense breast parenchyma. Architectural distortion and metallic clips in the central aspect of right breast are compatible with posttherapeutic changes. There is a group of suspicious microcalcifications in the upper outer quadrant of the right breast, superolateral to the previous surgical scar (white arrows).

Further evaluation with magnification views of the right breast for better assessment of the microcalcifications is recommended. An ultrasound should be performed to exclude underlying mass.

A3. Magnification views of the right breast in two orthogonal projections (Fig. 11.7c) show a large group of fine linear/branching microcalcifications seen in the outer central aspect of right breast (white arrows). Ultrasound (Fig. 11.7d) shows an

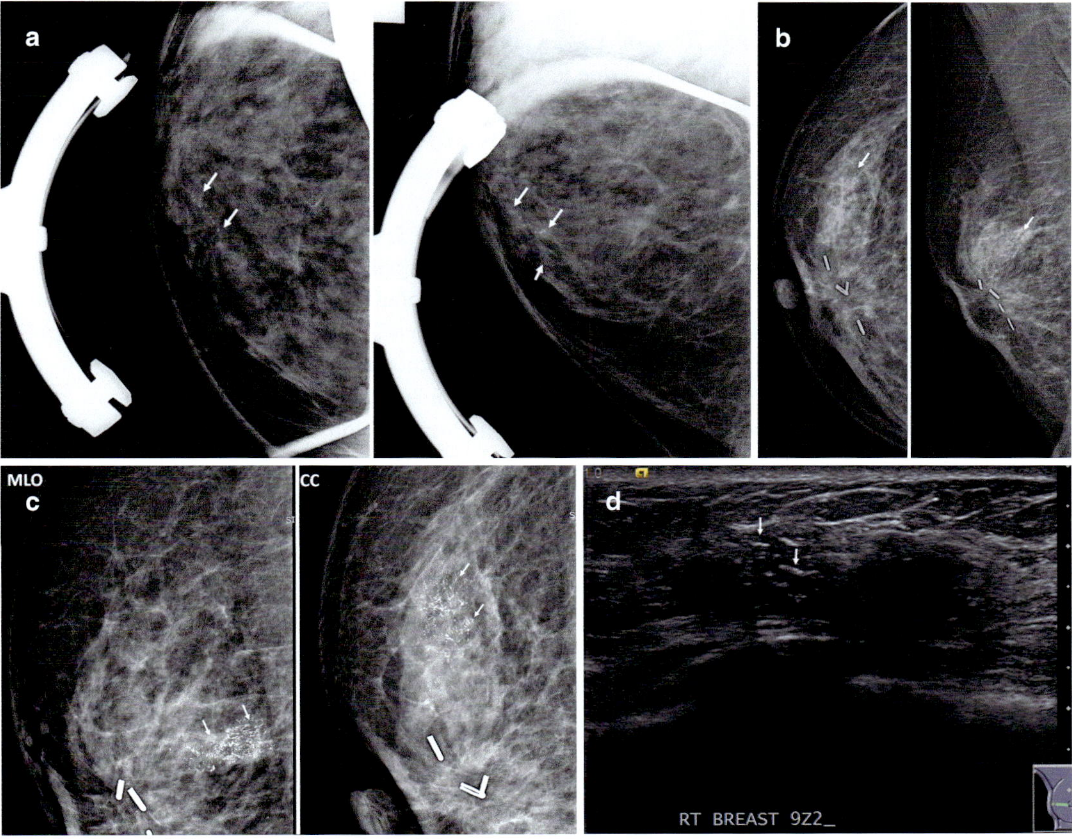

Fig. 11.7 (**a**) Right spot magnification views in orthogonal projections. (**b**) Right CC and MLO views. (**c**) Right spot magnification views in orthogonal projections. (**d**) Targeted right breast ultrasound

irregular hypoechoic mass with indistinct margins and parallel orientation at 9 o'clock in the right breast. The mass shows internal calcifications (white arrows). Mixed posterior features are noted. This mass corresponds to the mammographic microcalcifications in the right breast.

The findings are suspicious for recurrence of breast malignancy and categorized as BI-RADS 4C.

Ultrasound-guided biopsy was recommended with a post-biopsy specimen radiograph to ensure retrieval of the microcalcifications.

A4. There is radiological-pathological concordance. Findings confirm recurrent DCIS. Patient underwent right mastectomy.

Notes

Recurrent DCIS

There is high risk of local recurrence of DCIS in women who are young, have a family history of breast cancer, BRCA gene mutation, and history of mantle radiation in past. Tumor factors that increase the risk of recurrence include, large tumor size, micropapillary variant, high-grade DCIS with comedonecrosis, multifocal-multicentric disease, positive surgical margins, and triple negative subtype.

Radiological-Pathological (Rad-Path) Concordance

Imaging-guided needle biopsy is a reliable and accurate method of reaching a tissue diagnosis in benign or malignant breast conditions. Despite good technique, 0.3–8.2% of cancers can be missed on core biopsy. About 70% of these missed cancers are immediately identified due to discordant results. About 30% may be missed and are then identified on follow-up. It is therefore the responsibility of every radiologist to perform radiology-pathology correlation following all biopsies to avoid a delay in diagnosis. There are five different types of Rad-Path correlation:

Category 1: Concordant Malignancy

A lesion which appears suspicious for malignancy on imaging (BI-RADS category 4 or 5) undergoes needle biopsy to confirm malignancy is a concordant malignancy.

Category 2: Discordant Malignancy

A BI-RADS category 2 or 3 lesion with benign imaging features undergoing biopsy (new finding, palpable finding or interval growth) if proven malignant on histology is termed as discordant malignancy. The cancer is not missed in this case and hence management is similar to that for a concordant malignancy.

Category 3: Concordant Benign

A lesion which is initially thought to be benign radiologically (BI-RADS category 2, 3, or 4a) and also demonstrates benign pathology at needle biopsy is a concordant benign lesion.

Category 4: Discordant Benign

When a lesion has suspicious imaging features (BI-RADS category 4 or 5) but demonstrates benign histology results on needle biopsy, it is termed as discordant benign. The radiologist should carefully review the imaging features again and if the benign histology is still deemed discordant, then repeat biopsy or excision should be suggested to rule out false negative results. Some benign lesions that may mimic malignancy are sclerosing adenosis, fat necrosis, postsurgical scar, mastitis, granular cell tumor, diabetic mastopathy, desmoid tumor, and sarcoidosis. These may need excision biopsy to confirm benignity (true negative).

Discordant benign biopsies may also occur due to nontarget biopsy or faulty technique. These discordant benign lesions can lead to missed cancers at needle biopsy and should be carefully assessed to avoid a delay in diagnosis (false negative).

Category 5: Borderline or High Risk

Entities such as atypical ductal hyperplasia (ADH), lobular neoplasia (LN), and flat epithelial atypia (FEA) are not considered malignant but are known to increase lifetime risk for the development of breast cancer. These are termed as high-risk lesions. Management of these lesions is controversial, and a multidisciplinary approach is necessary. Women with high-risk lesions may also benefit from heightened screening and risk-reduction strategies.

Suggested Readings

ACR BI-RADS Atlas. 5th Edition. 2013.

Badruddoja M. Ductal carcinoma in situ of the breast: a surgical perspective. Int J Surg Oncol. 2012;2012:761364.

Binokay F, Soyupak S, Bicakci K, Bolat A. Wide spectrum of fibrocystic changes: MR findings.

Burstein HJ, Polyak K, Wong JS, Lester SC, Kaelin CM. Ductal carcinoma in situ of the breast. N Engl J Med. 2004;350(14):1430–41.

Dupont WD, Parl FF, Hartmann WH, Brinton LA, Winfield AC, Worrell JA, Schuyler PA, Plummer WD. Breast cancer risk associated with proliferative breast disease and atypical hyperplasia. Cancer. 1993;71(4):1258–65.

Foster MC, Helvie MA, Gregory NE, Rebner M, Nees AV, Paramagul C. Lobular carcinoma in situ or atypical lobular hyperplasia at core-needle biopsy is excisional biopsy necessary. Radiology. 2004;231(3):813–9.

Frappart L, Remy I, Lin HC, Bremond A, Raudrant D, Grousson B, Vauzelle JL. Different types of microcalcifications observed in breast pathology. Virchows Arch A. 1987;410(3):179–87.

Garreau JR, Nelson J, Look R, Walts D, Mahin D, Homer L, Johnson N. Risk counseling and management in patients with lobular carcinoma in situ. Am J Surg. 2005;189(5):610–5.

Georgian-Smith D, Lawton TJ. Calcifications of lobular carcinoma in situ of the breast: radiologic—pathologic correlation. Am J Roentgenol. 2001;176(5):1255–9.

Holland R, Stekhoven JS, Hendriks JH, Verbeek AL, Mravunac M. Extent, distribution, and mammographic/histological correlations of breast ductal carcinoma in situ. Lancet. 1990;335(8688):519–22.

Hyo Soon Lim MD, Su Jin Jeong MD, Ji Shin Lee MD, Min Ho Park MD, Jin Woong Kim MD, Sang Soo Shin MD, Jin Gyoon Park MD, Heoung Keun Kang MD. Paget disease of the breast: mammographic, US, and MR imaging findings with pathologic correlation. Radiographics. 2011;31:1973–87.

Kim SY, Kim HY, Kim EK, Kim MJ, Moon HJ, Yoon JH. Evaluation of malignancy risk stratification of microcalcifications detected on mammography: a study based on the 5th edition of BI-RADS. Ann Surg Oncol. 2015;22(9):2895–901.

Kohr JR, Eby PR, Allison KH, DeMartini WB, Gutierrez RL, Peacock S, Lehman CD. Risk of upgrade of atypical ductal hyperplasia after stereotactic breast biopsy: effects of number of foci and complete removal of calcifications. Radiology. 2010;255(3):723–30.

Kuhl CK, Schrading S, Bieling HB, Wardelmann E, Leutner CC, Koenig R, Kuhn W, Schild HH. MRI for diagnosis of pure ductal carcinoma in situ: a prospective observational study. Lancet. 2007;370(9586):485–92.

Narod SA, Iqbal J, Giannakeas V, Sopik V, Sun P. Breast cancer mortality after a diagnosis of ductal carcinoma in situ. JAMA Oncol. 2015;1(7):888–96.

Sickles EA. Breast calcifications: mammographic evaluation. Radiology. 1986;160(2):289–93.

Singh M, Rittenbach JV. Ductal and lobular proliferations: preinvasive breast disease. Early Diagnosis and Treatment of Cancer Series: Breast Cancer. 2011:11–20.

Sripathi S, Ayachit A, Kadavigere R, Kumar S, Eleti A, Sraj A. Spectrum of imaging findings in paget's disease of the breast—a pictorial review. Insight Imag. 2015;6(4):419–29.

Stomper PC, Connolly JL. Ductal carcinoma in situ of the breast: correlation between mammographic calcification and tumor subtype. Am J Roentgenol. 1992;159(3):483–5.

Stomper PC, Margolin FR. Ductal carcinoma in situ: the mammographer's perspective. Am J Roentgenol. 1994;162(3):585–91.

Tice JA, O'meara ES, Weaver DL, Vachon C, Ballard-Barbash R, Kerlikowske K. Benign breast disease, mammographic breast density, and the risk of breast cancer. J Natl Cancer Inst. 2013;105(14):1043–9.

Youk JH, Kim E-K, Kim MJ, Ko KH, Kwak JY, Son EJ, Choi J, Kang HY. Concordant or discordant? imaging-pathology correlation in a sonography-guided core needle biopsy of a breast lesion. Korean J Radiol. 2011;12(2):232–40.

12 Architectural Distortion and Asymmetry

12.1 Case 12.1

History: 77-year-old woman was referred to breast imaging for workup of incidental detection of enhancing left breast mass on a liver MRI.

Questions

Q1. Describe the abnormality on standard mammogram (Fig. 12.1a, b). What would you recommend next?

Q2. Describe the abnormality and give appropriate BI-RADS on additional views (Fig. 12.1c) and the ultrasound image (Fig. 12.1d) provided.

Q3. Provide possible differentials for this abnormality?

Answers

A1. Bilateral MLO (Fig. 12.1a) and CC (Fig. 12.1b) views show heterogeneously dense breast parenchyma. There is an isodense focal asymmetry seen in the central left breast (arrows). There is a small group of microcalcifications within this asymmetry (thick arrow). Bilateral vascular calcifications are noted. Skin, subcutaneous tissue, and nipple appear unremarkable (A metallic bead marker in upper half of right breast is to annotate a skin lesion).

Recommendations: Comparison to prior imaging and additional workup in the form of spot magnification views and a targeted ultrasound examination.

A2. Spot magnification views of the left breast in orthogonal planes (Fig. 12.1c) show the focal asymmetry to be persistent. There is a group of fine pleomorphic microcalcifications seen in this region (thick white arrows). There is no spiculated mass or architectural distortion identified in this region. Ultrasound (Fig. 12.1d) shows an irregular, hypoechoic mass at the 4 o'clock location in left breast. No internal vascularity is seen in this lesion. This mass correlates with the mammographic findings in the left breast. The findings are indeterminate to suspicious, especially in a 77-year-old woman. Category: BI-RADS 4. Ultrasound-guided biopsy of this lesion is recommended.

A3. Differential diagnosis for this case include:

- Invasive mammary carcinoma (ILC or IDC).
- DCIS.

Histopathology: Ultrasound-guided biopsy revealed high-grade DCIS. This is concordant based on imaging findings. Patient subsequently underwent left mastectomy.

N. Chotai, S. Kulkarni, *Breast Imaging Essentials*, https://doi.org/10.1007/978-981-15-1412-8_12

Notes

Asymmetries are often encountered in mammograms. As per the fifth edition of the BI-RADS lexicon, they are classified as follows:

1. **Asymmetry**: Asymmetry is defined as deposits of fibroglandular tissue, lacking the characteristics of a mass and usually seen in only one mammographic view. They demonstrate concave borders interspersed with fat and are usually unilateral. In almost 80% of cases an asymmetry represents summation artifacts from superimposition of normal breast structures. Invasive lobular carcinoma may present as an asymmetry.
2. **Focal Asymmetry**: When an asymmetry is seen on two standard views and has a similar shape on both views but not fitting the criteria of a mass, it is called a focal asymmetry. It occupies less than one quadrant in the breast. Although this usually represents an island of tissue, an ill-defined mass can present as a focal asymmetry, and hence requires further evaluation.
3. **Global Asymmetry**: When the asymmetry is greater in volume and involves a significant portion of the breast relative to the contralateral breast, without any associated mass or calcifications, it is termed global asymmetry. It usually represents a normal variant, many times with hormonal influence (Fig. 12.1e, *a–c*).
4. **Developing Asymmetry** (Case 12.2):
   A focal asymmetry which is either larger or denser than the previous examination is called a developing asymmetry. Comparison with prior mammograms is essential. In the absence of hormonal stimulation, trauma, surgery, or infection, the likelihood of malignancy ranges from 13–27% for the developing asymmetry and when seen should undergo biopsy.

12.2 Case 12.2

History: 70-year-old woman (average risk) underwent a routine screening mammogram.

Questions

Q1. Describe the abnormality on standard views (Fig. 12.2a, b). What would you advise next?

Q2. Describe the findings on additional mammogram (Fig. 12.2c) and ultrasound (Fig. 12.2d) provided. What would be appropriate BI-RADS?

Q3. What are the differentials for this abnormality?

Answers

A1. Serial left MLO (Fig. 12.2a) and CC (Fig. 12.2b) views from September 2006, 2008, and 2009 are available. Left breast shows heterogeneously dense breast parenchyma. There is a small, isodense developing asymmetry noted in the upper outer quadrant in the posterior third of the left breast (white arrow). It appears to be gradually increasing in size on serial mammograms. In 2009 it looks like a small mass on the MLO view. There are no associated suspicious microcalcifications or distortion.

Recommendation: Spot compression views for better evaluation of the developing asymmetry and targeted ultrasound of upper outer quadrant of left breast to look for a sonographic correlate.

A2. Additional spot compression views in orthogonal planes (Fig. 12.2c) show better margin depiction of the asymmetry which now can

Fig. 12.1 (**a**) Bilateral MLO views. (**b**) Bilateral CC views. (**c**) Left magnification views in orthogonal planes. (**d**) Targeted left breast ultrasound. (**e**) (*a–c*) Global asymmetry. Bilateral MLO (*a*) and CC (*b*) views show a large isodense asymmetry in upper outer quadrant of the left breast. No associated microcalcifications or architectural distortion is seen. Panoramic ultrasound image (*c*) reveals an island of normal appearing parenchyma in left breast conforming to the mammographic finding

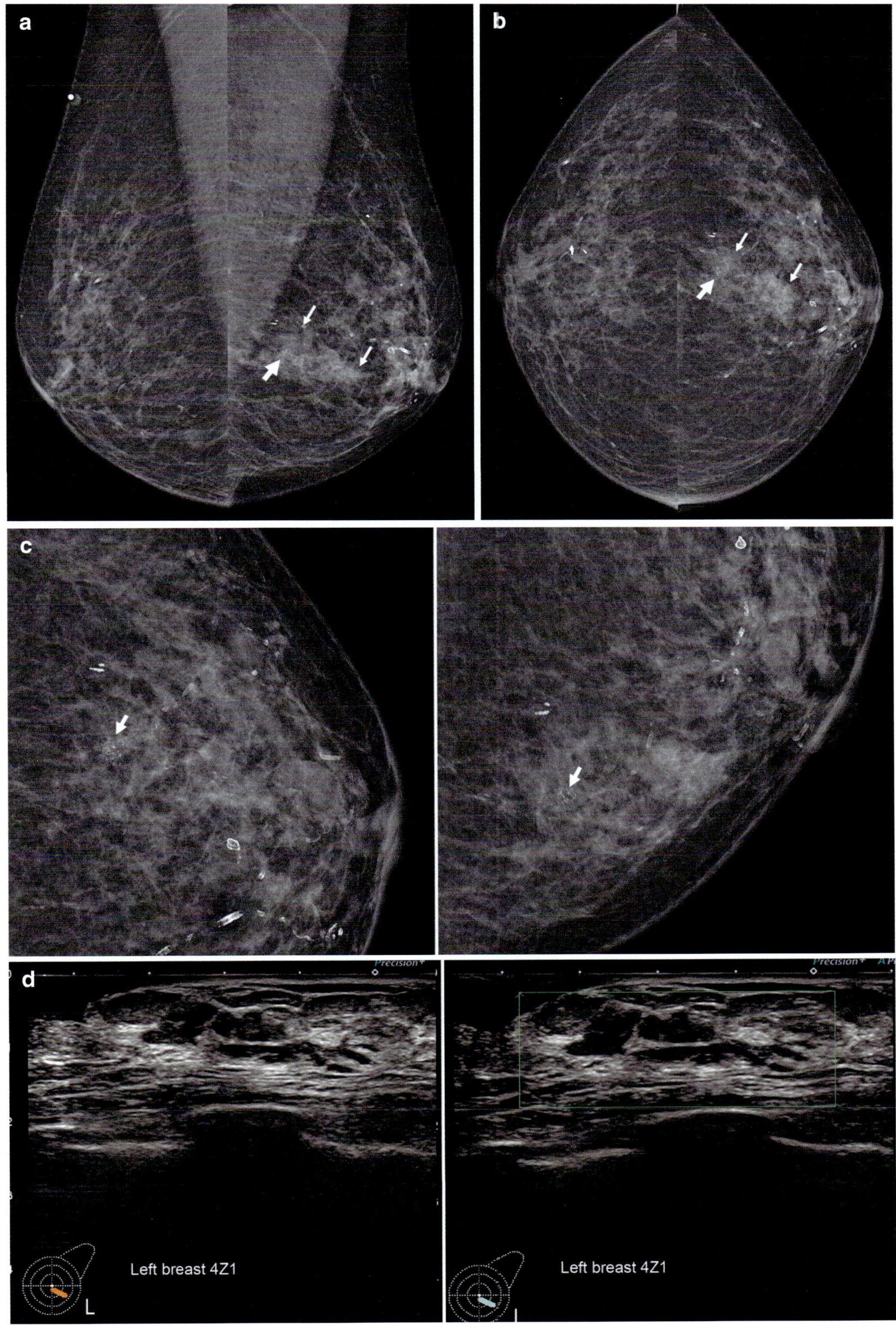
a
b
c
d
Left breast 4Z1
L
Left breast 4Z1

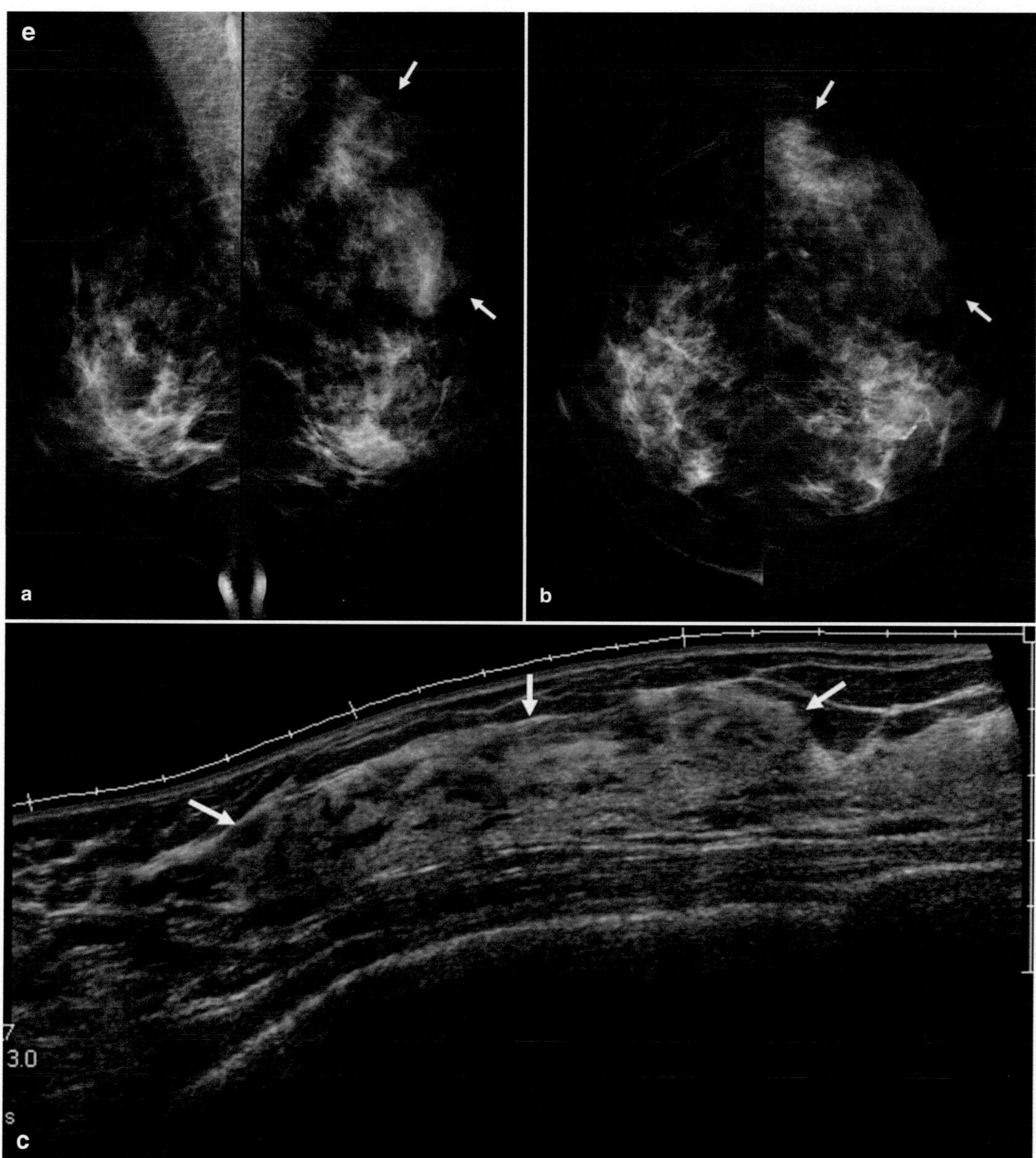

Fig. 12.1 (continued)

be reclassified as a mass (white arrows). No associated microcalcifications are seen. Ultrasound images (Fig. 12.2d) of the left breast at 2 o'clock location show a hyperechoic lesion with irregular margins laterally and a central hypoechoic nidus with minimal posterior shadowing (white arrows). It is likely to correlat with the mammographic finding.

Category: BI-RADS 4.

Ultrasound-guided biopsy is suggested. Insertion of a post-biopsy clip is suggested to mark the area as well as to correlate on two modalities to ensure that the correct area was biopsied.

Figure 12.2e shows the post biopsy marker clip in the targeted mammographic lesion (white arrows).

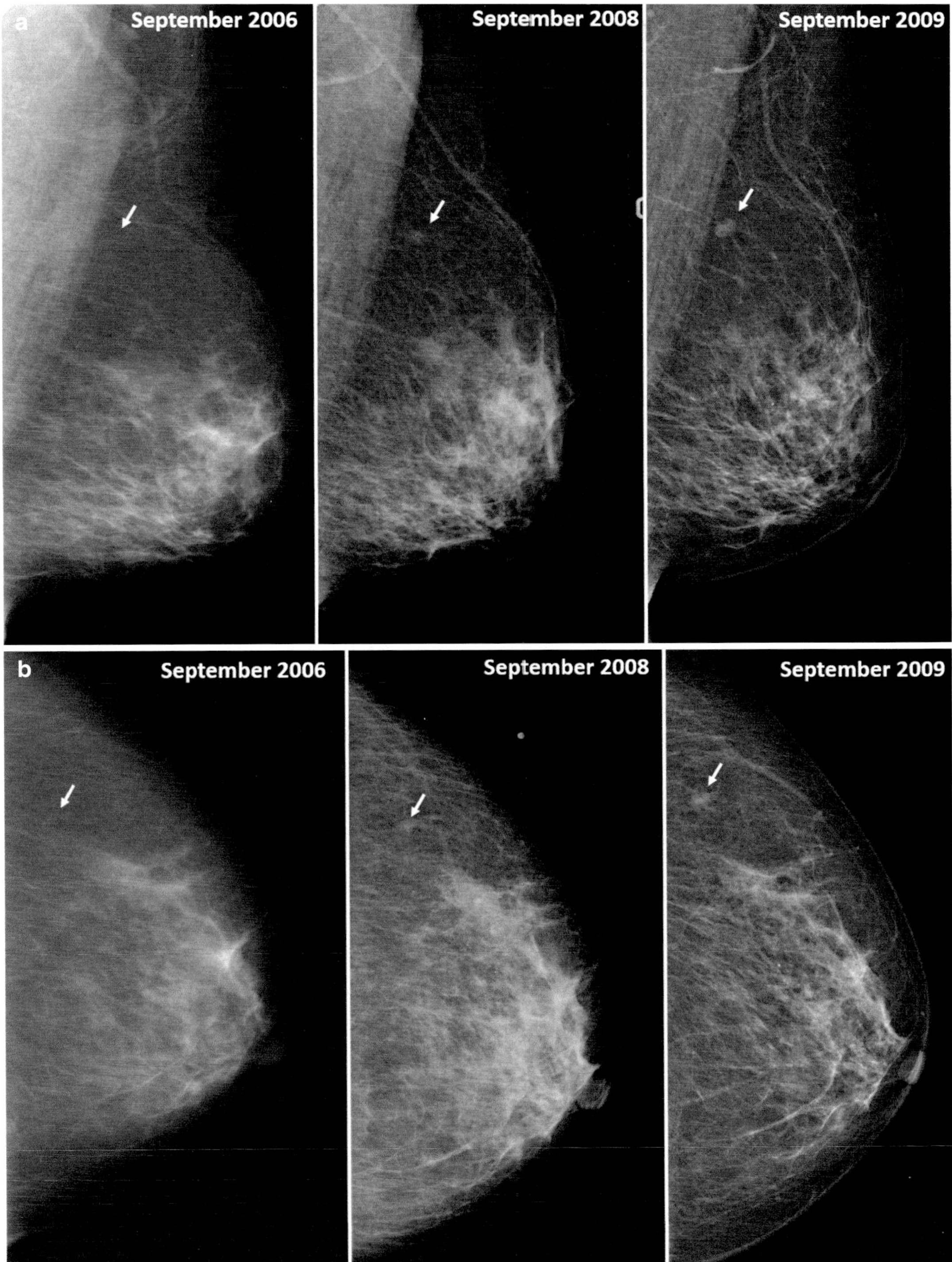

Fig. 12.2 (**a**) Serial left MLO views. (**b**) Serial left CC views. (**c**) Left spot compression views in orthogonal planes. (**d**) Targeted left breast ultrasound. (**e**) Left mammogram following post-biopsy clip placement

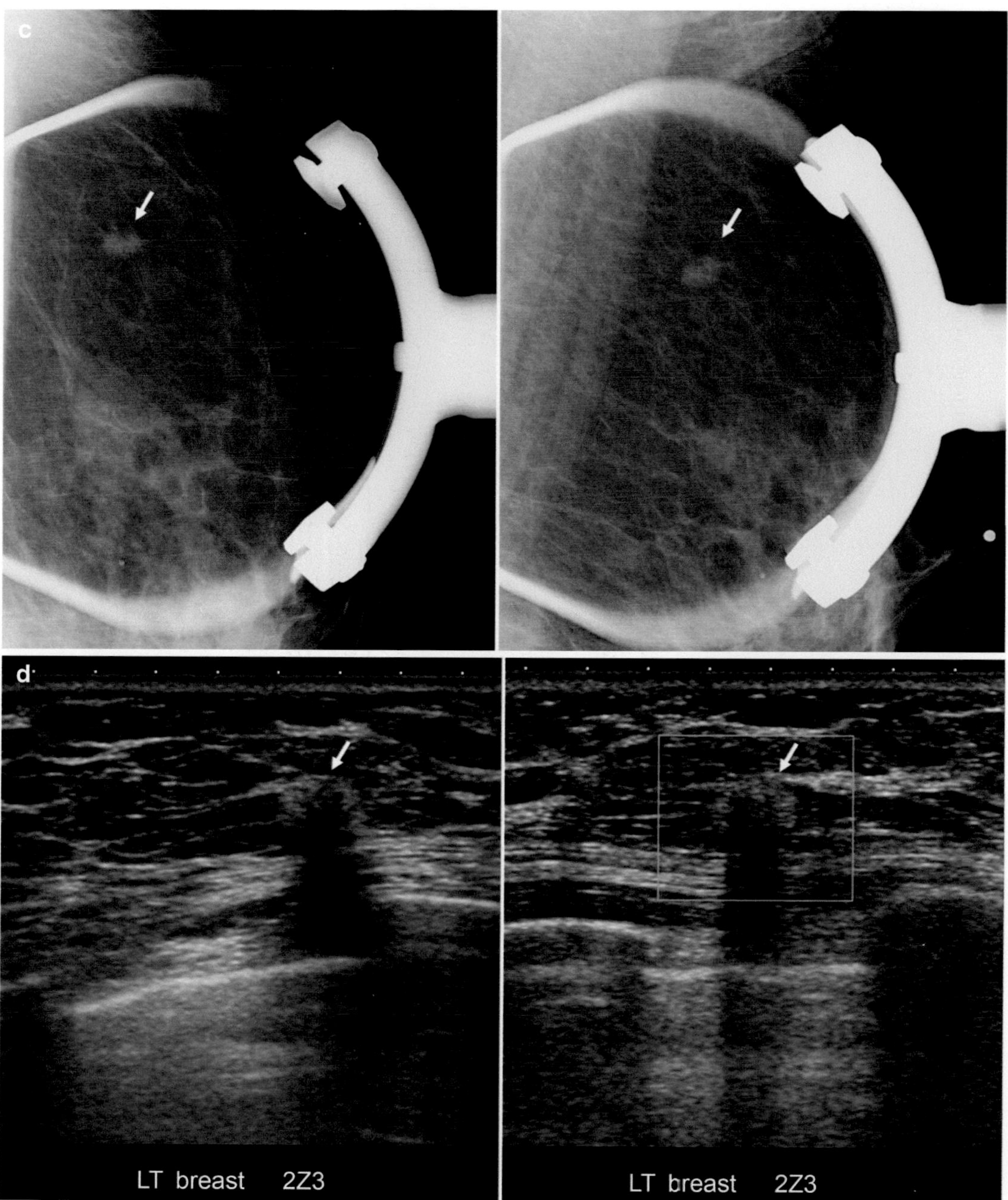

Fig. 12.2 (continued)

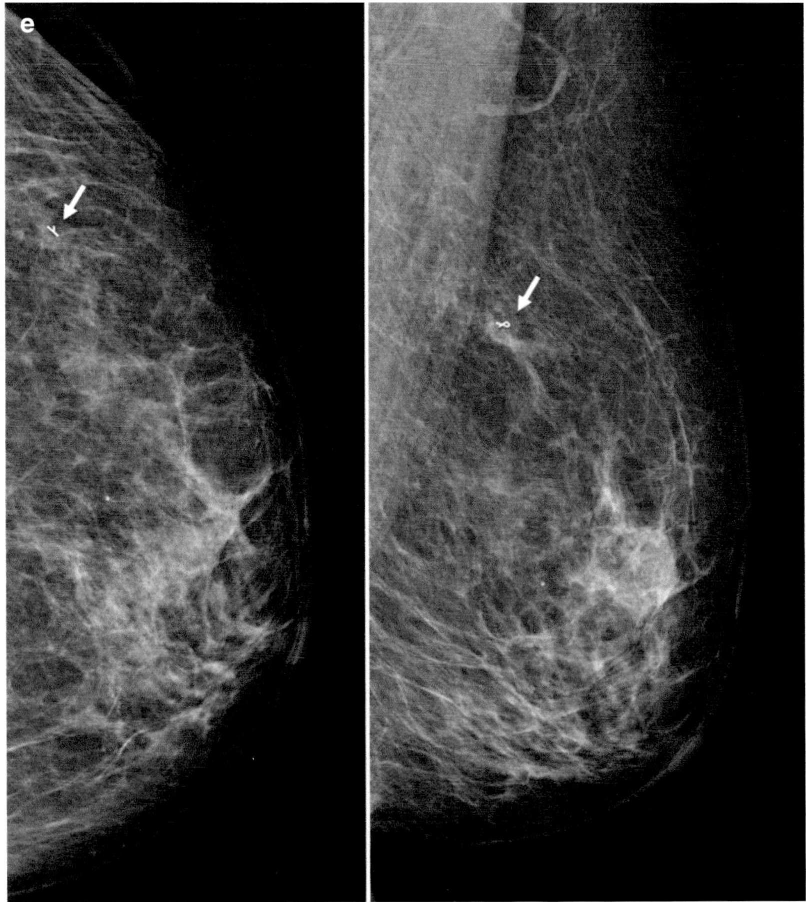

Fig. 12.2 (continued)

A3. Differential diagnosis includes: normal breast tissue (hormonal stimulation), invasive mammary carcinoma, infection, and postsurgical or posttraumatic changes.

Histopathology: Ultrasound-guided biopsy revealed Grade 2 invasive ductal carcinoma.

Notes

Echogenic Malignancies

Though malignant tumors are generally seen as hypoechoic masses on ultrasound, approximately 0.4% of malignant breast tumors are seen as hyperechoic lesions on sonography. A new hyperechoic lesion should be viewed with the same level of suspicion as a hypoechoic lesion and a careful scrutiny for concerning features should be made.

Small echogenic malignancies often show a small hypoechoic nidus. Stavros et al. first described this finding of a small isoechoic or hypoechoic central nidus with thick echogenic ill-defined halo. One should therefore be careful before dismissing a new echogenic lesion. Differential diagnosis would be IDC, ILC, DCIS, and rare lesions such as lymphoma, angiosarcoma, and metastasis.

12.3 Case 12.3

History: 55-year-old woman (average risk) underwent a routine screening mammogram.

Questions

Q1. Describe the abnormality on the provided mammogram (Fig. 12.3a–c).

Q2. Provide possible differentials in this case. What would you recommend next?

Q3. Describe the abnormality on ultrasound images (Fig. 12.3d) and give appropriate BI-RADS.

Q4. Ultrasound-guided biopsy of the mass was performed, and histopathology was reported as radial sclerosing lesion. What would you recommend next?

Answers

A1. Right MLO (Fig. 12.3a) and CC views (Fig. 12.3b) show heterogeneously dense breast parenchyma. There is an architectural distortion (white arrows) seen in the upper right breast associated with mild nipple retraction. A few punctate and coarse calcifications are seen in this region. Overlying skin is unremarkable.

Spot magnification views done in orthogonal planes (Fig. 12.3c) better depict the architectural distortion and exclude associated suspicious microcalcifications. It is important to exclude prior history of surgery and compare with prior imaging when available.

A2. Main differentials to be considered for architectural distortion in breast include: Invasive mammary carcinoma, DCIS,

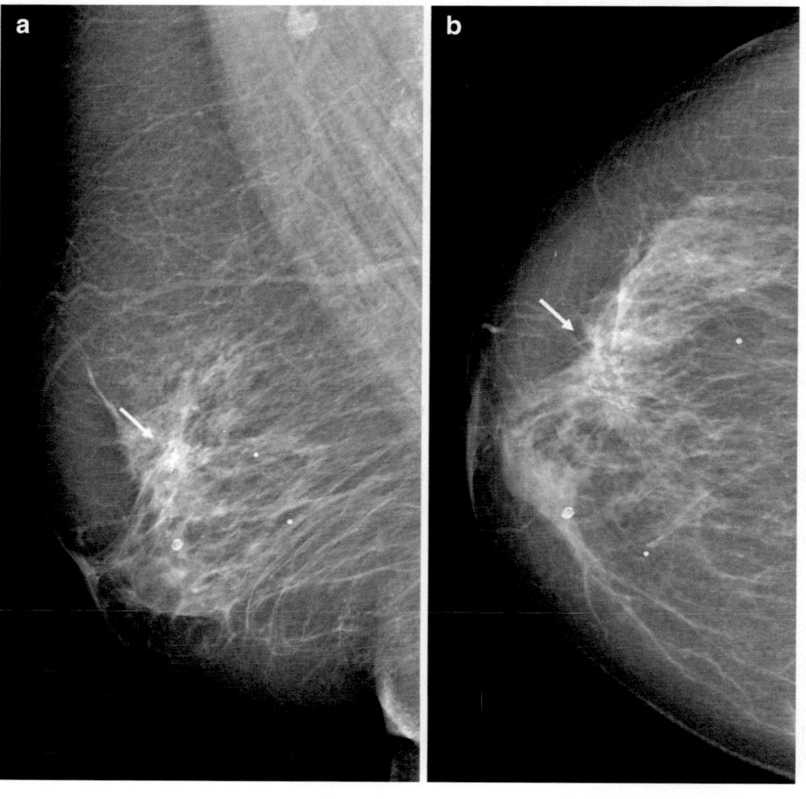

Fig. 12.3 (**a**) Right MLO view. (**b**) Right CC view. (**c**) Right spot compression views in orthogonal planes. (**d**) Automated breast volume ultrasound of central right breast

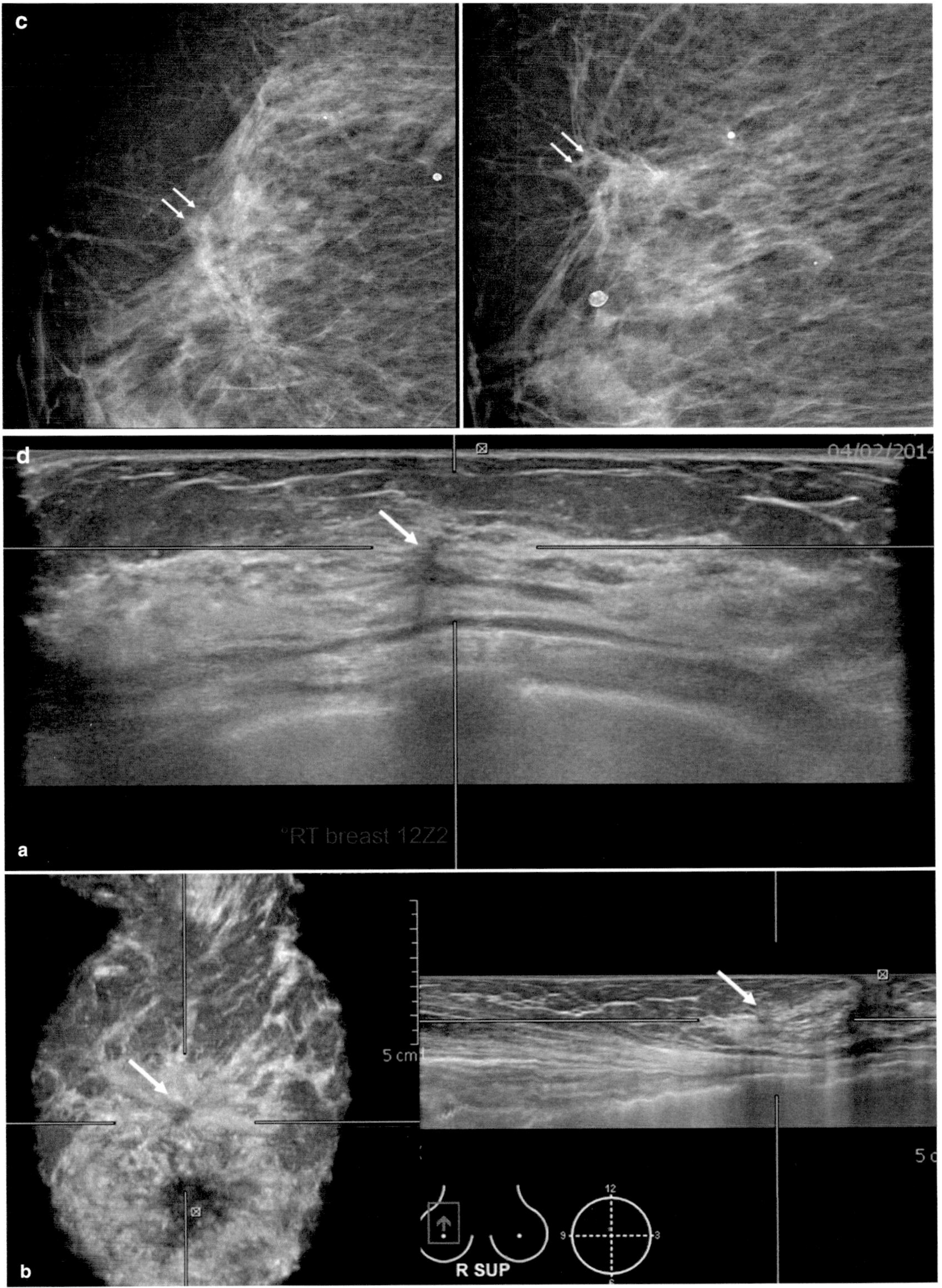

Fig. 12.3 (continued)

complex sclerosing lesion (radial scar) and post-operative change. In the absence of any prior breast surgery, the findings are considered suspicious. Further evaluation with ultrasound should be done.

A3. Axial (a), coronal (b), and sagittal (c) reconstructed images using automated breast volume ultrasound (Fig. 12.3d) shows an irregular, hypoechoic mass (white arrows) with dense posterior shadowing in the 12 o'clock location in the right breast. The mass shows antiparallel orientation, i.e., taller than wide. There is associated architectural distortion that is better appreciated on coronal image. The mass is felt to correlate with the mammographic architectural distortion. The findings are suspicious, and an ultrasound-guided biopsy is recommended. Category: BI-RADS 4.

A4. Histopathology of a radial sclerosing lesion could be concordant; however, a wire-guided excision is suggested to exclude further upgrade to malignancy.

Histopathology: Patient underwent right excision biopsy, and the final histopathology was radial sclerosing lesion with flat epithelial atypia. There was no upgrade to cancer.

Notes

Architectural Distortion

When normal architecture of breast is altered with thin spiculations radiating from a point without a definite mass, it is described as architectural distortion. Occasionally on mammography, it may appear as straightening at the anterior or posterior edge of the parenchyma. It may be associated with microcalcifications or asymmetry, which increases the risk of cancer. In the absence of appropriate history of surgery or trauma, architectural distortion is generally considered a suspicious finding, category BI-RADS 4 and histopathological correlation is warranted.

The risk of cancer in architectural distortion is deemed higher on a diagnostic mammogram versus screening mammogram (83% versus 67%). The presence of sonographic correlate is associated with higher risk of breast cancer (83%). On MRI, lack of enhancement is reassuring, nearly 100% NPV.

Complex Sclerosing Lesion (CSL) Or Radial Scar (RS)

These are benign proliferative lesions with central fibroelastosis and a spiculated appearance on imaging and histology. When a radial scar is more than 1 cm in size it is called a complex sclerosing lesion.

Mammogram generally shows architectural distortion with long radiating spicules and central lucency (Black star). They do not show skin retraction. There may be associated microcalcifications in 33–50% of cases that may suggest adenosis, ADH, or DCIS and sometimes low-grade tubular carcinomas.

These lesions are difficult to detect on ultrasound but occasionally may show tethering of a Cooper's ligament or a spiculated hypoechoic mass with shadowing.

On MRI, they may show a small spiculated enhancing mass or no enhancement at all.

They may show a 4–12% upgrade to more significant pathology on surgery and as high as 25–50% if biopsy shows associated ADH/LCIS/ALH. Hence excision biopsy is generally advised for a diagnosis of CSL or RS.

Occasionally, a stable RS may be documented over multiple years of screening. In these cases, it may be reasonable to forgo excision and just follow them. One may refer to their institutional guidelines.

Suggested Readings

Bahl M, Baker JA, Kinsey EN, Ghate SV. Architectural distortion on mammography: correlation with pathologic outcomes and predictors of malignancy. Am J Roentgenol. 2015;205(6):1339–45.

BIRADS® for: mammography and ultrasound (2013 updated version).

Linda A, Zuiani C, Lorenzon M, Furlan A, Girometti R, Londero V, Bazzocchi M. Hyperechoic lesions of the breast: not always benign. Am J Roentgenol. 2011;196:1219–24.

Resetkova E, Edelweiss M, Albarracin CT, Yang WT. Management of radial sclerosing lesions of the breast diagnosed using percutaneous vacuum-assisted core needle biopsy: recommendations for excision based on seven years' of experience at a single institution. Breast Cancer Res Treat. 2011;127(2):335–43.

Sickles EA. Findings at mammographic screening on only one standard projection: outcomes analysis. Radiology. 1998;208(2):471–5.

Stavros AT, Thickman D, Rapp CL, Dennis MA, Parker SH, Sisney GA. Solid breast nodules: use of sonography to distinguish between benign and malignant lesions. Radiology. 1995;196:123–34.

Youk JH, Kim E-K, Ko KH, Kim MJ. Asymmetric mammographic findings based on the fourth edition of BI-RADS: types, evaluation, and management. RadioGraphics. 2009; https://doi.org/10.1148/rg.e33.

13 Benign Breast Diseases

13.1 Case 13.1

History: 57-year-old woman with occasional spontaneous blood-stained left nipple discharge. No family history of breast cancer.

Questions

Q1. Describe the lesion on mammogram (Fig. 13.1a–c).
Q2. Describe the lesion on ultrasound (Fig. 13.1d) and give appropriate BI-RADS.
Q3. Provide possible differentials.

Answers

A1. Bilateral MLO (Fig. 13.1a) and CC (Fig. 13.1b) views show heterogeneously dense breast parenchyma. There is an isodense mass in the left retroareolar breast with partially obscured margins (white arrow). No associated microcalcifications or architectural distortion is noted. Right breast is unremarkable.

Spot compression views of the left retroareolar region (Fig. 13.1c) show the mass to be oval with partially circumscribed margins (white arrows). The surrounding parenchymal tissues obscure the posterior margin. No microcalcifications are noted.

A2. Ultrasound images (Fig. 13.1d) show a complex (solid cystic) mass in the left retroareolar region at the 3 o'clock location corresponding to the mammographic abnormality. It is associated with a mildly dilated duct distal to the mass (white arrows), suggesting its intraductal location. The solid component shows internal vascularity.

DIAGNOSIS: Intraductal papillary lesion categorized as BI-RADS 4.

An ultrasound-guided biopsy of the solid component should be performed to exclude an intracystic papillary carcinoma. Some pathologists may prefer complete excision of a suspected papillary mass without a biopsy. The argument being that a core biopsy may traverse the fibrovascular stalk leading to the necrosis of the entire lesion, precluding accurate pathological diagnosis of invasive disease. Refer to your institutional guidelines.

A3. Possible differentials: Simple intraductal papilloma, intraductal papilloma with atypia, intracystic papillary carcinoma, atypical intraductal epithelial proliferation, and a less likely possibility of a complex benign cyst with thick contents.

N. Chotai, S. Kulkarni, *Breast Imaging Essentials*, https://doi.org/10.1007/978-981-15-1412-8_13

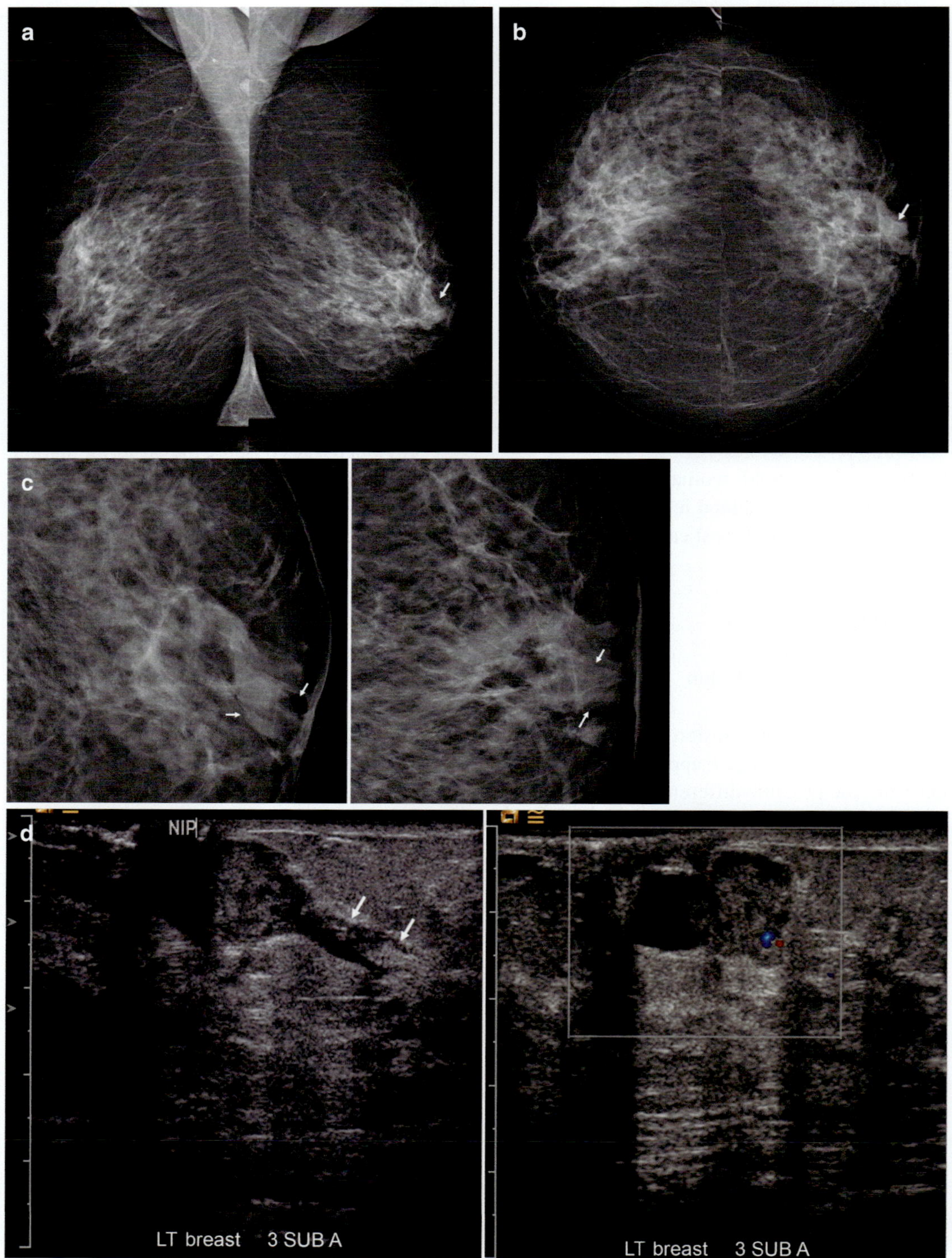

Fig. 13.1 (**a**) Bilateral MLO views. (**b**) Bilateral CC views. (**c**) Left spot compression views in orthogonal projections. (**d**) Targeted left breast ultrasound

Notes

Intraductal Papilloma

Intraductal papilloma (IDP) is a benign intraductal mass that commonly presents as a spontaneous blood-stained or straw-colored nipple discharge. It constitutes about 10% of all benign breast neoplasms. Histopathology reveals epithelial and myoepithelial cell proliferation with a fibrovascular stalk. They occur in women in the 40–50 years' age group. They may be central or peripheral.

The central variety is more common (almost 80%) and is usually solitary. They are typically noted in large lactiferous ducts centrally located near nipple. They may lead to a focal distention of the duct giving it an intracystic papillary appearance. These present with spontaneous straw-colored discharge from a single duct orifice.

Peripheral variety are generally multiple, arise in TDLUs and may present as multiple small peripheral masses and may be associated with RS, ADH, DCIS, or IDC.

Imaging Appearances

Mammography: Many lesions are occult on mammography and when seen they are circumscribed, round or oval masses. Papillomas may have associated clustered punctate or amorphous microcalcifications.

Ultrasound appearance of a periareolar dilated duct with intraductal mass is common and the fibrovascular stalk may be visible on color Doppler. They may present as a complex solid-cystic mass with a variable solid component ranging from tiny mural nodules to masses.

On MRI, T2W images may show a dilated hyperintense duct with a hypointense intraductal mass. On DCE, variable enhancement, washout kinetics, and associated ductal enhancement may be noted.

The risk of breast cancer is two- to fourfold if the papilloma is associated with atypia. It is higher in multiple peripheral papillomas compared to single central papilloma. Reported upgrade rate to carcinoma is about 12–14% and to ADH/other high-risk lesions is about 20%.

Generally, a papilloma on biopsy, especially one associated with atypia, is excised.

13.2 Case 13.2

History: 51-year-old woman with a routine screening mammogram.

Questions

Q1. Describe the findings on mammogram (Fig. 13.2a–c).

Q2. Describe the findings on ultrasound (Fig. 13.2d) and give appropriate BI-RADS.

Q3. Provide possible differentials for a circumscribed mass on a mammogram.

Answers

A1. Bilateral MLO (Fig. 13.2a) and CC views (Fig. 13.2b) show heterogeneously dense breast parenchyma. There is an oval, circumscribed, isodense mass in the lower inner quadrant of the left breast (white arrow). There is another smaller, round, circumscribed, isodense mass with internal calcification in the central aspect of the right breast (double white arrows). Both these masses have benign imaging features. Additionally, there is a small spiculated mass in the upper outer quadrant of the left breast (thick white arrow). This needs further evaluation with spot compression views. No other abnormalities are noted.

Spot compression views of left breast in orthogonal planes (Fig. 13.2c) show a small spiculated mass with fine pleomorphic microcalcifications (thick white arrows) within the confines of the mass.

A2. Select ultrasound images of both breasts (Fig. 13.2d) show an irregular hypoechoic mass (thick white arrow) with angular margins, posterior acoustic shadowing and antiparallel orientation in the left breast at 12 o'clock (a). There is architectural distortion seen around the mass. This correlates with the spiculated mass seen on mammogram. This lesion has suspicious features on both modalities and histological correlation from this mass would be recommended. Category BI-RADS 4.

There are oval, circumscribed, hypoechoic masses with parallel orientation seen in the right breast at the 8 (b) and in the left breast at the 6–7 (c) o'clock positions. No posterior acoustic features noted. They correlate with the circumscribed masses seen on mammogram. They have typical benign imaging features likely representing fibroadenomata. In the absence of any other concern, these are both categorized as BI-RADS 3.

A3. Differential for a well-circumscribed mass on mammography includes: cysts, fibroepithelial lesions (fibroadenoma, phyllodes, and rarely lactational adenoma, tubular adenoma), pseudoangiomatous stromal hyperplasia (PASH), intramammary LN, and well-circumscribed malignancies (mucinous tumor, IDC, papillary carcinoma, triple negative cancer, and metastasis)

Notes

Fibroadenoma

A fibroadenoma is the most common benign breast neoplasm in premenopausal young women (age 25–45 years). It is also the most common

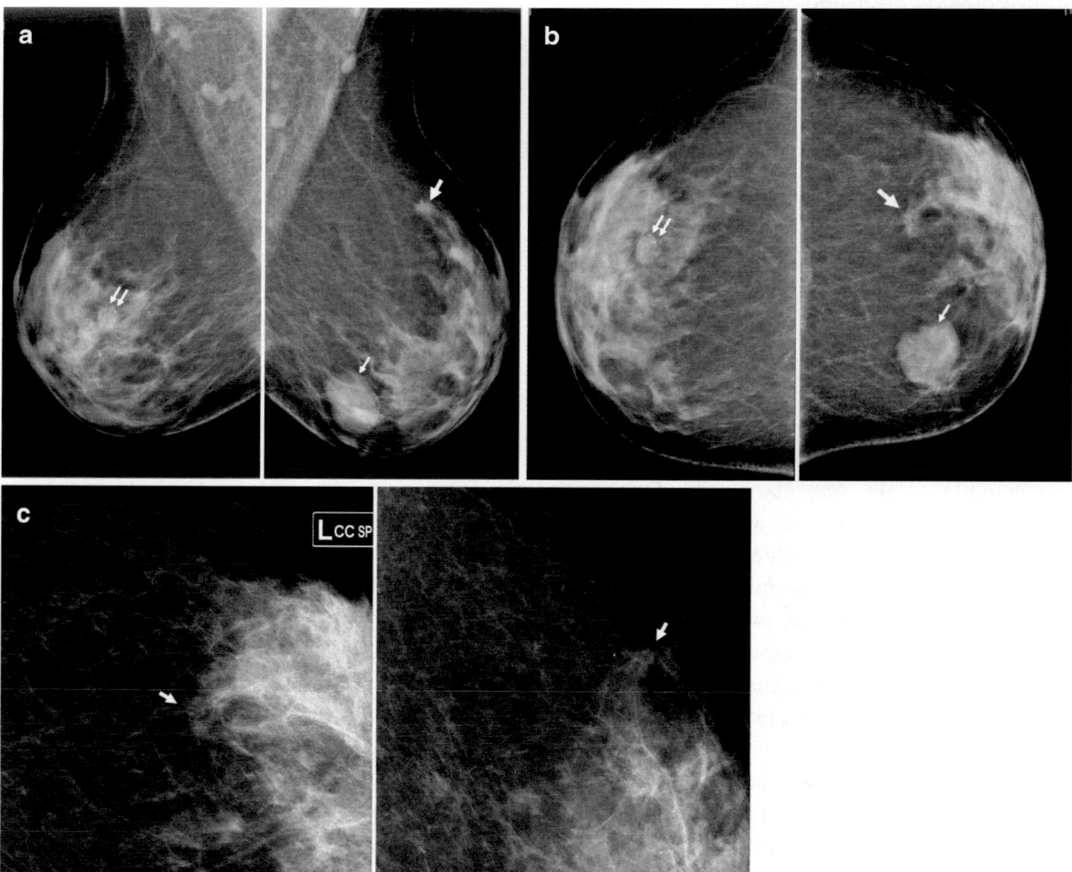

Fig. 13.2 (**a**) Bilateral MLO views. (**b**) Bilateral CC views. (**c**) Left spot compression views in orthogonal projections. (**d**) Targeted bilateral breast ultrasound images

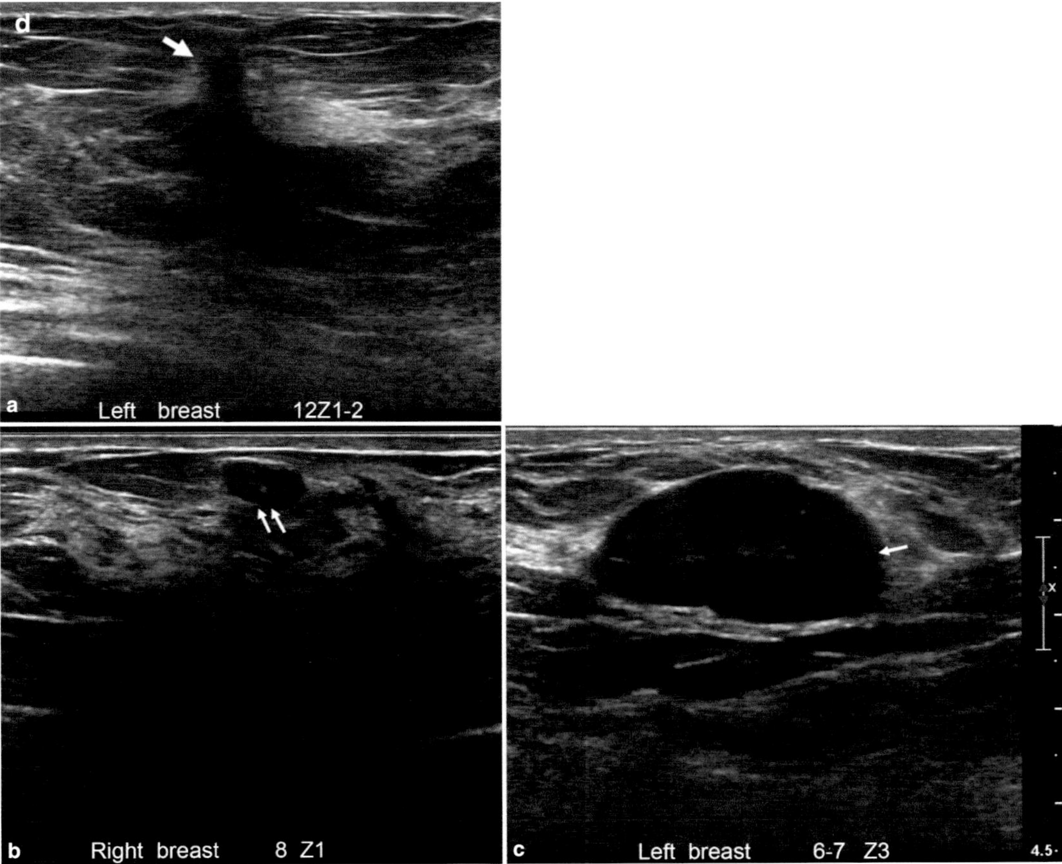

Fig. 13.2 (continued)

benign breast tumor in women of all ages. These are mixed stromal and epithelial tumors.

Fibroadenoma may present clinically as a painless, palpable, highly mobile, firm breast mass. It may be detected incidentally on a screening mammogram in asymptomatic women.

Mammogram may show circumscribed, round to oval, isodense mass with coarse heterogeneous calcifications or the classic popcorn coarse calcifications (especially in involuting fibroadenoma).

Ultrasound shows oval, circumscribed, isoechoic to homogeneously hypoechoic lesion with internal echogenic septum and may show internal calcifications and vascularity.

MRI appearance of fibroadenomata may be varied. They are generally seen as a circumscribed, round or oval, isointense on T1WI and hyperintense of T2WI images. Sclerotic, densely hyalinized, or fibrotic fibroadenomata may lose their T2 hyperintensity and may appear iso- to hypointense on T1WI and T2WI.

Following contrast injection, fibroadenomata generally shows homogeneous internal enhancement with nonenhancing dark septae and a progressively increasing or a plateau type of enhancement. A densely hyalinized fibroadenoma may not show any enhancement on post-contrast images.

Management

Fibroadenomata may involute after menopause and some show slow growth during pregnancy. Stable fibroadenomata can be left alone and may be followed during the patient's routine screening. Some of them get excised based on their clinical symptoms, radiological growth, or the patient's preference. Generally, for an incidentally detected asymptomatic fibroadenoma in a premenopausal woman a 6-, 12-, and 18 (or 24)-month targeted ultrasound follow-up is recommended to establish 2-year stability after which patient can return to the routine screening interval. Any interval change (i.e., >20% growth in 6 months) should trigger an ultrasound core biopsy or excision. Any fibroadenoma that shows increased cellularity on core biopsy should be excised due to the underlying likelihood of phyllodes tumor.

Excision can be surgical or via vacuum-assisted devices as per institutional preference.

13.3 Case 13.3

History: 53-year-old average-risk women presents for a screening mammogram.

Questions

Q1. Describe the abnormality on the provided mammogram (Fig. 13.3a) and ultrasound image (Fig. 13.3b).

Q2. What history would you like to confirm? Provide the appropriate BI-RADS category.

Answers

A1. Right MLO and CC views (Fig. 13.3a) show heterogeneously dense breast parenchyma. There is a round, circumscribed, lucent (fat density) mass seen in the upper central right breast (white arrows). There are no associated calcifications. No spiculated mass or architectural distortion is seen. Skin, subcutaneous tissue, and nipple appear unremarkable. Ultrasound images of right breast (Fig. 13.3b) show a 1.2 × 1.1 × 1.0 cm round, circumscribed, anechoic mass with low-level echoes at the 1 o'clock location, about 3–4 cm from the nipple. No internal vascularity is seen. This is felt to correlate with the fat density lesion seen on mammogram and likely represents fat necrosis.

A2. This finding may be secondary to trauma and upon enquiry, this patient did confirm history of trauma to right breast a few weeks before mammogram. This has typically benign features and would be assigned category BI-RADS 2. Routine mammographic screening would be suggested.

Notes

Fat Necrosis

This is a benign nonsuppurative process involving ischemia of breast fat and may happen as a sequela of trauma, surgery, or radiation.

Mammogram is the best imaging modality for diagnosis. A circumscribed, round, lucent-centered (fat density) lesion, with or without peripheral calcification (Fig. 13.3c), is generally noted on mammogram. Occasionally there may be surrounding increased density secondary to reactive edema or tissue fibrosis.

On ultrasound, the findings show progressive stages starting with tissue edema, anechoic cystic lesion, complex echogenic (solid cystic) mass (Fig. 13.3d) to eventually a heavily calcified lesion. Posterior features may change from enhancement in early cystic phase to shadowing in delayed calcified phase. Differentiation from a malignancy can be hard on ultrasound and correlation with mammography is helpful.

MRI typically shows fat intensity lesion- high signal on T1WI that gets suppressed on fat-saturated sequences often helping clinch the diagnosis. A variable appearance is noted on T2WI based on the stage of evolution. DCE-MRI may show peripheral enhancement, which may mimic a rim enhancing tumor.

Occasionally, if fat necrosis is seen as a densely fibrotic inflammatory mass, it may mimic invasive cancer and may need a biopsy for differentiation. In early calcification stage, the calcifications may be quite pleomorphic and may mimic DCIS and may require a biopsy to differentiate.

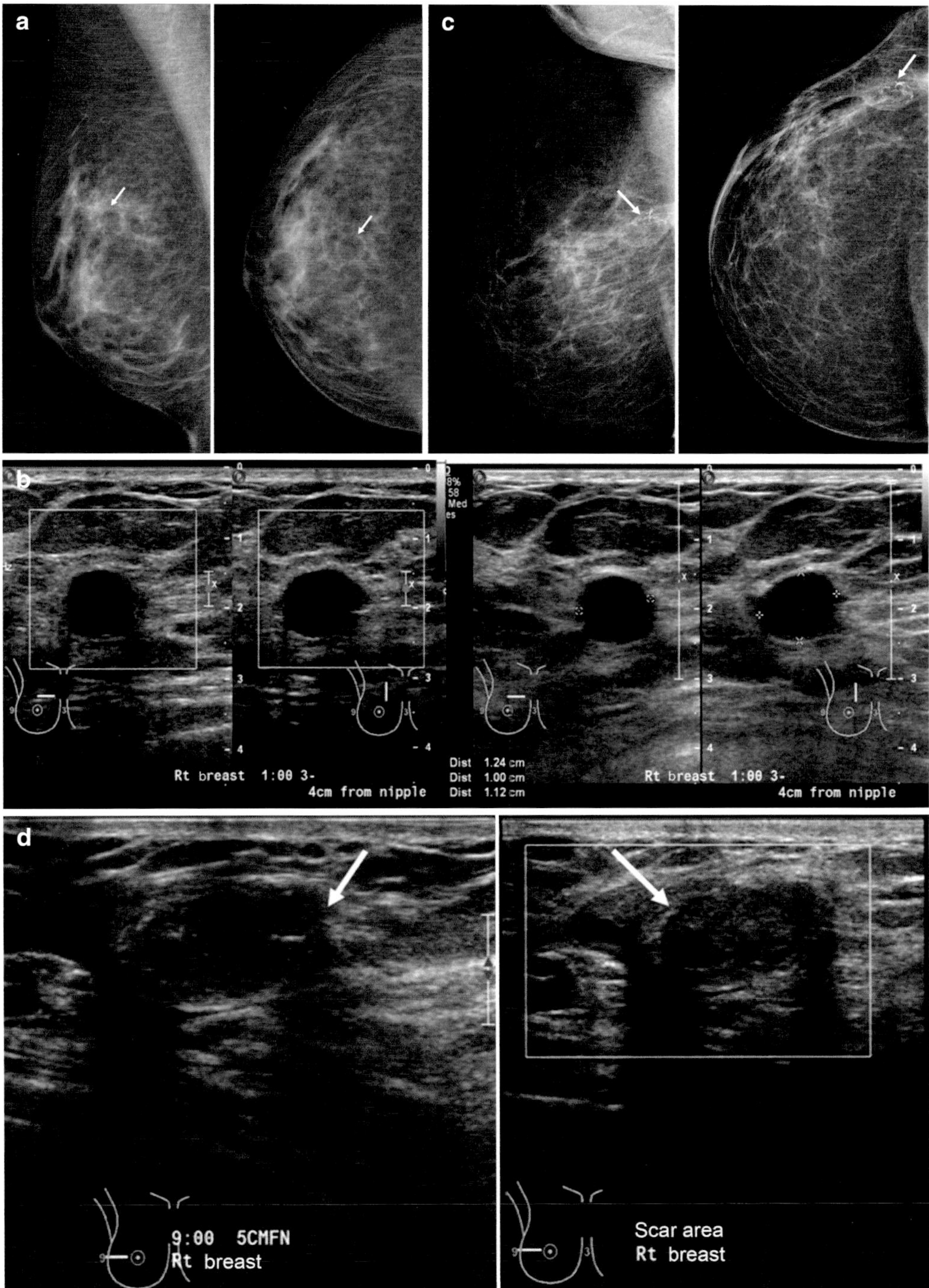

Fig. 13.3 (**a**) Right mammogram in MLO and CC projections. (**b**) Targeted right breast ultrasound. (**c**) Right mammogram—companion case. Right mammogram in MLO and CC projections show architectural distortion in upper outer quadrant of the right breast. This was a post-surgical change. Oval, circumscribed fat-density lesion (white arrows) in the operative bed with peripheral calcification suggests fat necrosis. (**d**) Targeted right breast ultrasound—companion case. Ultrasound images of right breast at the 9 o'clock location, about 5 cm from nipple shows an oval, circumscribed, thick-walled isoechoic lesion with mixed posterior features (white arrows). This correlates with the fat necrosis seen on mammogram and is seen commonly in postoperative bed

Postoperative fat necrosis at the operative bed generally shows calcifications after 1.5–2.0 years of intervention. If calcification is seen earlier than that, then local recurrence should be excluded, especially if the primary tumor was calcified.

13.4 Case 13.4

History: 51-year-old woman presents with a palpable right breast lump, gradually increasing in size. Two mammograms 2 years apart are provided. No significant family history.

Questions

Q1. Describe the mammographic abnormality (Fig. 13.4a) and subsequent 2-year follow up mammogram (Fig. 13.4b).
Q2. Describe the abnormality on Ultrasound (Fig. 13.4c). What would be appropriate BI-RADS?
Q3. Provide possible differentials.
Q4. Ultrasound-guided biopsy of the mass was reported as benign phyllodes tumor. What would you recommend next?

Answers

A1. Right MLO and CC views (Fig. 13.4a) show heterogeneously dense breast parenchyma. A metallic bead marker is seen in upper outer quadrant of the right breast to annotate the site of clinically palpable lump. Underneath the marker is seen a partially defined high-density mass in posterior third depth of the right breast (white arrows). No suspicious microcalcifications are noted.

The follow-up mammogram of the right breast after 2 years (Fig. 13.4b) shows significant increase in the size of the mass (white arrows). The mass still shows circumscribed border and high density. There is no associated architectural distortion or microcalcifications.

A2. Ultrasound images of right breast (Fig. 13.4c) from 2012 (a) at the 10 o'clock region shows a circumscribed, oval, hypoechoic mass with parallel orientation corresponding to the mammographic abnormality. Mild irregularity is seen along the anterior margin.

On follow-up ultrasound after 2 years (b), the palpable mass has significantly increased in size. Its internal echotexture has changed and is now heterogeneous with internal vascularity and cystic changes. The mass has suspicious features, and histological correlation is recommended. Category: BI-RADS 4.

A3. Main differentials to be considered are growing fibroadenoma, phyllodes, invasive mammary carcinoma, and primary sarcoma of breast.

A4. Histology of phyllodes is concordant. Surgical excision of the mass with wide excision margins is recommended.

Notes

Phyllodes Tumor (PT)

Phyllodes tumors have two main components: epithelial tissue and stromal or mesenchymal tissue. The name is derived from its histological appearance simulating a leaf-like architecture with cleft-like spaces lined by epithelium, and hypercellular stroma. Various synonyms have been used for this tumor including cystosarcoma phyllodes, cellular fibroadenoma, and juvenile fibroadenoma. In 1838, the name *cystosarcoma phyllodes* was first introduced by Müller, from Greek word *sarcoma*, meaning flesh appearance, and *phyllon*, meaning leaf-like. The term sarcoma is a misnomer as majority of PTs are benign. A cellular fibroadenoma is a fibroadenoma that shows prominent cellular stroma on histology. Juvenile fibroadenomas also show cellular stroma with a gynecomastoid pericanalicular growth pattern. They occur commonly in adolescent girls and may grow to enormous sizes. A juvenile fibroadenoma larger than 5 cm is termed as a giant fibroadenoma.

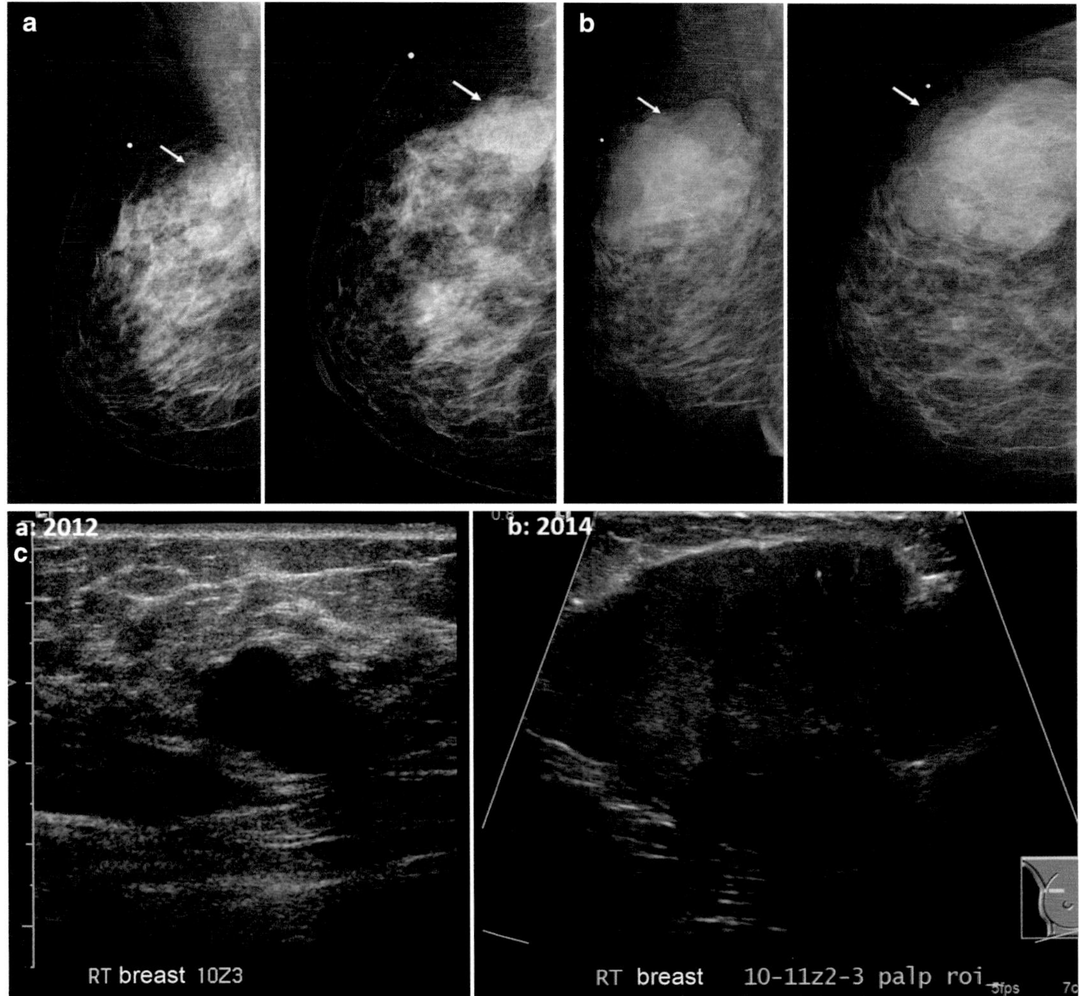

Fig. 13.4 (**a**) Right mammogram in MLO and CC views. (**b**) Right mammogram in MLO and CC views 2 years later. (**c**) Targeted right breast ultrasound: 2012 and 2014

Clinically, PTs are commonly seen between 40–55 years of age. Most tumors present as large, rapidly growing, circumscribed mass without microcalcifications and tend to be locally aggressive and have an increased tendency to recur.

There are three varieties of phyllodes tumors: benign (56–60%), borderline (about 20%), and malignant (about 15–20%). These tumors frequently show local recurrence as follows: benign variety (5–15%), borderline variety (10–25%), malignant variety (25–40%). Doubling time of malignant variety can be as low as 36 days and of benign variety up to 116 days.

Malignant phyllodes tend to show hematogenous metastasis (20%) to the lung and bones and have a 5-year survival rate of about 55–75%.

Mammogram shows circumscribed, high density, round/oval mass. Microcalcifications are rare. Indistinct margin may favor malignant etiology.

On ultrasound, PTs are generally circumscribed tumors with round to oval shape and sometimes indistinct to irregular margins. They show heterogeneous internal echotexture, cystic components, horizontal linear clefts, and echogenic septae. They tend to be highly vascular and show variable posterior features. Microcalcifications are generally absent in phyllodes.

MRI appearance may include heterogeneous, low to isointense signal on T1WI. Internal high intensity may suggest hemorrhage. On T2WI, phyllodes tumors generally appear as mixed-intensity, heterogeneous mass with internal cystic spaces and clefts and hyperintense surrounding tissue in 20% cases. Postcontrast imaging show rapidly enhancing, round/oval mass, with nonenhancing cystic areas in some tumor. Nonenhancing internal septae may be seen in about 45% lesions.

Management

Wide local surgical excision is generally recommended for PT, with wider margins in malignant variety to avoid local recurrence. As there is no lymphatic spread ALND or SLNB is not performed. Adjuvant radiotherapy may be associated with reduced local recurrence rates.

13.5 Case 13.5

History: 43-year-old woman presents with non-tender, palpable lump in right outer breast.

Questions

Q1. Describe the abnormality on the mammogram (Fig. 13.5a, b).

Q2. Describe the abnormality on ultrasound (Fig. 13.5c) and give differential and appropriate BI-RADS.

Answers

A1. Bilateral MLO (Fig. 13.5a) and CC views (Fig. 13.5b) show extremely dense breast parenchyma. There is a 1.5–2 cm, circumscribed, round, fat-containing lesion noted in upper outer quadrant of the right breast (white arrows). There is no associated architectural distortion or suspicious microcalcifications seen in this region. No suspicious feature is identified in the left breast. Skin, subcutaneous tissue, and nipple appear unremarkable.

A2. Ultrasound images (Fig. 13.5c) show an oval, circumscribed, isoechoic lesion with central echogenic component and poor internal vascularity at the 9 o'clock location in the right breast corresponding to the palpable mass and the mammographic finding. Differential diagnosis of a fat-containing benign mass is a hamartoma or galactocele or a lipoma.
Category: BI-RADS 2.
In the absence of history of recent lactation, possibility of lipoma/hamartoma would be considered more likely. Comparison with prior mammograms would be helpful to assure benign etiology and stability.

Notes

Fibroadenolipoma (Hamartoma)

A hamartoma is a focal developmental pseudotumor composed of normal breast parenchyma. It is encapsulated with varying degrees of fat, fibroglandular, and fibrous tissue components. A pseudocapsule is formed by the compressed parenchyma. Hamartomas make about 3–4% of benign breast tumors. They are more accurately called fibroadenolipoma. The imaging appearance depends on which component is prominent (fibro, adeno, or lipomatous tissue).

Clinically, it may present as a painless palpable lump in 4th–5th decade or it may be detected incidentally on a screening mammogram in asymptomatic women. Estrogen and progesterone receptors in hamartomas are similar to the normal breast tissue and hence they may grow in size during pregnancy and lactation.

Mammogram is the best imaging tool. It is generally seen as a round to oval, circumscribed, varying-density mass with pseudocapsule. It shows the classic "breast within breast" appearance.

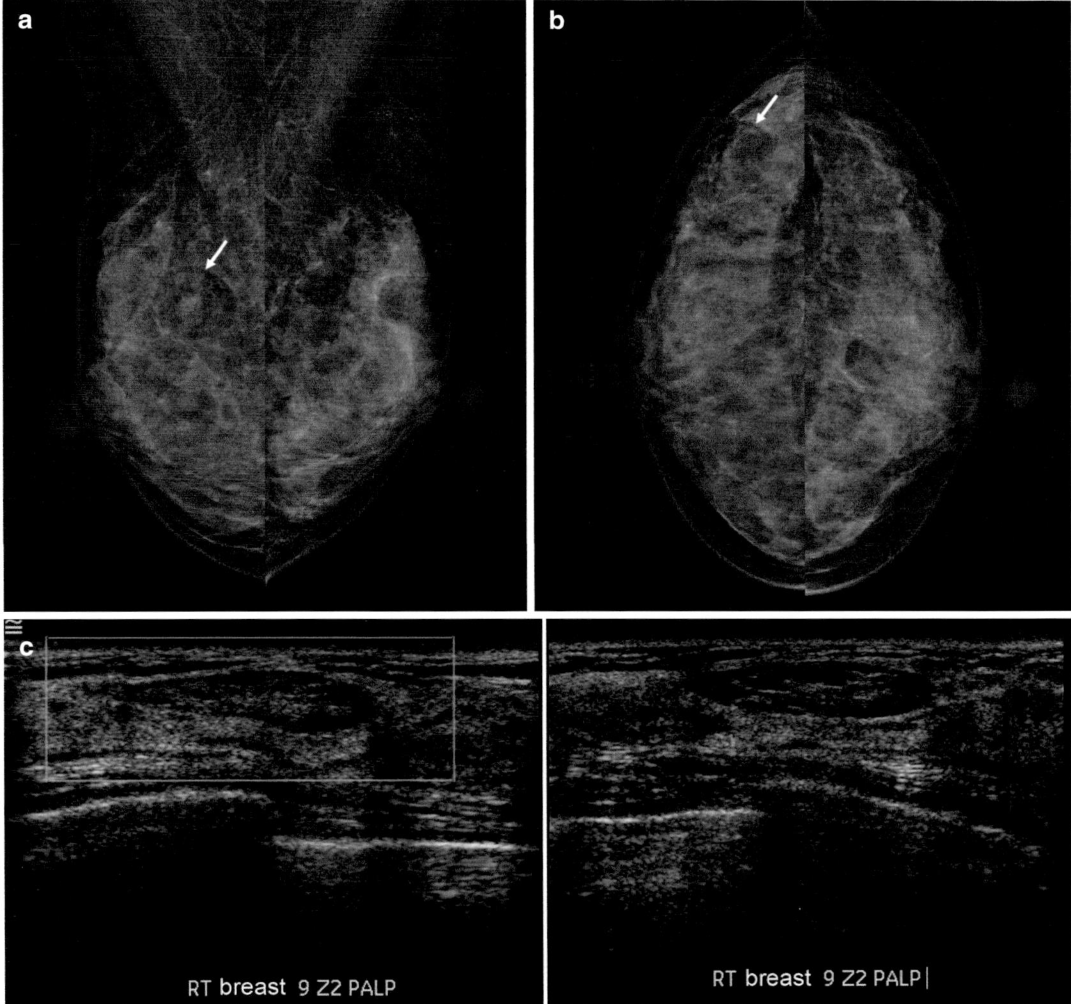

Fig. 13.5 (**a**) Bilateral MLO views. (**b**) Bilateral CC views. (**c**) Targeted right breast ultrasound

On ultrasound, it generally appears as an oval, mixture of hypoechoic fat and echogenic glandular element with variable posterior features. Pseudocapsule may/may not be identified and it may show minimal internal vascularity. It may be compressible similar to normal parenchyma.

MRI may show an encapsulated glandular and fat-containing lesion that shows enhancement similar to rest of the breast parenchyma.

On histology, the lobular distribution and presence of fat distinguishes hamartoma from fibroadenoma. Rarely malignancy, DCIS, or IDC may arise within the fibroglandular tissue of the hamartoma.

Suggested Readings

Chala LF, de Barros N, de Camargo Moraes P, Endo É, Kim SJ, Pincerato KM, Carvalho FM, Cerri GG. Fat necrosis of the breast: mammographic, sonographic, computed tomography, and magnetic resonance imaging findings. Curr Probl Diagn Radiol. 2004;33(3):106–26.

El-Wakeel H, Umpleby HC. Systematic review of fibroadenoma as a risk factor for breast cancer. Breast. 2003;12(5):302–7.

Franceschini G, Masetti R, Brescia A, Mulè A, Belli P, Costantini M, Magistrelli A, Picciocchi A. Phyllodes tumor of the breast: magnetic resonance imaging findings and surgical treatment. Breast J. 2005;11(2):144–5.

Francis A, England D, Rowlands D, Bradley S. Breast papilloma: mammogram, ultrasound and MRI appearances. Breast. 2002;11(5):394–7.

Gatta G, Pinto A, Romano S, Ancona A, Scaglione M, Volterrani L. Clinical, mammographic and ultrasonographic features of blunt breast trauma. Eur J Radiol. 2006;59(3):327–30.

Gordon PB, Gagnon FA, Lanzkowsky L. Solid breast masses diagnosed as fibroadenoma at fine-needle aspiration biopsy: acceptable rates of growth at long-term follow-up. Radiology. 2003;229(1):233–8.

Gutman H, Schachter J, Wasserberg N, Shechtman I, Greiff F. Are solitary breast papillomas entirely benign? Arch Surg. 2003;138(12):1330.

Kurz KD, Roy S, Saleh A, Diallo-Danebrock R, Skaane P. MRI features of intraductal papilloma of the breast: sheep in wolf's clothing? Acta Radiol. 2011;52(3):264–72.

Lee EH, Wylie EJ, Bourke AG, De Boer WB. Invasive ductal carcinoma arising in a breast hamartoma: two case reports and a review of the literature. Clin Radiol. 2003;58(1):80–3.

Liberman L, Bonaccio E, Hamele-Bena D, Abramson AF, Cohen MA, Dershaw DD. Benign and malignant phyllodes tumors: mammographic and sonographic findings. Radiology. 1996;198(1):121–4.

Lu Q, Tan EY, Ho B, Chen JJ, Chan PM. Surgical excision of intraductal breast papilloma diagnosed on core biopsy. ANZ J Surg. 2012;82(3):168–72.

Sperber F, Blank A, Metser U, Flusser G, Klausner JM, Lev-Chelouche D. Diagnosis and treatment of breast fibroadenomas by ultrasound-guided vacuum-assisted biopsy. Arch Surg. 2003;138(7):796–800.

Wahner-Roedler DL, Sebo TJ, Gisvold JJ. Hamartomas of the breast: clinical, radiologic, and pathologic manifestations. Breast J. 2001;7(2):101–5.

Williams HJ, Hejmadi RK, England DW, Bradley SA. Imaging features of breast trauma: a pictorial review. Breast. 2002;11(2):107–15.

14 Invasive Mammary Carcinoma

14.1 Case 14.1

History: 50-year-old woman with palpable right breast lump. Family history of postmenopausal breast cancer in a maternal aunt. No prior breast surgery or intervention.

Questions

Q1. Describe the abnormality on the mammogram and spot compression views (Fig. 14.1a–c). What would be your next suggestion?

Q2. Describe the abnormality on ultrasound (Fig. 14.1d).

Q3. Provide possible differentials.

Q4. Describe the role of MRI in this diagnosis.

Answers

A1. Bilateral MLO (Fig. 14.1a) and CC views (Fig. 14.1b) show extremely dense breast parenchyma. There is a metallic marker placed over the inner half of right breast to annotate the site of clinically palpable lump. Underneath the marker is seen a high-density mass (white arrows) with indistinct margins in the posterior third of the breast. Distortion and some spiculation is demonstrated along the medial margin. There is associated skin retraction. Spot compression views of the right breast (Fig. 14.1c) show a high-density mass (white arrows) with spiculated margin. Few microcalcifications are noted in and around the mass. Left breast is unremarkable. No enlarged axillary nodes are noted. An ultrasound examination is suggested, followed by a core biopsy.

A2. Ultrasound (Fig. 14.1d) shows an irregular, hypoechoic mass in the right breast at the 2 o'clock location. The mass shows microlobulated margins, parallel orientation, minimal internal vascularity, and mixed posterior features. This mass correlates with the spiculated mass seen on mammogram. The imaging features are suspicious on mammogram as well as ultrasound for invasive breast malignancy. There is abnormal right axillary node (white arrow) noted with thickened cortex and compressed fatty hilum. Category: BI-RADS 5. Histological correlation from the right breast mass and right axillary node would be recommended. In the context of dense breast tissue a contralateral screening ultrasound may be considered along with complete assessment of the ipsilateral breast to exclude additional disease.

An ultrasound-guided biopsy was performed.

Histopathology: Grade 2 invasive lobular carcinoma

N. Chotai, S. Kulkarni, *Breast Imaging Essentials*, https://doi.org/10.1007/978-981-15-1412-8_14

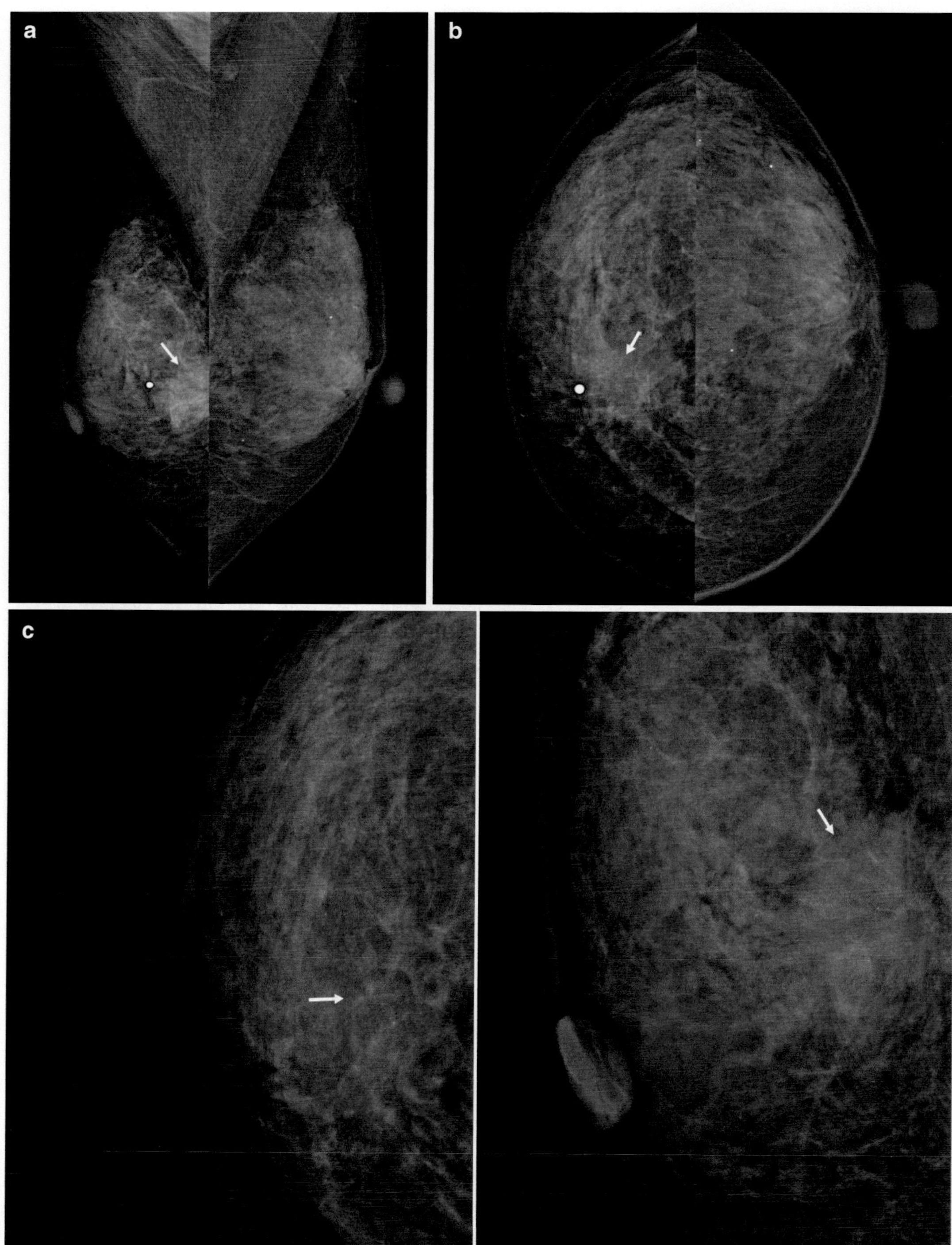

Fig. 14.1 (**a**) Bilateral MLO views. (**b**) Bilateral CC views. (**c**) Right spot compression views in orthogonal views. (**d**) Targeted right breast and axillary ultrasound. (**e**) Companion case. 45-year-old woman with grade 2 ILC. MRI MIP shows a large heterogeneously enhancing mass (white arrow) in outer half of right breast. Multiple enhancing foci seen in the other part of the right breast (thick white arrows) raises the possibility of multifocal-multicentric disease. Post mastectomy histopathology confirmed multicentric ILC

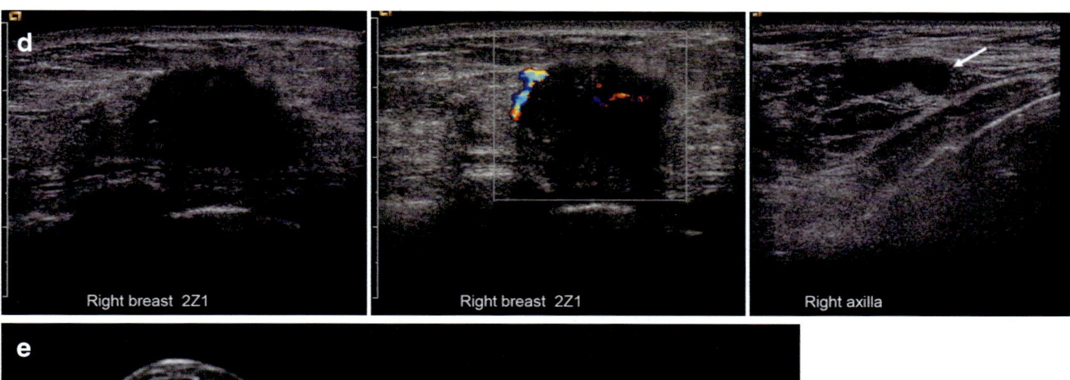

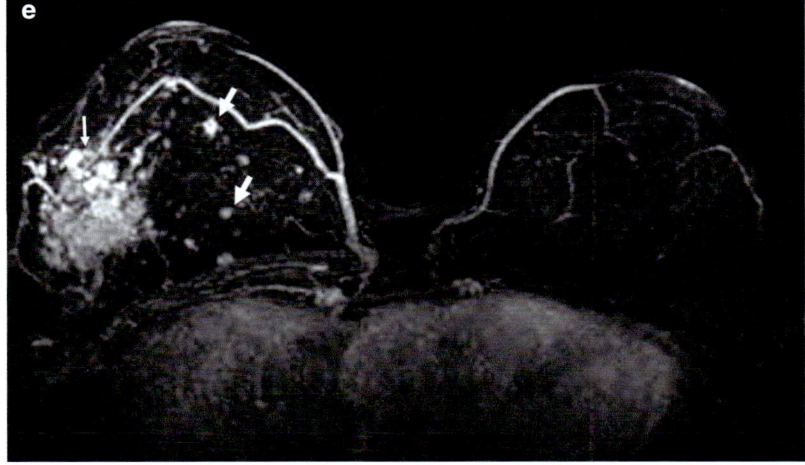

Fig. 14.1 (continued)

A3. The main differentials to be considered for a spiculated mass in breast include: invasive mammary carcinoma, fat necrosis, postsurgical changes, radial scar, rarely DCIS, or fibrotic lesions like fibromatosis (desmoid tumor). (The positive predictive value of a spiculated mass on ultrasound for breast malignancy is about 91%).

Rare benign causes of spiculated lesion include granulomatous mastitis, diabetic mastopathy, and sarcoidosis. Imaging may not be able to differentiate between these conditions and histopathological confirmation may be needed.

A4. A newly diagnosed ILC is an indication for staging MRI. ILC tends to be underestimated with conventional imaging and MRI helps in assessing the true extent, multifocality and multicentricity of ILC. It also helps in axillary staging and excluding contralateral synchronous malignancies. MRI is especially useful in young women who have dense breast tissue and/or are genetically high risk. Some ILCs may show very mild or no enhancement, but biopsy should be still considered when other suspicious features are evident.

Notes

Invasive Lobular Carcinoma (ILC)

ILC is more common in older age group and represents about 8–10% of all breast cancers. ILC invades surrounding breast tissue in "single cell fashion" without invoking much desmoplastic tissue reaction and often coexists with lobular neoplasia (LCIS and ALH). It has been postulated that one of the risk factors for developing ILC is hormone replacement therapy (HRT) in postmenopausal women.

Multifocal/multicentric (Fig. 14.1e) or bilateral disease is more common with ILC compared to IDC. It tends to be larger at presentation but generally has equal to better stage matched outcome. Most ILC are ER/PR positive and HER2 negative.

On mammography, ILC commonly presents as a spiculated mass and occasionally as an isolated architectural distortion or developing asymmetry on a single view. Microcalcifications are relatively less common with ILC. Sensitivity of mammography for ILC varies between 35–70%.

On ultrasound, irregular mass with intense shadowing is the commonest appearance on ultrasound. Sensitivity of ultrasound for ILC varies between 80–94% and is higher than mammography.

MRI is the best imaging tool for ILC and should be offered for staging for the reasons described previously. Preoperative MRI also reduces the risk of positive surgical margin in breast conservation surgery.

14.2 Case 14.2

History: 53-year-old woman presented with history of a palpable right breast lump since a few months. No prior study was available for comparison. No family history of breast cancer.

Questions

Q1. Describe the abnormality on the mammogram (Fig. 14.2a, b).

Q2. Describe the abnormality on ultrasound (Fig. 14.2c) and MRI (Fig. 14.2d). Provide appropriate BI-RADS.

Q3. What is the role of Tamoxifen in such a condition?

Answers

A1. Right MLO and CC views (Fig. 14.2a) along with tomosynthesis images (Fig. 14.2b) show a spiculated mass in the upper inner quadrant of the right breast (white arrows). There are no associated microcalcifications within the mass. Right breast skin and nipple appear unremarkable. No enlarged right axillary nodes are noted on mammogram.

A2. Ultrasound images (Fig. 14.2c) of the right breast at the 1 o'clock location, 3 cm from nipple, shows an irregular hypoechoic mass with microlobulated margin and minimal internal vascularity. No significant posterior features noted. This mass correlates with the spiculated mass seen on mammogram.

MRI images of right breast (Fig. 14.2d) show a suspicious mass (white arrow) in the upper inner quadrant of the right breast. Color angiomap image (a) shows washout kinetics in the mass; postcontrast image (b) shows a heterogeneously enhancing, irregular mass with spiculated margin in the mid third of the breast. DWI (c) and ADC (d) images show restricted diffusion within the mass. The overlying skin and underlying muscle are not involved by the mass. Overall, the imaging features on all modalities are highly suspicious for invasive mammary carcinoma and histology would be suggested. Category BI-RADS 5.

A3. Tamoxifen is a selective estrogen receptor modulator (SERM) drug that is used in the treatment of estrogen-positive breast cancer. It works by reducing the growth of breast cancer cells and acting as an anti-angiogenetic agent. It is shown to reduce the recurrence rate as well as reduce the risk of cancer in contralateral breast. It has some side effects like increased risk of endometrial cancer, increased risk of deep venous thrombosis, and pulmonary embolism.

Histopathology: Grade 2 IDC of no special type. The tumor was ER/PR and HER2/neu positive. Patient underwent lumpectomy followed by radiation. Sentinel node was negative. Tamoxifen and Herceptin (Trastuzumab) were then given to the patient to reduce the risk of recurrence.

Notes

Infiltrating Ductal Carcinoma (IDC)

Invasive ductal carcinomas show invasion of tumour cells beyond basement membrane. The commonest variety is the no special type (NST) or not otherwise specified (NOS). Special types like medullary, mucinous, tubular carcinoma are seen in 10%.

Clinically, the patient may present with a firm, palpable mass, nipple or skin tethering or retraction. When the size of the breast cancer (Tsize) is >5 cm or there is involvement of surrounding structures such as skin/chest wall or invasion or extensive axillary metastases, it is termed as locally advanced breast cancer (LABC).

Mammographically, the commonest appearance is that of an irregular or spiculated, high-density mass. Associated architectural distortion and microcalcifications are common findings. Occasionally, the tumor may present as a focal

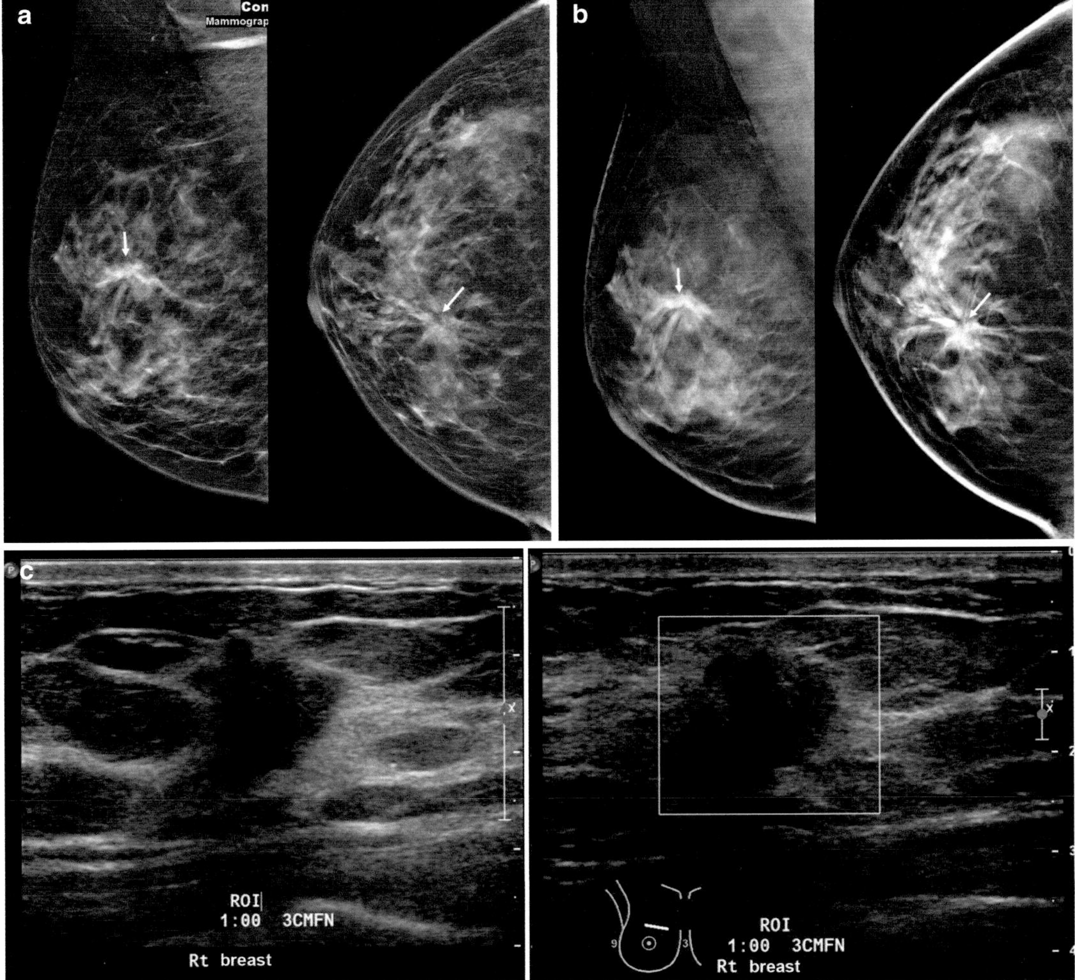

Fig. 14.2 (**a**) Right MLO and CC views. (**b**) Right DBT MLO and CC views. (**c**) Targeted right breast ultrasound with color doppler. (**d**) (*a–d*) Right breast MRI. (*a*) Color angiomap; (*b*) DCE; (*c*) DWI; (*d*) ADC

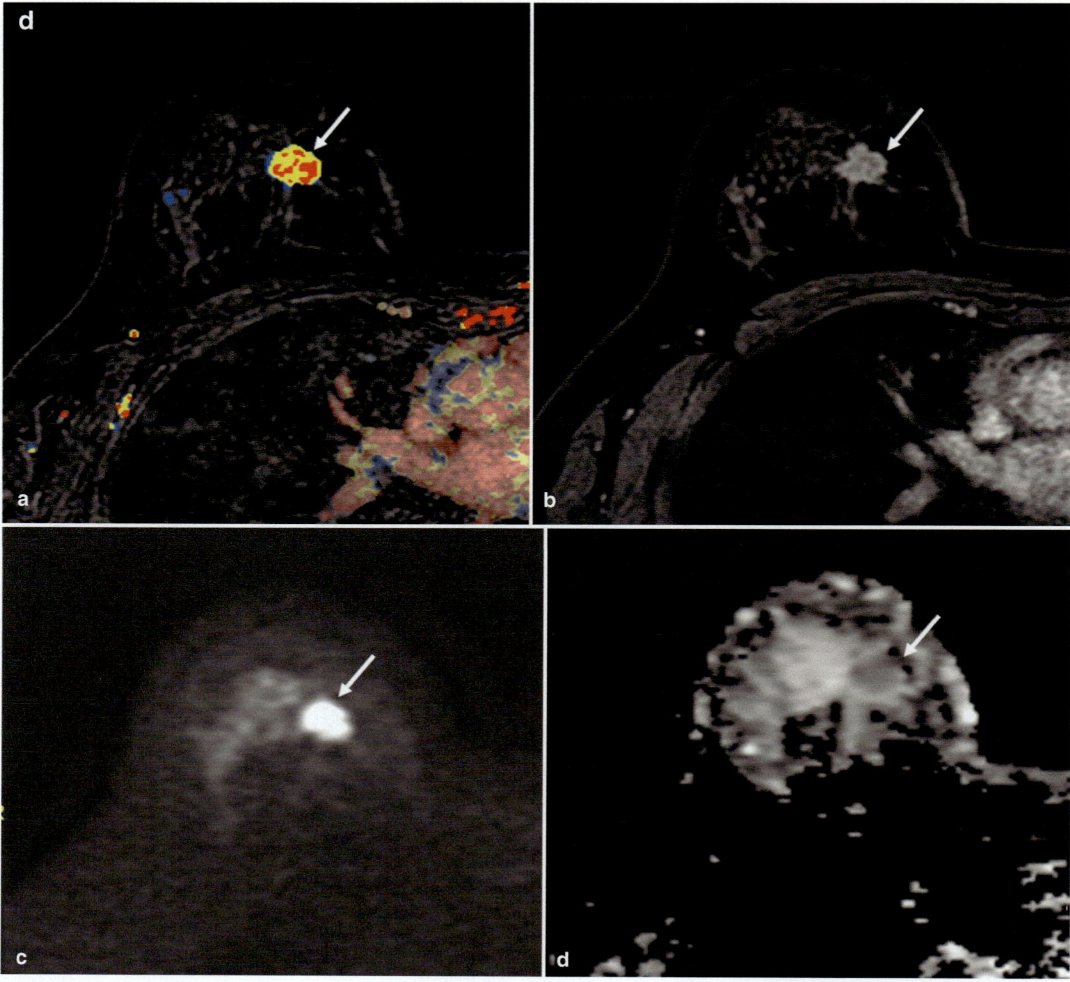

Fig. 14.2 (continued)

asymmetry, developing density or circumscribed mass.

Ultrasound shows the classic spiculated mass that is taller than wide (antiparallel), posterior shadowing, growth along the Cooper's ligament, distortion, ductal extension, and microcalcifications. Ultrasound also helps in axillary staging and guided intervention. Special types of IDC such as triple-negative cancers or mucinous cancers can appear as very benign-looking masses on ultrasound.

MRI has about 92% sensitivity for the detection of invasive disease and the negative predictive value is almost 98%. A classical IDC shows an irregular enhancing mass with washout. It may show rim enhancement, tumor heterogeneity, associated intraductal disease, involvement of surrounding structures and axillary disease. MRI is the best modality for staging and detection of contralateral synchronous cancer. It is also used in the assessment of response to neoadjuvant treatment.

Breast Conservation Therapy (BCT)

The National Surgical Adjuvant Breast and Bowel Project (NSABP) B 06 compared total mastectomy (TM) to lumpectomy, with or without radiation therapy, in the treatment of stages I and II breast cancer. Long-term follow-up (5–6 years) showed similar disease-free, distant disease-free, and overall survival rates for lumpectomy, with or without radiation therapy, when compared to total mastectomy cases. The incidence of ipsilateral breast cancer recurrence (in-breast recurrence), however, was higher in the lumpectomy group that did not receive radiation therapy. The goal of BCT is not only to preserve the breast, but also have a cosmetically acceptable outcome without compromising local tumor control.

Contraindications to BCT include prior radiotherapy to the breast or chest wall, persistent positive resection margins, multicentric breast cancer, pregnancy, and diffuse malignant-appearing mammographic microcalcifications.

Complications of breast cancer treatment include seroma, arm swelling, nerve injury and pain, arm stiffness, shoulder stiffness/pain and phantom breast syndrome. Other known complications include delayed cellulitis and pain along chest wall, axilla, and upper extremity. The incidence of arm morbidity is seen to be less in BCT compared to mastectomy, and less frequent with sentinel lymph node biopsy than after axillary lymph node dissection.

Adjuvant Treatment

Adjuvant chemotherapy is given for node-positive cases. Presurgical chemotherapy is termed as neo-adjuvant chemotherapy (NAC) and is generally given for stage III tumor, locally advanced tumor, and inflammatory breast cancer.

Adjuvant hormonal therapy is given for hormone-receptor-positive cases.

Adjuvant radiotherapy (RT) is given following breast conserving surgery (BCS) performed for high-grade DCIS and invasive mammary carcinoma. Radiotherapy may be withheld for women undergoing BCS for low-grade DCIS. Postmastectomy radiation is given when ≥4 positive axillary lymph nodes, T3 and T4 (skin/chest wall involved), LABC, and close or positive surgical margins. Most trials have shown moderate reduction in cancer deaths and improvement in 15-year overall survival with adjuvant RT. Contraindications of RT: Collagen vascular disease (active SLE, Scleroderma), prior irradiation to breast/chest, pregnancy.

14.3 Case 14.3

History: 52-year-old average-risk woman presents for a screening mammogram.

Questions

Q1. Describe the abnormality on mammogram (Fig. 14.3a–c). What is the appropriate BI-RADS? What would you advise next?
Q2. Describe the abnormality on ultrasound (Fig. 14.3d).
Q3. Describe the findings on MRI (Fig. 14.3e). What is the role of MRI in this patient?

Answers

A1. Bilateral MLO (Fig. 14.3a) and CC views (Fig. 14.3b) show heterogeneously dense breast parenchyma. There is a high-density mass with spiculated margins noted in the posterior left breast along the PNL (double white arrows). There are loosely grouped, fine pleomorphic microcalcifications (thick white arrows) seen in the lower inner quadrant of the left breast in anterior to mid third with underlying distortion and focal asymmetry. The magnification views of the left breast (Fig. 14.3c) show the spiculated mass (double white arrows) with fine pleomorphic microcalcifications in segmental distribution (thick white arrows). Right breast is unremarkable. No enlarged axillary nodes are noted. Ultrasound of breast and axilla is suggested, followed by a biopsy.

A2. Ultrasound (Fig. 14.3d) shows an irregular, hypoechoic mass in the left breast in the lower outer quadrant (a) that correlates with the mammographic mass. The mass shows microlobulated margins. There is no significant internal vascularity (b) and mixed posterior features noted. There is smaller, irregular hypoechoic mass seen in the lower inner quadrant of the left breast (c and d). This likely correlates with the area of microcalcifications seen on mammogram. The imaging features may suggest invasive mammary cancer with a possible in situ component involving two quadrants.

Category: BI-RADS 5.

A3. MRI images in postcontrast T1W fat-suppressed and color angiomap are available. There is a heterogeneously enhancing mass with irregular margins seen in the posterior central aspect of left breast (thick white arrow). It shows wash out kinetics on color angiomap. This correlates with the suspicious mass seen on conventional imaging. There is linear non-mass enhancement seen in the lower inner quadrant of the left breast (white arrows). It shows plateau kinetics on color angiomap. This correlates with the area of microcalcifications seen on mammogram. Both the lesions are suspicious and histological correlation is suggested.

Histopathology: Ultrasound-guided biopsy of both masses was performed. The histology from the mass in the lower outer quadrant of left breast revealed mixed grade 2 invasive ductal and lobular carcinoma and the mass in the lower inner quadrant revealed high-grade DCIS.

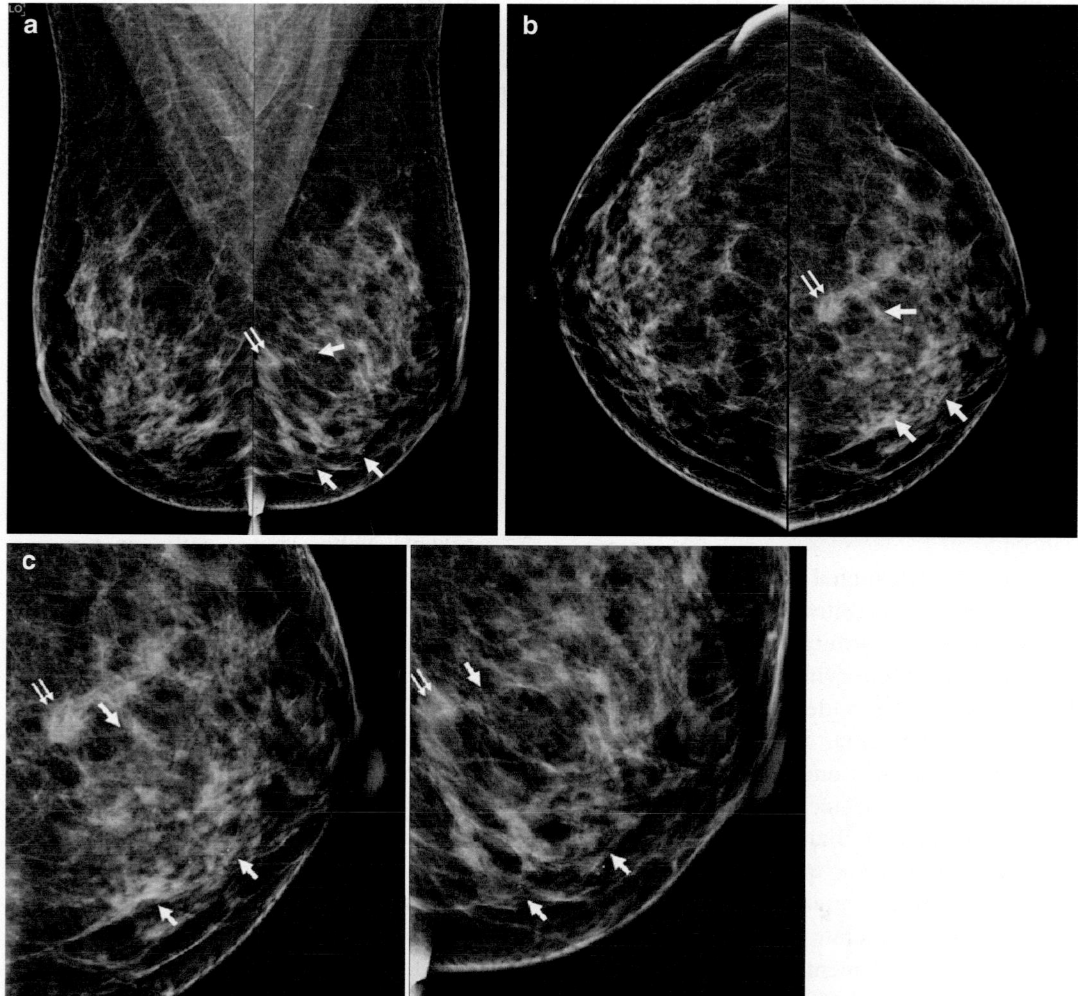

Fig. 14.3 (**a**) Bilateral MLO views. (**b**) Bilateral CC views. (**c**) Left breast spot magnification views in orthogonal projections. (**d**) (*a–d*): Targeted left breast ultrasound. (**e**) (*a*, *b*): Breast MRI (*a*) DCE and (*b*) Color angiomap

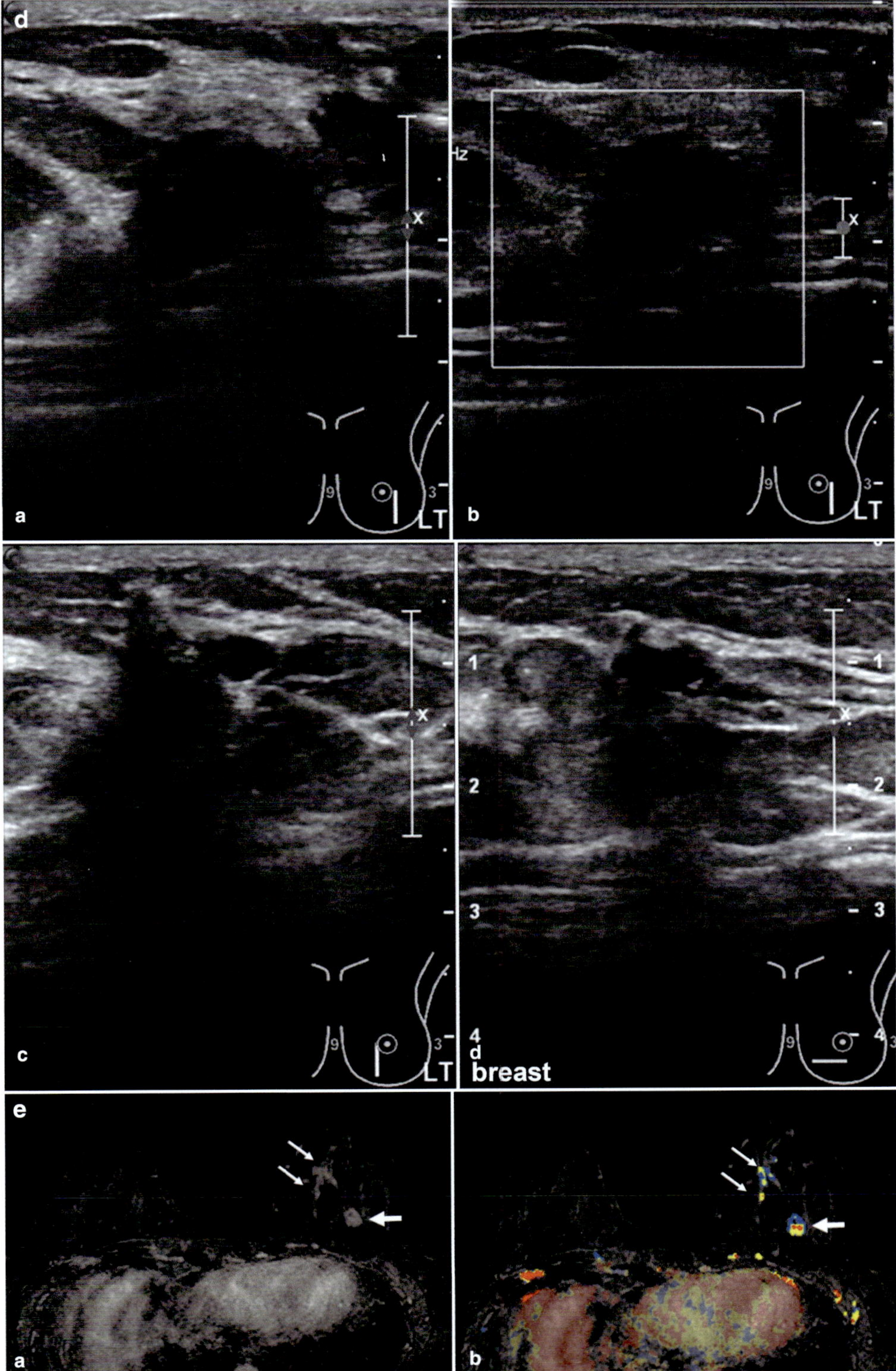

Fig. 14.3 (continued)

The patient underwent left mastectomy. Postop adjuvant chemotherapy was given.

Notes

Mixed Invasive Ductal and Lobular Carcinomas

This is a heterogeneous group of invasive mammary carcinomas with ductal as well as lobular features. Clinical and imaging features are not distinguishable from any other invasive mammary carcinomas. The ductal component is no specific type (NOS) comprising of 10–49% of the tumor with remaining part having lobular features. Hormone replacement therapy (HRT) is more strongly associated with ILC and mixed ductal-lobular carcinoma.

Tumor Grading

Grading of invasive mammary carcinoma is based on tubule formation, nuclear pleomorphism, and mitotic activity—each scored on a scale of 1–3.

Grade 1 tumor: Score 3–5.
Grade 2 tumor: Score 6–7.
Grade 3 tumor: Score 8–9.

TNM Staging

The American Joint Committee on Cancer (AJCC) has developed TNM classification for all cancers, including breast cancer. It stages the cancer based on size of the tumor (**T status**), nodal metastasis (**N status**), and distant metastasis beyond breast and axilla (**M status**). Latest AJCC classification for breast cancer was revised in the eighth edition produced in January 2018. The new classification, along with TNM status, also includes biological factors of tumor for countries where testing is available. The new factors included are:

1. Tumor grade.
2. Hormone receptor status (Estrogen Receptor Positive/Negative ER+/ER-, Progesterone Receptor Positive PR+/PR-).
3. Human epidermal growth factor: positive/negative (HER2+/HER2-).
4. Gene expression panels like Oncotype DX and Mamma Print (tests that help predict the likelihood of recurrence of a tumor after treatment, especially in early-stage breast cancer).

TNM class	Criteria
T0	No evidence of primary tumor
T1a	Carcinoma in situ
T1	<or = 2 cm
T1m1c	microinvasion 0.1 cm or less
T1a	>0.1–0.5 cm
T1b	>0.5–1 cm
T1c	>1–2 cm
T2	>2–5 cm
T3	>5 cm
T4	Any size tumor with direct extension to: (a) chest wall or (b) skin
T4a	Chest wall, not including the pectoralis muscle
T4b	Skin edema, ulceration, satellite skin nodule
T4c	4a and 4b
T4d	Inflammatory carcinoma
Nx	Regional lymph nodes cannot be removed
N0	No regional lymph node metastasis
N1	Metastasis to movable ipsilateral axillary lymph nodes
N2	Metastases in ipsilateral level I, II axillary lymph nodes that are clinically fixed or matted(N2a) ; or in clinically detected ipsilateral internal mammary nodes in the absence of clinically evident axillary lymph node metastases (N2b)
N3	Metastases in ipsilateral infraclavicular lymph nodes (N3a) or clinically apparent ipsilateral internal mammary lymph nodes (N3b) or ipsilateral supraclavicular lymph nodes (N3c)
MX	Distant metastasis cannot be assessed
M0	No distant metastasis
M1	Distant metastasis

Breast cancer stages	Classification criteria based on TNM
Stage 0	Tis, N0, M0
Stage I	T1, N0, M0
Stage IIA	T0, N1, M0 or T1, N1, M0 or T2, N0, M0
Stage IIB	T2, N1, M0 or T3, N0, M0

Breast cancer stages	Classification criteria based on TNM
Stage IIIA	T0, N2, M0 or T1, N2, M0 or T2, N2, M0 or T3, N1, M0 or T3, N2, M0
Stage IIIB	T4, N0, M0 or T4, N1, M0 or T4, N2, M0
Stage IIIC	any T, N3, M0
Stage IV	any T, any N, M1

14.4 Case 14.4

History: 59-year-old woman with palpable right breast lump. No other contributing history.

Questions

Q1. Describe the abnormality on mammogram (Fig. 14.4a) and ultrasound (Fig. 14.4b) with appropriate BI-RADS.

Q2. Describe the abnormality on MRI (Fig. 14.4c).

Q3. Provide possible differentials in this case.

Answers

A1. Right MLO and CC views (Fig. 14.4a) show heterogeneously dense breast parenchyma. There is an oval, circumscribed, high-density mass noted in the central aspect of the right breast in the mid third depth (white arrows). There is no architectural distortion or suspicious microcalcifications in this region. No enlarged axillary nodes are noted. Ultrasound (Fig. 14.4b) shows an oval, isoechoic mass in the right breast with microlobulated margins (white arrows). The mass shows parallel orientation, moderate internal vascularity, and posterior enhancement. This mass correlates with the high-density mass seen on mammogram. The imaging features are indeterminate and an ultrasound core biopsy would be recommended. Category: BI-RADS 4.

A2. MRI images are available in T1WI (a), T2WI (b), DCE T1WI subtracted image (c), DWI(d) and ADC(e) sequences. There is an oval, circumscribed, mass (white arrows) in the central aspect of the right breast. The mass is isointense on T1WI, is partially hyperintense on T2WI, and shows peripheral, rim enhancement on DCE T1WI subtracted image. It is hyperintense on DWI images as well as ADC, suggesting T2 shine through with no restricted diffusion. Although the mass is oval, circumscribed, T2 shows bright signal with no restriction, other features are suspicious, and the possibly benign features should not deter the reader from tissue sampling. Patient is postmenopausal and the likelihood of her developing a new benign solid mass is low.

A3. Differential diagnosis based on imaging findings: fibroadenoma, phyllodes, mucinous carcinoma, invasive ductal carcinoma, mucocele like lesion.

Histopathology: Ultrasound core biopsy revealed intermediate-grade node-negative mucinous carcinoma; ER/PR positive and HER2/neu negative. Patient underwent BCT.

Notes

Invasive Mucinous Carcinoma

Mucinous carcinoma is a special type of invasive breast cancer that is associated with a large component of the tumor (>50%) involved in secretion of extracellular mucin. The pure mucinous variety shows >90% mucin-producing component and is rare comprising of about 2% of all breast neoplasms. The mixed variety shows 50–90% mucin-producing component and also shows an invasive ductal epithelial component. Pure variety of mucinous carcinoma is more commonly better differentiated (lower grade) and less commonly node positive. Hence it has a more favorable prognosis compared to IDC. A 10-year survival for pure variety mucinous carcinoma is more than 90%. Some mixed mucinous cancers may be associated with DCIS and lobular neoplasia.

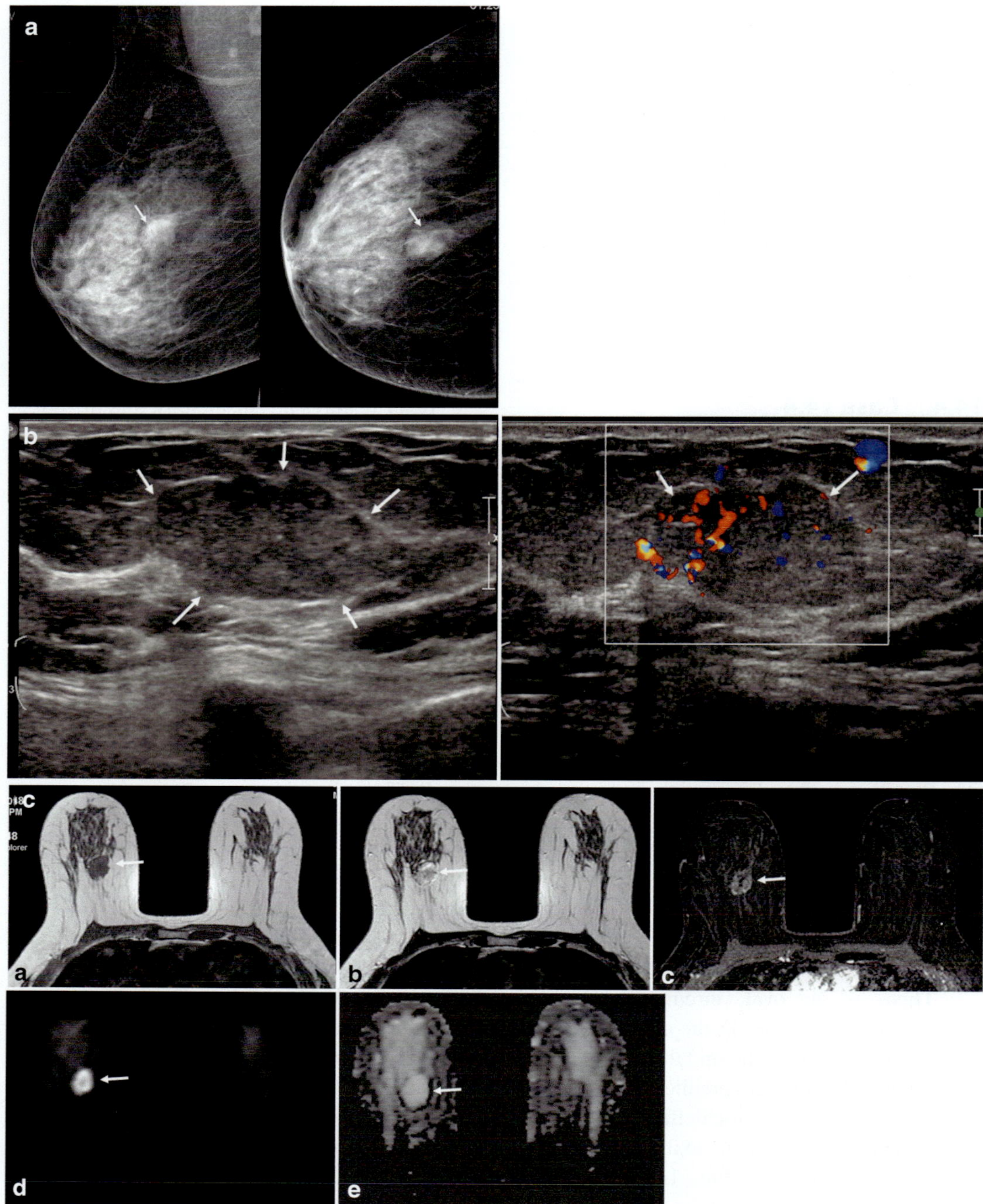

Fig. 14.4 (**a**) Right mammogram in MLO and CC views. (**b**) Targeted right breast ultrasound. (**c**) (*a–d*) MRI breast images of the same patient

Mucinous carcinoma is frequently hormone receptor positive, lacks HER2/neu expression, and has increased expression of MUC2 and MUC5 (mucin core proteins).

Clinically, it generally presents as a slow-growing, palpable mass in nearly 50% of cases. It more frequently is seen in the older age group, about 50–60 years. Pure variety of mucinous tumor is common in older postmenopausal women while mixed variety is more common in younger women.

On examination, it may feel soft to firm and may be fixed to chest wall/skin if large.

On mammography, mucinous tumor generally presents as round to oval, circumscribed to partially circumscribed, iso- to high-density mass. Microcalcifications are rare – relatively more common in mixed type. Twenty percent of mucinous cancers may be occult on mammogram.

Ultrasound generally shows round to oval (rarely irregular), isoechoic to fat (especially when small) to hypoechoic mass with partially circumscribed to microlobulated margins, posterior enhancement in 50%, internal vascularity in about 35% cases. They are likely to be misdiagnosed as benign masses due to overlap with benign features.

On MRI, this tumor typically shows high signal intensity on T2WI and shows variable signal intensity on T1WI. Commonly, postcontrast images show slow to rapid initial enhancement with persistent or plateau kinetics on delayed imaging. Pure mucinous carcinomas show low DWI and high ADC values, which help to differentiate them from benign lesions.

14.5 Case 14.5

History: 80-year-old-woman with a palpable right breast lump and serosanguinous right nipple discharge since a few months. No other contributory history.

Questions

Q1. Describe the abnormality on mammogram (Fig. 14.5a, b) and ultrasound (Fig. 14.5c) with appropriate BI-RADS.

Q2. Please provide possible differentials.

Q3. What care would you recommend for biopsy of this lesion?

Answers

A1. Bilateral MLO (Fig. 14.5a) and CC views (Fig. 14.5b) of both breasts show predominantly fatty breast parenchyma. There is a metallic marker placed over the lower inner quadrant of the right breast to annotate the site of clinically palpable lump. Underneath the marker is seen a high-density mass with circumscribed margins in the posterior third of the right breast. There is no associated architectural distortion or suspicious microcalcifications noted. No suspicious features are noted in the left breast. Bilateral breast skin, subcutaneous tissue, and nipple appear unremarkable. No enlarged axillary nodes are noted. Ultrasound (Fig. 14.5c) shows an oval, circumscribed, complex solid-cystic mass in the right breast at the 4 o'clock location that correlates with the clinically palpable lump. There is an intracystic irregular solid component with internal vascularity. The cystic component of the mass shows internal echoes/debris and posterior enhancement. This complex cystic mass correlates with the high-density palpable mass seen on mammogram. The imaging features are suspicious, and a core biopsy is necessary. Category: BI-RADS 4.

A2. Differentials of a complex solid-cystic breast mass include: intraductal papillary lesion (papilloma or papillary carcinoma), invasive ductal carcinoma, complex degenerating fibroadenoma, abscess, hematoma, fat necrosis, galactocele, and phyllodes.

A3. Image-guided biopsy of the solid component is necessary to obtain the correct diagnosis. This may require prior aspiration of the cystic component to collapse the mass. This aspirate can also be sent for cytology. Non-image-guided biopsies in outpatient clinic may yield a false negative result due to inadequate sampling of the solid component.

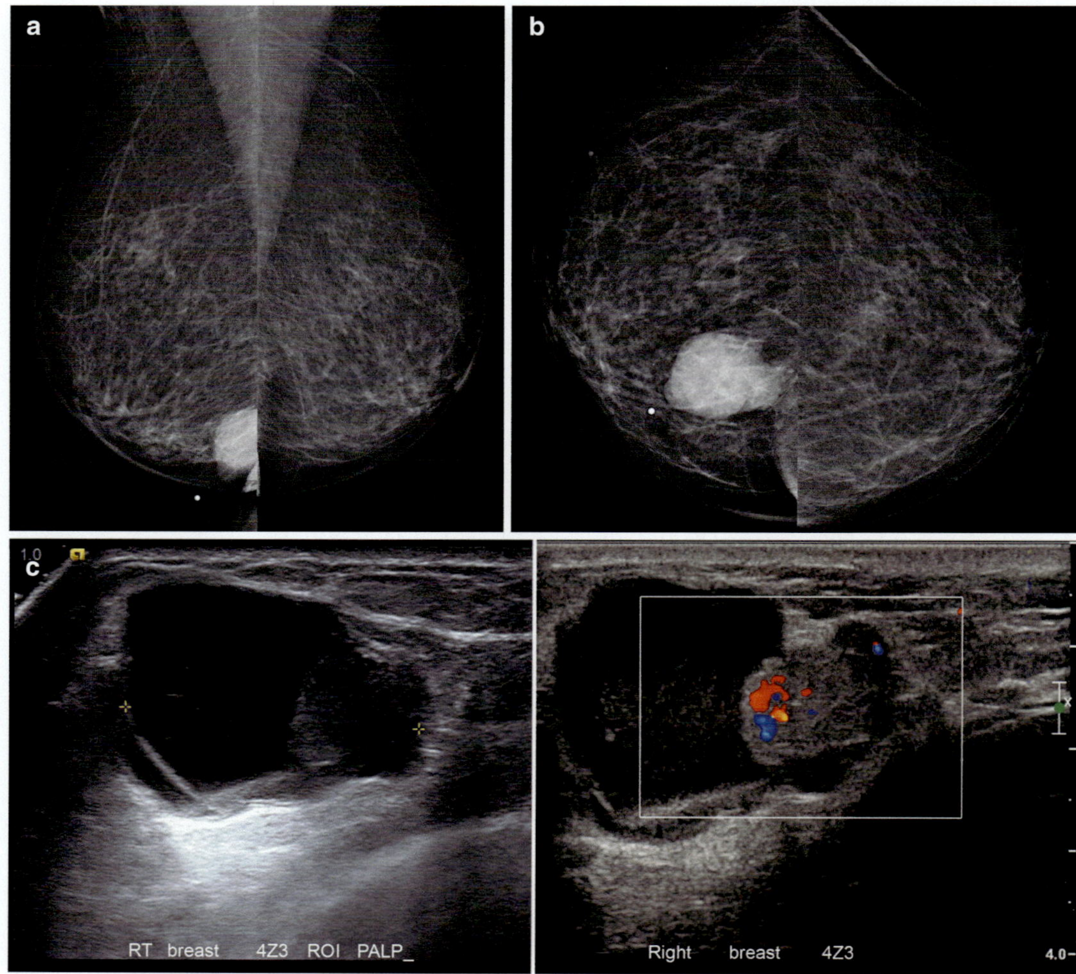

Fig. 14.5 (**a**) Bilateral MLO views. (**b**) Bilateral CC views. (**c**) Targeted right breast ultrasound

Histopathology: Invasive papillary carcinoma; ER/PR positive and HER2/neu negative. Patient underwent right mastectomy.

Notes

Invasive Papillary Carcinoma

Invasive papillary carcinoma constitutes about 1–2% of invasive breast cancer. It is usually seen in postmenopausal women. Common clinical presentation is a firm mobile palpable mass and about one-third patients may have nipple discharge (bloody or serosanguinous).

On pathology they show a papillary architecture and hence called invasive papillary carcinoma. The invasive component is generally focally present and hence may be missed on core biopsy. It is often accompanied by DCIS in the surrounding breast. As compared to invasive ductal carcinoma, they have better prognosis. Most tumors are hormone receptor positive and lack HER2/neu overexpression.

On mammography, it commonly presents as a dense mass which is round to oval with circumscribed to partially obscured margins. There may be associated amorphous to pleomorphic microcalcifications. Rarely may present as a spiculated mass.

Common sonographic appearances include solid or complex solid-cystic mass, intracystic mass or intraductal lesion, presence of papillary projections, internal vascularity, and posterior enhancement.

MRI shows heterogeneously enhancing, circumscribed intracystic mass or a complex cystic enhancing mass. Axillary nodal metastasis is rare.

Management consists of local therapy (lumpectomy and adjuvant radiotherapy or mastectomy) and systemic therapy based on tumor features. Most tumors are hormone receptor positive and lack HER2/neu overexpression.

14.6 Case 14.6

History: 51-year-old woman was recalled following a screening mammogram. Family history of breast cancer in second-degree cousin. No prior breast intervention.

Questions

Q1. Describe the findings on right tomosynthesis images (Fig. 14.6a) and magnification views (Fig. 14.6b) provided.

Q2. Describe the finding on ultrasound (Fig. 14.6c) with appropriate BI-RADS category.

Q3. Provide possible differentials.

Answers

A1. Right DBT MLO and CC views show extremely dense breast parenchyma. There is a small spiculated mass with architectural distortion in the upper outer quadrant of the right breast in middle third (white arrows). Magnification views show a few associated microcalcifications in this lesion (white arrows). No other suspicious finding is noted in the right breast. No enlarged axillary nodes are noted.

A2. Ultrasound image of the right breast shows an irregular, hypoechoic mass in the right breast at the 11 o'clock location. It appears taller than wide. There is no significant posterior feature noted. The mass correlates with the spiculated mass shown on mammogram. The imaging features are suspicious and histological correlation from the mass would be suggested. Category: BI-RADS 4.

A3. The differentials to be considered are complex sclerosing lesion/radial scar, invasive ductal carcinoma, invasive lobular carcinoma, DCIS, postsurgical/traumatic scar or fat necrosis and sclerosing adenosis.

Histopathology: Grade 1 IDC with tubular features. The tumor was ER/PR positive and HER2/neu negative. Patient underwent lumpectomy. Nodes were negative for metastasis. No adjuvant treatment was advised. Patient was advised Tamoxifen.

Notes

Invasive Tubular Carcinoma

Invasive tubular carcinoma is a type of invasive ductal carcinoma. On microscopy, it shows well-differentiated tubular structures with open lumina lined by a single layer of epithelium. It contributes to 1–2% of female breast cancer and is a most frequent carcinoma found with radial scar. Clinically, more than 50% of tubular carcinoma are diagnosed at screening with the mean age of about 50 years. Some may present with a palpable mass. This tumor is generally slow growing with favorable prognosis and up to 95–98% 5-year survival.

Pathologically, pure variety shows >90% tubular structures on histology while mixed variety shows 50–89% tubular structures on histology.

On mammography, common appearance includes small, irregular spiculated mass, associated amorphous or pleomorphic microcalcifications (in 50%) and some may have associated architectural distortion.

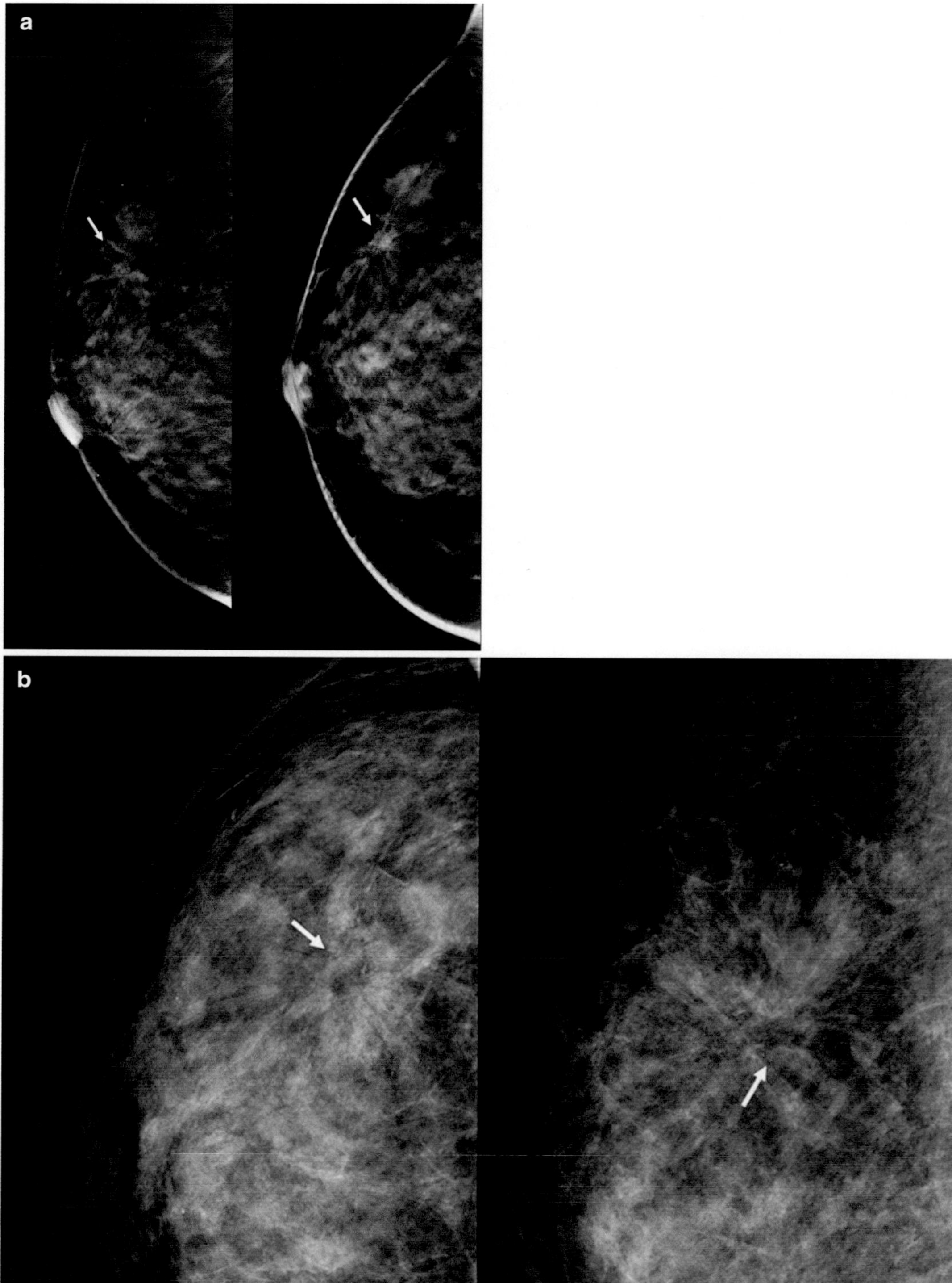

Fig. 14.6 (**a**) Right DBT MLO and CC views. (**b**) Right spot compression views in orthogonal projections. (**c**) Targeted right breast ultrasound

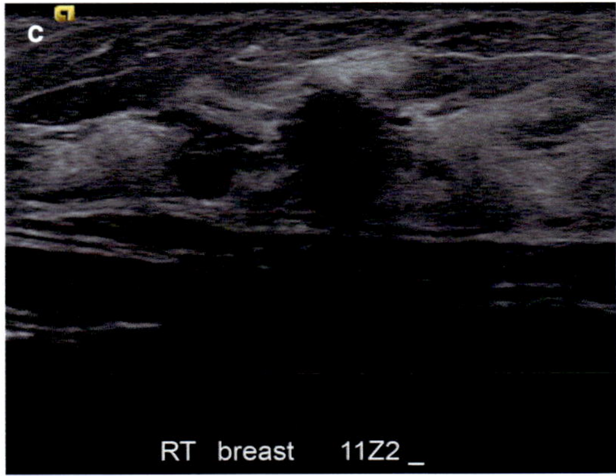

Fig. 14.6 (continued)

Ultrasound generally shows a spiculated hypoechoic mass with architectural distortion, may be antiparallel orientation, and posterior shadowing in some cases.

MRI shows typical features of a breast cancer. The tumor is generally iso- to slightly hypointense on T1 and T2WI and shows enhancing spiculated mass with rapid initial phase and delayed washout dynamic on postcontrast images. It is important to know that occasionally, tubular carcinoma may show mild or absent enhancement leading to false negative results.

Lumpectomy/breast conservative surgery with clear margin is the recommended treatment (except for multifocal disease). The role of radio and chemotherapy is controversial. Adjuvant hormonal therapy is generally given as most of these tumors are estrogen receptor positive.

14.7 Case 14.7

History: 81-year-old woman with history of left breast palpable lump. No family history of breast cancer.

Questions

Q1. Describe the abnormality on mammogram (Fig. 14.7a–c).

Q2. Describe the abnormality on ultrasound (Fig. 14.7d) with appropriate BI-RADS category.

Q3. What is the difference between multifocal and multicentric tumor?

Answers

A1. Bilateral MLO (Fig. 14.7a) and CC views (Fig. 14.7b) show scattered fibroglandular breast parenchyma. There is a metallic marker placed over the lower inner quadrant of the left breast to annotate the site of clinically palpable lump. Underneath the marker is seen an irregular, high-density mass with microlobulated margins in the mid third of the breast (white arrows). On spot compression views of the left breast (Fig. 14.7c), the margins of this mass appear partly indistinct. There is another smaller high-density spiculated mass seen in the upper inner quadrant in the posterior third of the left breast (thick white arrows). No suspicious microcalcifications are seen in the left breast. No suspicious feature is identified in the right breast. Skin, subcutaneous tissue, and nipple appear unremarkable. No enlarged axillary nodes are noted. Findings are suspicious for multicentric left breast cancer.

A2. Ultrasound of left breast (Fig. 14.7d) shows an irregular, palpable mass at the 6 o' clock location, with microlobulated margins, heterogeneous internal echotexture, anti-parallel orientation, mixed posterior features, and moderate internal vascularity. There is another, smaller hypoechoic mass at the 10 o'clock location, with indistinct margins and posterior shadowing. Both these masses correlate with the mammographic findings Category: BI-RADS 5.

Ultrasound-guided biopsy of both these masses should be suggested to confirm multicentricity.

A3. When there are more than one tumor foci, separated by benign breast tissue, in the ipsilateral breast it is termed as synchronous

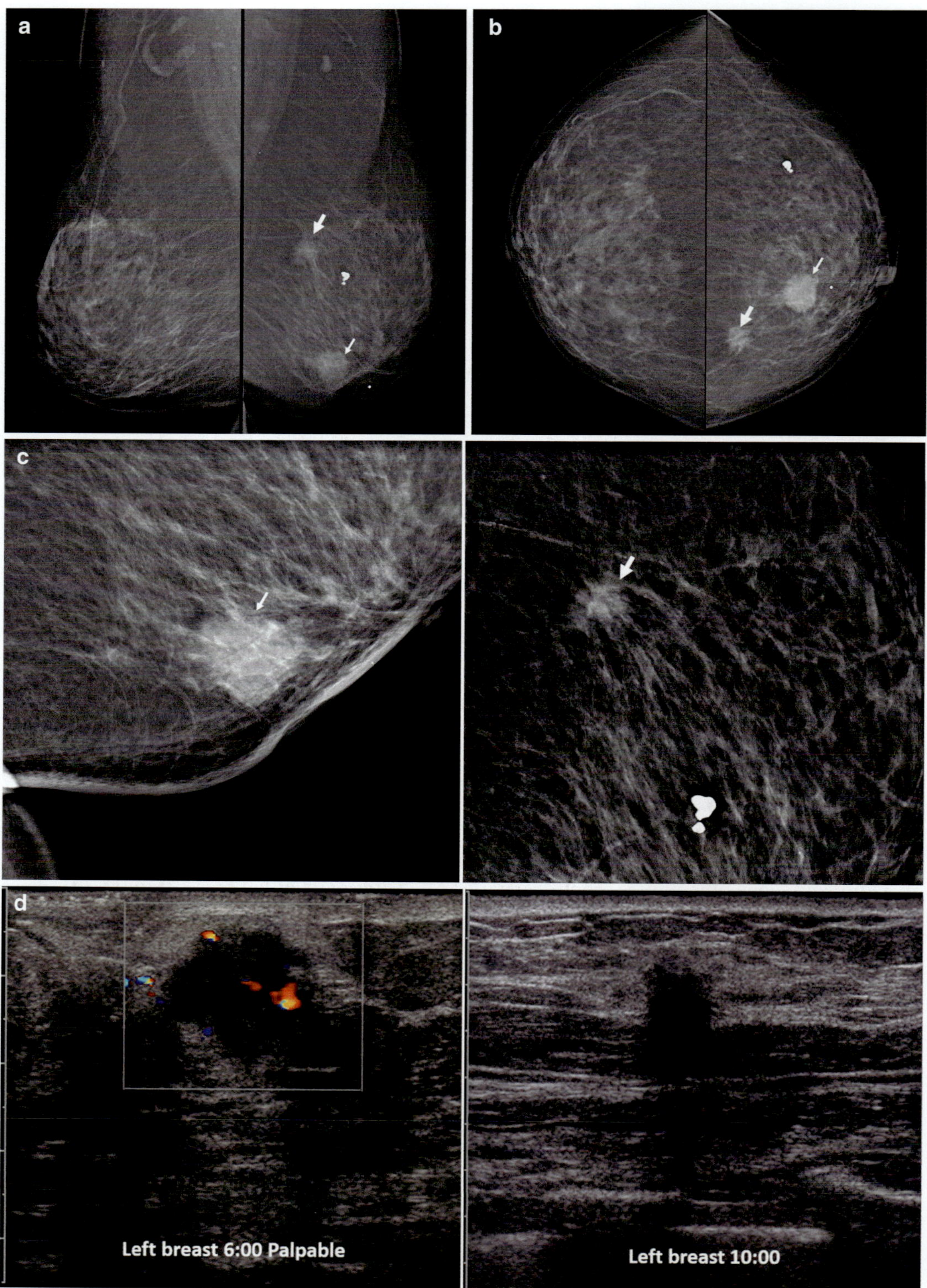

Fig. 14.7 (**a**) Bilateral MLO views. (**b**) Bilateral CC views. (**c**) Left breast spot compression views in orthogonal projections. (**d**) Targeted left breast ultrasound. (**e**) Companion case: Multifocal multicentric breast cancer. DCE-MRI shows multiple heterogeneously enhancing masses (white arrows) in the right breast. Enlarged right level 2 axillary node is seen posterior to the pectoralis minor muscle (thick white arrow)

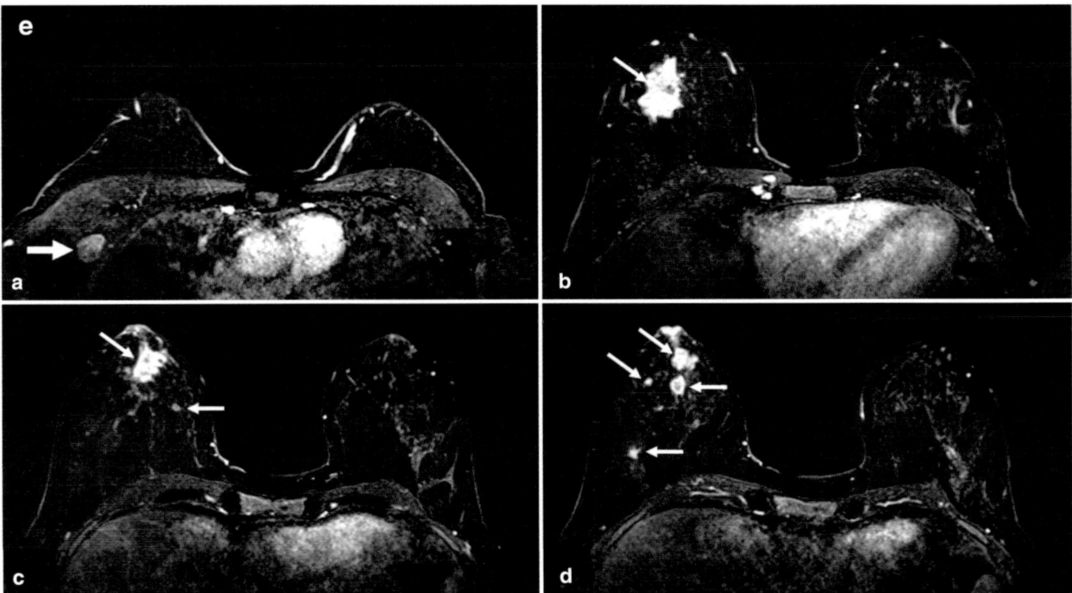

Fig. 14.7 (continued)

tumor. If the tumor foci are located within the same quadrant of breast, it is termed as multifocal (MF) breast cancer and are believed to be arising in the same ductal system. If the tumor foci are separated by more than 5 cm or are located in different breast quadrants, it is termed as multicentric (MC) breast cancer and are believed to arise in separate duct systems.

Notes

Multifocal and Multicentric Carcinoma

About 15–35% breast cancers are multifocal/multicentric (MF/MC). The incidence of MF/MC is higher now because of increased detection due to the use of adjuvant USG and MRI in staging. MF/MC cancers are common with young age, large tumor size, lobular carcinoma, and the presence of peritumoral lymphovascular invasion. They are also associated with higher incidence of locoregional (lymph node) and distant metastases. MRI is the best modality for detection of MF/MC and hence is a very powerful staging tool (Fig. 14.7e).

MF/MC cancers depending on the extent are still amenable to breast conservation surgery if adequate breast tissue can be preserved with acceptable cosmetic results.

Suggested Readings

Bitencourt AG, Graziano L, Osório CA, Guatelli CS, Souza JA, Mendonça MH, Marques EF. MRI features of mucinous cancer of the breast: correlation with pathologic findings and other imaging methods. Am J Roentgenol. 2016;206(2):238–46.

Evans WP, Warren Burhenne LJ, Laurie L, O'Shaughnessy KF, Castellino RA. Invasive lobular carcinoma of the breast: mammographic characteristics and computer-aided detection. Radiology. 2002;225(1):182–9.

Ingle SB, Murdeshwar HG, Siddiqui S. Papillary carcinoma of breast: minireview. World J Clin Cases. 2016;4(1):20.

Lacroix-Triki M, Suarez PH, MacKay A, Lambros MB, Natrajan R, Savage K, Geyer FC, Weigelt B, Ashworth A, Reis-Filho JS. Mucinous carcinoma of the breast is genomically distinct from invasive ductal carcinomas of no special type. J Pathol. 2010;222(3):282–98.

Lamb PM, Perry NM, Vinnicombe SJ, WELLS CA. Correlation between ultrasound characteristics, mammographic findings and histological grade in patients with invasive ductal carcinoma of the breast. Clin Radiol. 2000;55(1):40–4.

Leonard CE, Howell K, Shapiro H, Ponce J, Kercher J. Excision only for tubular carcinoma of the breast. Breast J. 2005;11(2):129–33.

Livi L, Paiar F, Meldolesi E, Talamonti C, Simontacchi G, Detti B, Salerno S, Bianchi S, Cardona G, Biti GP. Tubular carcinoma of the breast: outcome and loco-regional recurrence in 307 patients. Eur J Surg Oncol. 2005;31(1):9–12.

Lynch SP, Lei X, Chavez-MacGregor M, Hsu L, Meric-Bernstam F, Buchholz TA, Zhang A, Hortobagyi GN, Valero V, Gonzalez-Angulo AM. Multifocality and multicentricity in breast cancer and survival outcomes. Ann Oncol. 2012;23(12):3063–9.

Mann RM, Hoogeveen YL, Blickman JG, Boetes C. MRI compared to conventional diagnostic work-up in the detection and evaluation of invasive lobular carcinoma of the breast: a review of existing literature. Breast Cancer Res Treat. 2008;107(1): 1–4.

Memis A, Ozdemir N, Parildar M, Ustun EE, Erhan Y. Mucinous (colloid) breast cancer: mammographic and US features with histologic correlation. Eur J Radiol. 2000;35(1):39–43.

Menezes GL, Knuttel FM, Stehouwer BL, Pijnappel RM, van den Bosch MA. Magnetic resonance imaging in breast cancer: a literature review and future perspectives. World J Clin Oncol. 2014;5(2):61.

Menezes GL, van den Bosch MA, Postma EL, El Sharouni MA, Verkooijen HM, van Diest PJ, Pijnappel RM. Invasive ductolobular carcinoma of the breast: spectrum of mammographic, ultrasound and magnetic resonance imaging findings correlated with proportion of the lobular component. Springerplus. 2013;2(1):621.

Mitnick JS, Vazquez MF, Harris MN, Schechter S, Roses DF. Invasive papillary carcinoma of the breast: mammographic appearance. Radiology. 1990;177(3):803–6.

Neri A, Marrelli D, Megha T, Bettarini F, Tacchini D, De Franco L, Roviello F. Clinical significance of multifocal and multicentric breast cancers and choice of surgical treatment: a retrospective study on a series of 1158 cases. BMC Surg. 2015;15(1):1.

Newstead GM, Baute PB, Toth HK. Invasive lobular and ductal carcinoma: mammographic findings and stage at diagnosis. Radiology. 1992;184(3):623–7.

Nijenhuis MV, Emiel JT. Conservative surgery for multifocal/multicentric breast cancer. Breast. 2015;24:S96–9.

Pal SK, Lau SK, Kruper L, Nwoye U, Garberoglio C, Gupta RK, Paz B, Vora L, Guzman E, Artinyan A, Somlo G. Papillary carcinoma of the breast: an overview. Breast Cancer Res Treat. 2010;122(3):637–45.

Rotstein AH, Neerhut PK. Ultrasound characteristics of histologically proven grade 3 invasive ductal breast carcinoma. Australas Radiol. 2005;49(6):476–9.

Sheppard DG, Whitman GJ, Fornage BD, Stelling CB, Huynh PT, Sahin AA. Tubular carcinoma of the breast: mammographic and sonographic features. Am J Roentgenol. 2000;174(1):253–7.

Soo MS, Williford ME, Walsh R, Bentley RC, Kornguth PJ. Papillary carcinoma of the breast: imaging findings. AJR. Am J Roentgenol. 1995;164(2):321–6.

Sullivan T, Raad RA, Goldberg S, Assaad SI, Gadd M, Smith BL, Powell SN, Taghian AG. Tubular carcinoma of the breast: a retrospective analysis and review of the literature. Breast Cancer Res Treat. 2005;93(3):199–205.

The AJCC Cancer Staging Manual, Eighth Edition (2018).

15 Neoadjuvant Chemotherapy and Biomarkers

15.1 Case 15.1

History: 57-year-old woman presents with a palpable right breast mass and right skin changes.

Questions

Q1. Describe the abnormality on provided images and give the BI-RADS category.
Q2. Does involvement of the pectoralis muscle (major and minor) make the breast cancer inoperable?
Q3. What is the significance of internal mammary lymph nodes?

Answers

A1. Imaging findings are as follows:

Mammogram: Bilateral MLO (Fig. 15.1a) and CC (Fig. 15.1b) views show grossly abnormal right breast mammogram with a large area of asymmetry in the upper outer quadrant (white arrows) and associated skin thickening. There are increased reticular markings throughout the breast with minimal retraction of the nipple. There are no associated calcifications noted in the right breast. Enlarged, dense right axillary node is seen. Left mammogram appears unremarkable.

Ultrasound: Panoramic ultrasound view of the right breast (Fig. 15.1c) reveals a hypoechoic irregular mass with diffuse skin thickening (white arrows). There is an abnormally thickened hypoechoic right axillary lymph node seen in Fig. 15.1d.

MRI: Post-contrast MRI T1W subtracted image (Fig. 15.1e) reveals an irregular enhancing mass in the outer half of right breast, associated skin enhancement, and an enhancing tumor deposit within the body of the pectoralis major muscle (white arrow). There is a small internal mammary lymph node (thick white arrow).

(also note inhomogeneous fat suppression in the contralateral breast). The findings are suggestive of right locally advanced breast cancer (LABC).

Category: BI-RADS 5.

Histopathological correlation from the mass and axillary node is suggested.

A2. Adherence or extension of tumor into the pectoralis muscles does NOT count as involvement of chest wall and can be treated by radical surgery (following neoadjuvant treatment) with removal of the involved muscle. Involvement of intercostal muscles and underlying structures is considered involvement of chest wall and is classified as T4.

N. Chotai, S. Kulkarni, *Breast Imaging Essentials*, https://doi.org/10.1007/978-981-15-1412-8_15

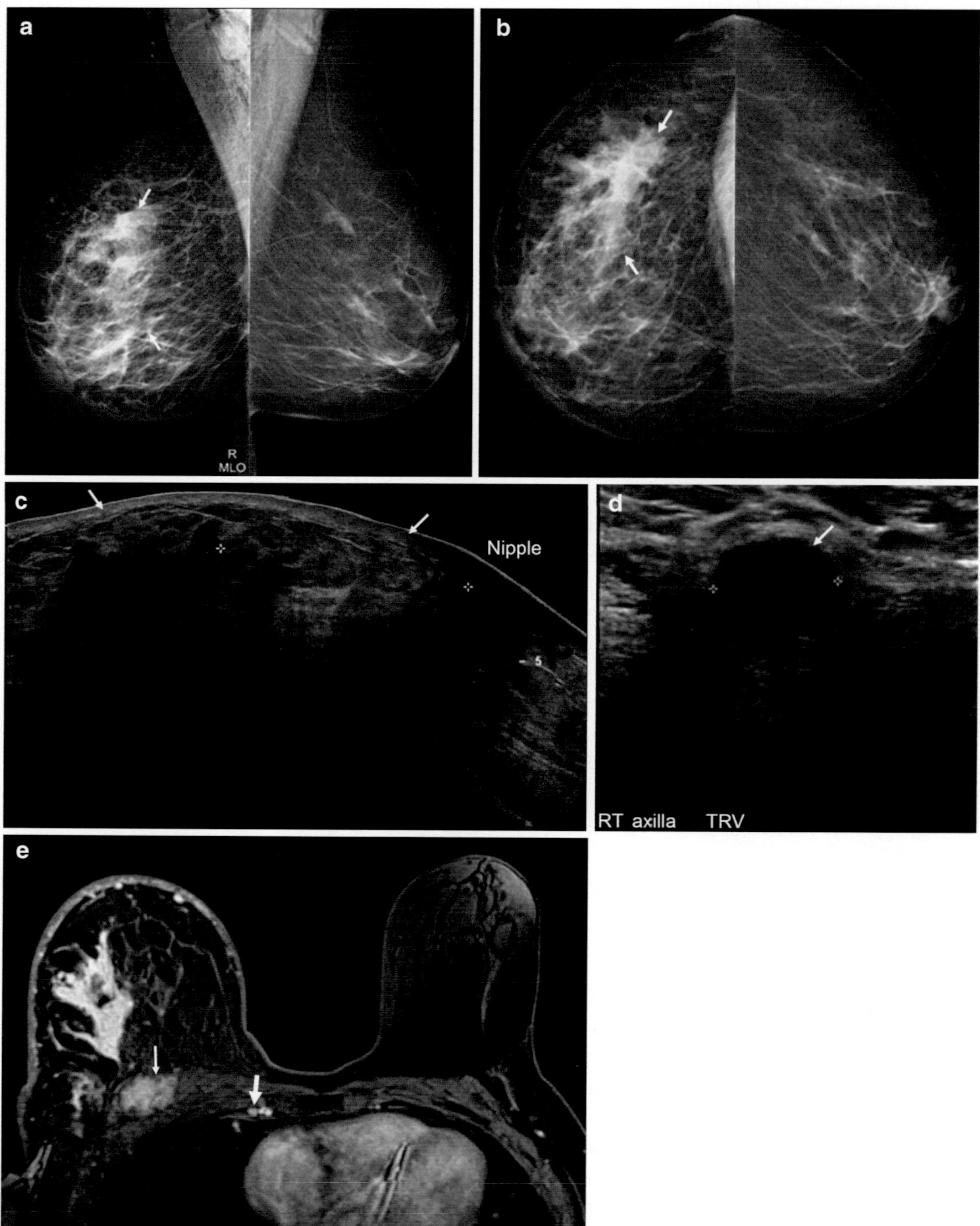

Fig. 15.1 (**a**) Bilateral MLO views. (**b**) Bilateral CC views. (**c**) Panoramic ultrasound image of right breast. (**D**) Targeted right axillary ultrasound. (**e**) Axial DCE MRI T1WI with fat suppression

A3. The therapeutic implications of internal mammary (IM) and supraclavicular (SC) nodal involvement in locally advanced breast cancer are unclear. Hence, the therapeutic choices in cases where IM and/ or SC lymph nodes are involved are still not uniformly defined. IM nodes detected on imaging are not necessarily excised. Small-sized IM may be difficult to biopsy. Usually radiotheraphy fields are adjusted to include the IM in the radiation field. Failure to offer combined-modality treatments may lead to loco-regional failure of disease control.

Notes

Locally Advanced Breast Cancer

It is estimated that about 10% of breast cancers are locally advanced breast cancer (LABC) at the time of diagnosis. They have higher recurrence risk compared to early-stage disease for obvious reasons.

According to the National Comprehensive Cancer Network (NCCN), the definition of LABC includes:

1. Tumors more than 5 cm in size (T3) with regional lymphadenopathy (N1–3).
2. Tumors of any size with direct extension to the chest wall or skin, or both (including ulcer or satellite nodules), regardless of regional lymphadenopathy.
3. Presence of regional lymphadenopathy (clinically fixed or matted axillary lymph nodes, or any of infraclavicular, supraclavicular, or internal mammary lymphadenopathy) regardless of tumor stage.

Traditionally, LABC was treated palliatively with extensive surgery; however, more recently, novel targeted therapies based on tumor biomarkers have become available. These are given as preoperative neoadjuvant chemotherapy, which downgrade the tumor size and volume allowing less disfiguring and less extensive surgery. The molecular subtype of breast cancer (luminal versus nonluminal variety) determines the response rate, pathologic complete response (pCR), and overall survival rate after neoadjuvant chemotherapy. For example, triple negative tumors and HER2+ tumors have a higher rate of pCR compared to the luminal A or B subtypes.

15.2 Case 15.2

History: 37-year-old woman presents with a palpable right breast mass.

Questions

Q1. Describe the imaging findings.

Q2. Given the morphology of the cancer, and what type of cancer is it likely to be?

Q3. What are TNBCs?

Q4. How are TNBCs treated?

Answers

A1. **Mammography:** Synthetic views of bilateral breast tomosynthesis in MLO (Fig. 15.2a) and CC (Fig. 15.2b) views show a partially circumscribed mass (white arrow) in the right upper outer periareolar region causing retraction of the nipple. No associated calcifications are noted. Multiple small rounded and dense axillary lymph nodes are seen in the right axilla. Left mammogram is unremarkable.

Ultrasound: Ultrasound image (Fig. 15.2c(*a*)) shows a hypoechoic microlobulated complex solid-cystic mass (thick white arrow) in the right retroareolar region. Figure 15.2c(*b*) shows abnormal lobulated hypoechoic axillary lymph nodes (double white arrows).

MRI: Axial DCE MRI (Fig. 15.2d(*a*)) and colorangio MIP (Fig. 15.2d(*b*)) images show malignant mass in right central breast with washout kinetic (white arrow). There is nipple retraction noted but no direct invasion of the nipple is identified. Multiple smaller enhancing foci noted laterally in the breast are raising possibility of a multifocal malignancy.

Final imaging diagnosis is multifocal invasive mammary carcinoma with possible involvement of ipsilateral axillary nodes. BI-RADS 5. Ultrasound guided core biopsy is suggested.

Histopathology: 14G core biopsy: Triple negative grade 3 adenocarcinoma with metastatic lymph node involvement.

A2. The young age of presentation and a vascular complex solid-cystic morphology indicates that it could be a triple negative breast cancer (TNBC). They may also mimic well circumscribed benign masses.

A3. TNBC is a subtype of breast cancer which is negative for estrogen receptor (ER), progesterone receptor (PR), and human epidermal growth factor receptor 2 (HER2). It is characterized by a unique molecular profile and tends to be more aggressive compared to other subtypes with distinct metastatic pattern. Due to the absence of the above-mentioned receptors there is no targeted therapies available for this subtype. This subtype of breast cancers are more common in African American and Hispanic women and women with BRCA 1 gene mutations and generally occur in younger women. They account for 10–20% of invasive breast cancers. Given their aggressive nature, they generally show more cystic components, rounded margins, and rapid growth.

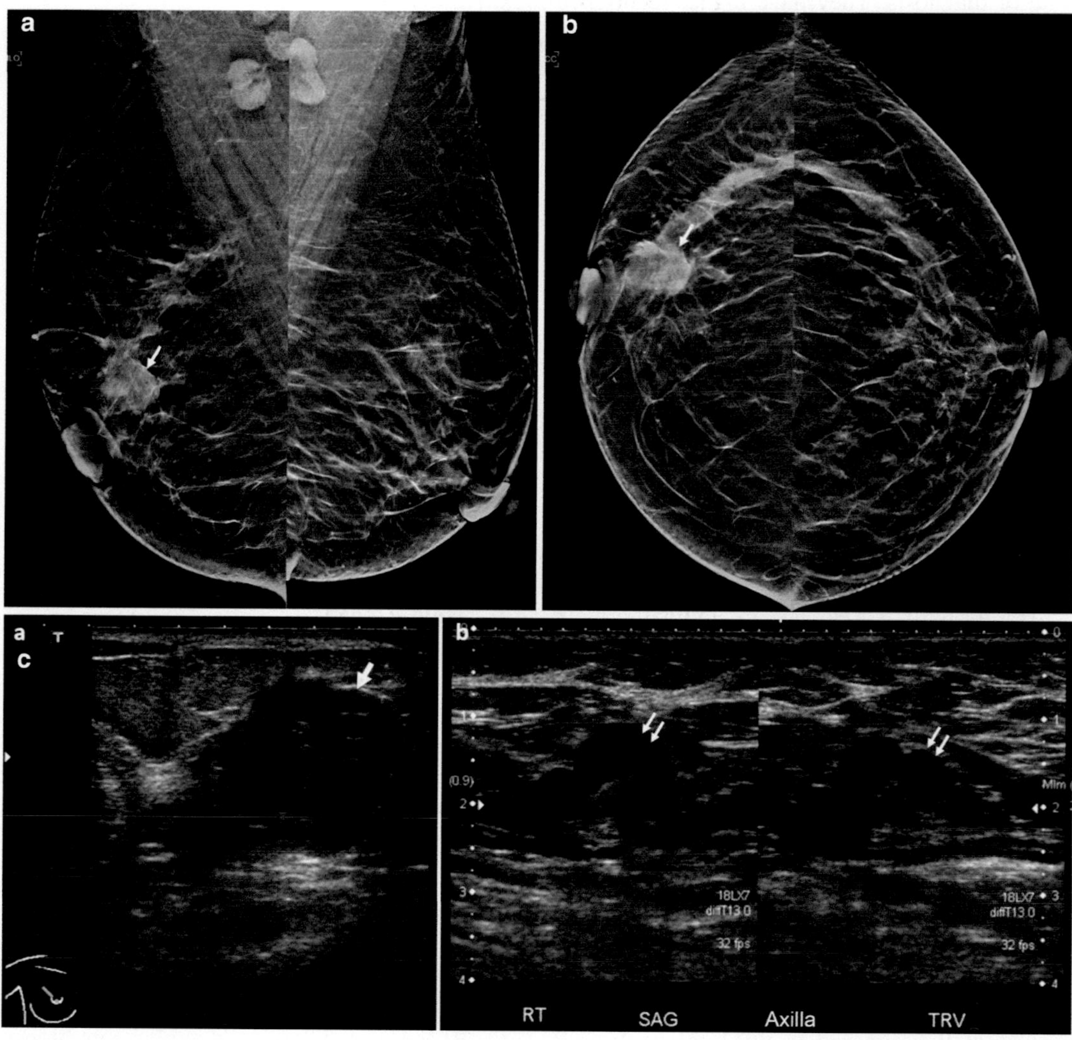

Fig. 15.2 (**a**) Bilateral MLO views. (**b**) Bilateral CC views. (**c**) Targeted right breast and axillary ultrasound. (**d**) Pre- and post-neoadjuvant chemotherapy axial DCE MRI subtracted T1WI

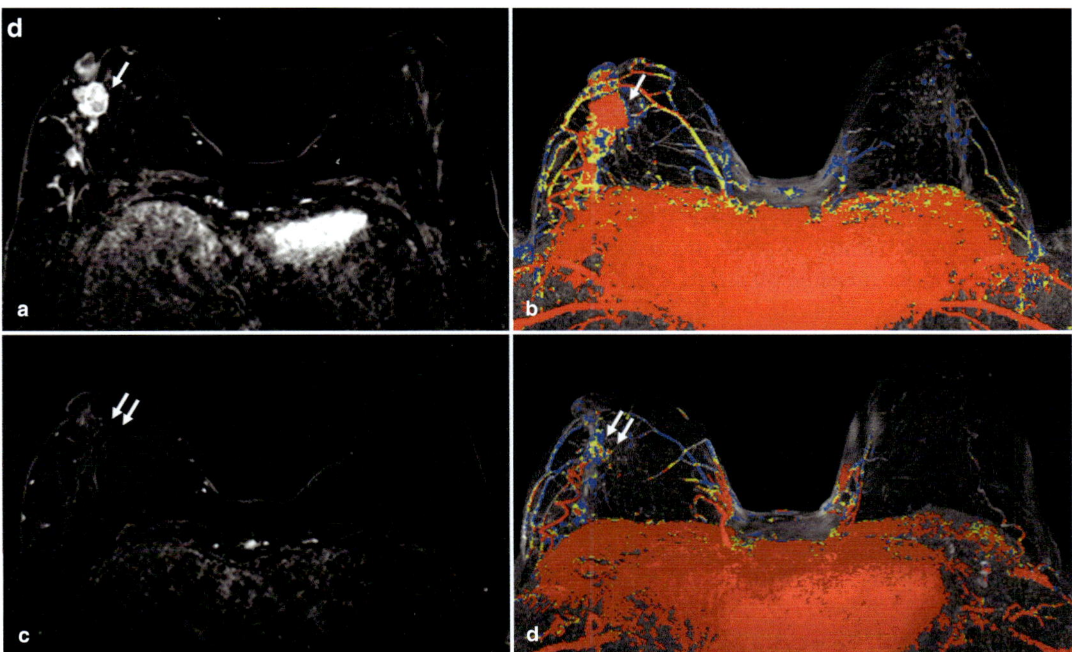

Fig. 15.2 (continued)

A4. Although these cancers are highly aggressive, they are highly responsive to neoadjuvant therapies. In this case in Fig. 15.2d(*c*, *d*) post-neoadjuvant treatment shows significant concentric reduction of the tumor mass with a smaller volume of residual tumor tissue (double white arrows). This is categorized as partial response to treatment.

Notes

Neoadjuvant Therapy

Neoadjuvant or presurgical therapy refers to the administration of therapy before surgery and has been used for over two decades to downstage locally advanced and unresectable primary breast cancers to make them operable. Several studies, including the landmark NSABP 18 trial, have demonstrated that administration of the same chemotherapy in the neoadjuvant versus adjuvant setting is associated with similar outcomes. While traditionally neoadjuvant chemotherapy has been used to downstage locally advanced and unresectable primary breast cancers, a number of studies have highlighted the role of neoadjuvant endocrine therapy as an alternative option to chemotherapy in HR-positive tumors, particularly for postmenopausal women. The goal of neoadjuvant therapy is to improve surgical outcomes by causing tumor shrinkage by providing effective systemic therapy. Neoadjuvant chemotherapy is preferred frequently in women with aggressive breast cancers like luminal B, triple-negative, and *HER2*-positive subtypes.

When patients are treated with neoadjuvant chemotherapy, efficacy is monitored by the extent of tumor shrinkage. *RECIST* (Response Evaluation Criteria In Solid Tumors) is a set of published rules that define this response, when cancer patients improve ("respond"), stay the same ("stable"), or worsen ("progression") during treatments.

RECIST response criteria to assess for residual disease are as follows:

1. **Complete Response (CR)**: Complete disappearance of all target lesions and any pathological lymph nodes (whether target or nontarget) is considered as CR. The lymph node size should be less than 10 mm in short axis.

2. **Partial Response (PR)**: When the tumor foci are still seen, but show at least 30% decrease in the sum of diameters of target lesions, taking as reference the baseline sum diameters, it is termed as PR.
3. **Progressive Disease (PD)**: When there is increase in the sum of diameters of target lesions by at least 20% with at least 5 mm increase in the absolute diameter, it is termed as PD. Appearance of one or more new lesions is also considered PD.
4. **Stable Disease (SD)**: When there is neither shrinkage to qualify for PR nor sufficient increase to qualify for PD, it is termed as SD.

15.3 Case 15.3

History: 69-year-old woman presented with a palpable mass in the right retroareolar region. She presented for diagnostic work up which included a mammogram, ultrasound, and a bilateral breast MRI.

Questions

Q1. Describe the findings in the provided images (Fig. 15.3a–e). What would be the next step?
Q2. What is the purpose of using post-biopsy clips in a neoadjuvant setting?
Q3. Describe the findings in Fig. 15.3f.
Q4. What is the complete radiological response?

Answers

A1. Imaging findings are as follows:

Mammography: Right MLO and CC projections (Fig. 15.3a) show a radio-opaque marker that annotates the site of palpable lump. Underneath the marker is seen an irregular mass in the right retroareolar region (white arrow). There is retraction of the nipple and no associated calcifications. A single right axillary LN is noted with eccentrically thickened cortex.

Ultrasonography: Ultrasound image (Fig. 15.3b) shows a hypoechoic, irregular mass in the right breast at the 6 o'clock retroareolar region that correlates with the palpable area of concern. Peripheral vascularity is seen around the mass. It is associated with tissue stiffness around the mass on shear wave elastography (Fig. 15.3c) in keeping with malignant features. No retroareolar shadowing is seen.

MRI: Single postcontrast T1w subtracted axial MRI image (Fig. 15.3d) shows a heterogeneously enhancing solid unifocal retroareolar mass in the right breast (white arrow).

Imaging features are suggestive of a solid right retroareolar unifocal mass with nipple retraction suggestive of invasive mammary carcinoma (BI-RADS 5).

Ultrasound-guided core biopsy of the mass is recommended. Post biopsy, a marker clip may be deployed within the tumor following the biopsy. Surgical oncology referral is suggested.

A2. All cancers selected for neoadjuvant treatment undergo clip placement in the index mass in order to document the location of the mass. In the event of complete response following neoadjuvant chemotherapy, the clip indicates where the original index mass was located. This aids imaging-guided excision and also aids the pathologist to locate the tumor bed in the postsurgical specimen.

Some centers also place clips in biopsy positive axillary lymph nodes in order to minimize surgical dissection in the axilla and to ensure that the prechemotherapy positive lymph node gets excised at final surgery. In this particular case, a prominent axillary lymph node underwent a fine needle aspiration and was positive. Figure 15.3e shows a post clip right mammogram in MLO projection which demonstrates clip in the index lesion as well as in the axilla (white arrows). Reticulation of soft tissue in breast and axilla is secondary to recent biopsy procedure.

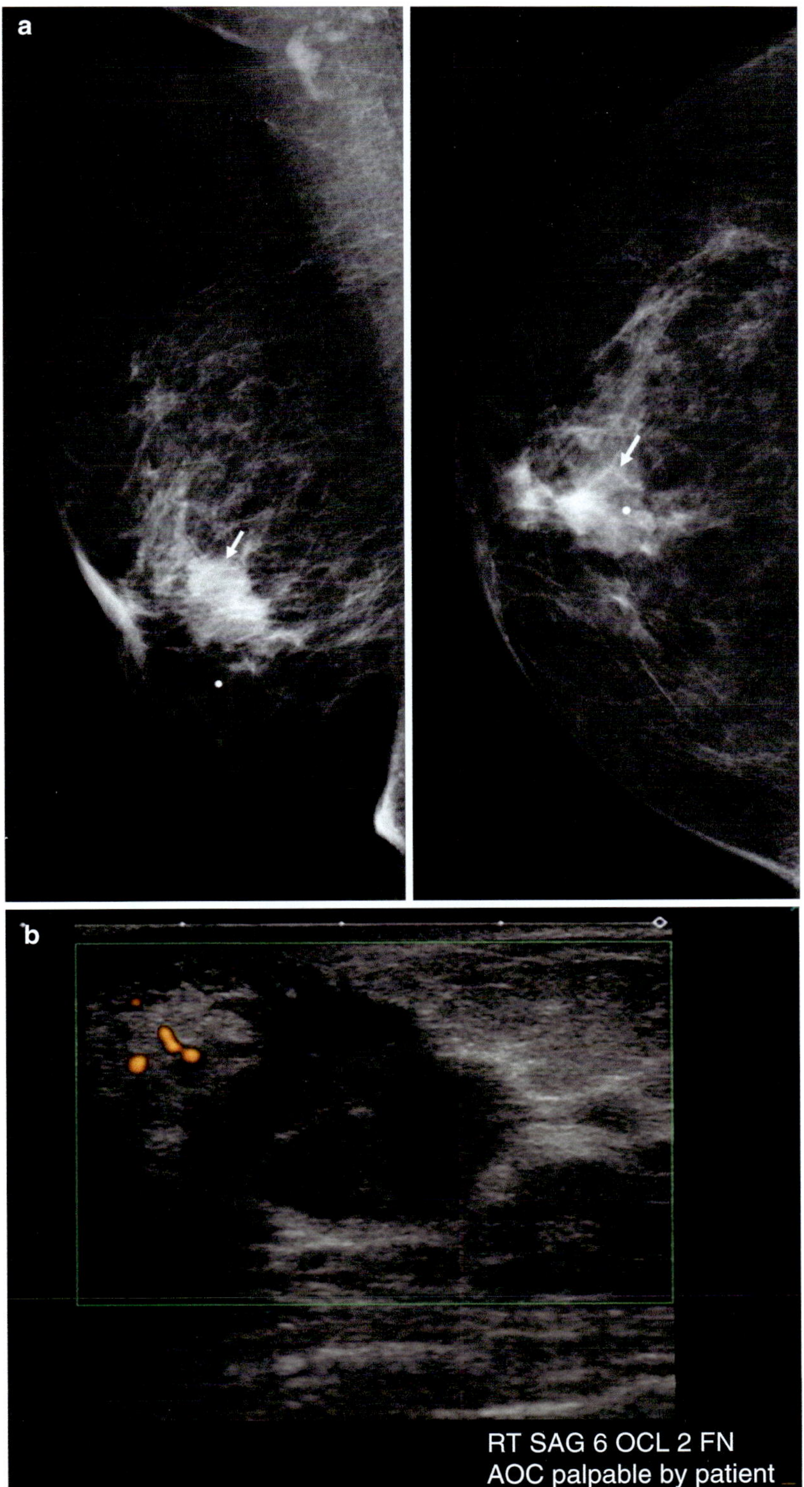

Fig. 15.3 (**a**) Right mammogram. (**b**) Targeted right breast ultrasound. (**c**) Shear wave elastography image of right breast mass. (**d**) Axial DCE MRI. (**e**) Post-biopsy right MLO to document clip position. (**f**) Post neoadjuvant chemotherapy re-staging axial DCE MRI

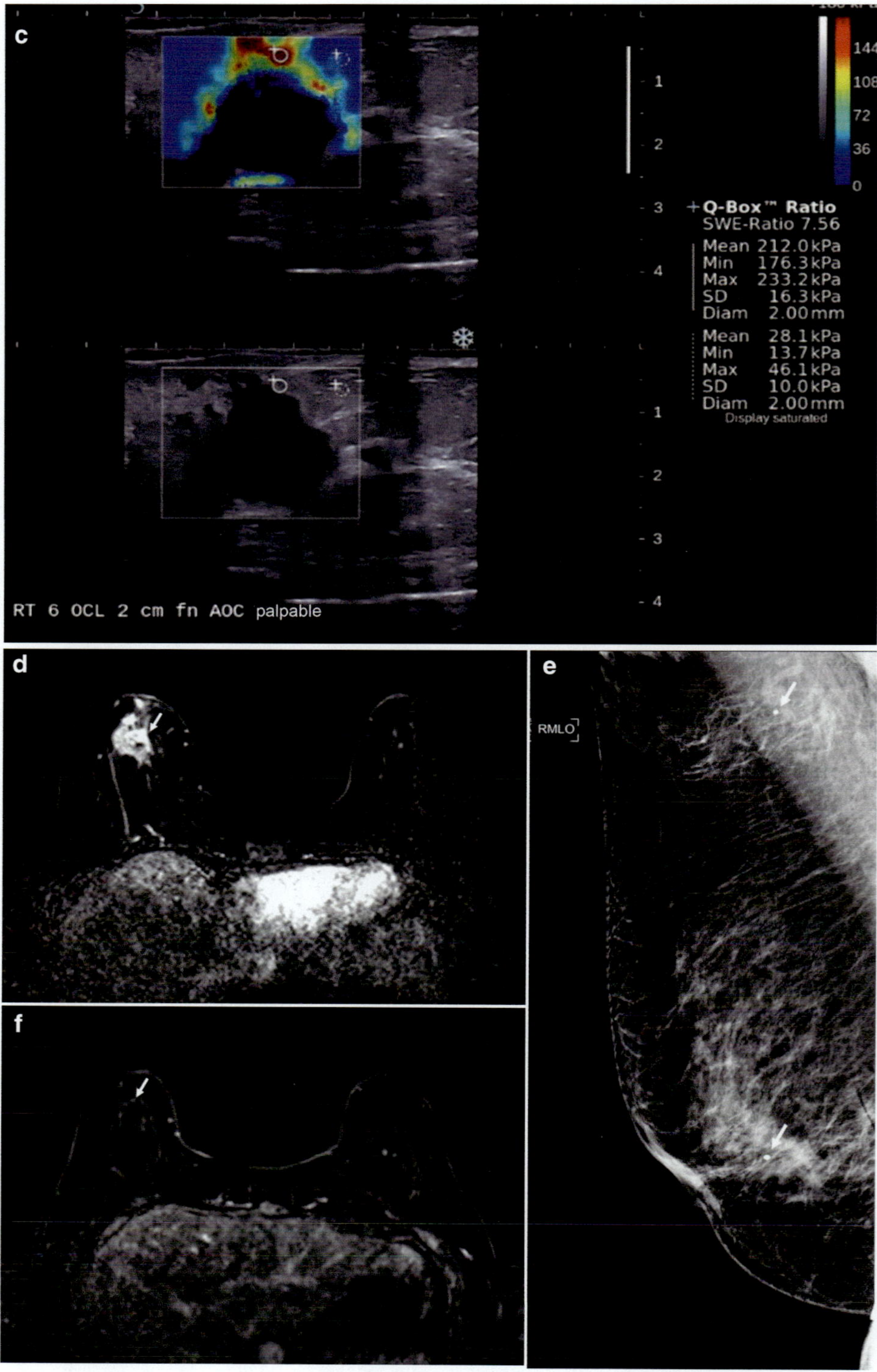

Fig. 15.3 (continued)

A3. Fig. 15.3f shows axial DCE T1WI subtraction of the post-neoadjuvant restaging MRI. Image reveals complete imaging resolution of the enhancing mass (white arrow) previously documented which indicates good response to neoadjuvant chemotherapy and provides a favorable postsurgical outcome to the patient.

A4. Complete radiological response is when there is no residual mass noted on post neoadjuvant treatment imaging. It is important to note the difference between complete radiological response and complete pathological response.

Complete radiological response is when there is no residual enhancing mass noted; however, there may still be residual nonenhancing or hypoxic solid tumor tissue within the tumor bed, which may be occult to imaging but will be seen on the final pathology of the tumor bed. A *complete pathological response* is when no residual tumor is seen on final postsurgical pathology.

Histopathology: Post-neoadjuvant right mastectomy revealed a 0.2 cm maximum dimension of invasive ductal carcinoma. Negative SLNB.

Notes

Biomarkers and Genomic Testing

It has been demonstrated that some breast cancer cells have receptors on their outer wall that catch specific hormone and stimulate unrestricted tumor growth. The commonly tested immunohistochemistry (IHC) biomarkers are estrogen receptors, progesterone receptors, and HER2.

Estrogen receptor (ER) positive. Breast cancer cells with estrogen receptors grow in the environment of circulating estrogen. By using antiestrogen hormone therapy (endocrine therapy), the tumor growth can be blocked.

Progesterone receptor (PR) positive. These breast cancer cells have receptors sensitive to progesterone that in turn stimulate cell overgrowth. Endocrine therapy can block the growth of the cancer cells in this type of tumor.

Hormone receptor negative. These tumor cells lack hormone receptors and hence are not benefited by endocrine therapy.

***HER2* gene.** Cancer cells positive for *HER2* receptors have overexpression of the HER2 gene, thereby producing excessive growth-producing protein called HER2. Herceptin and Trastuzumab are drugs that target the HER2 protein blocking it and thereby controlling the growth and killing the cancer cells.

Other biomarkers such as *Ki 67, p53, and C kit* overexpression are also used in clinical practice where available.

Based on the presence or absence of the receptors and additional genetic profiling of breast cancers they are divided into different types, the more common ones being Luminal A, Luminal B, HER2 overexpression, Basal-like, etc.

Luminal A subtype of breast cancer cells are ER and PR positive and HER2 negative. They benefit from endocrine therapy and may also benefit from chemotherapy.

Luminal B subtype of breast cancer cells are positive for ER and PR as well as for HER2. They are likely to benefit from endocrine therapy, HER2 targeted therapy, and chemotherapy.

HER2 positive cancer subtype cells are ER and PR negative, but HER2 positive. They benefit from chemotherapy and treatment targeted toward HER2.

Basal-like cancer subtype cells are negative for ER, PR, and HER2 receptors and are also called triple-negative breast cancer. They are likely to benefit from chemotherapy.

Genomic testing provides tests such as Oncotype Dx, Mammaprint, etc., which are predictive biomarkers and can help calculate risk of recurrence. Gene expression profiling tests analyze a number of different genes within cancer cells to predict risk of cancer recurrence. Women with a high score of risk of recurrence potentially benefit from adjuvant chemotherapy and those with low risk of recurrence may forgo adjuvant chemotherapy.

If standard methods predict the chance of recurrence is very small, then gene expression profiling tests probably aren't necessary. Nor are these tests necessary in an aggressive cancer in which there is clearly benefit from using chemotherapy. For cancers that fall between these two categories, where a decision needs to be made about whether to use chemotherapy, gene expression profiling can be particularly helpful.

15.4 Case 15.4

History: 67-year-old woman with a left retracted nipple and a palpable finding underwent a bilateral mammogram, ultrasound, and a bilateral MRI.

Questions

Q1. Describe the imaging findings (Fig. 15.4a–d).

Q2. Figure 15.4e represents post neoadjuvant chemotherapy. Describe imaging findings and discuss its clinical implications.

Q3. What is inflammatory carcinoma?

Answers

A1. Imaging findings are as follows:

Mammography: Bilateral MLO (Fig. 15.4a) and CC views (Fig. 15.4b) show diffuse increased interstitial markings with some spiculation in the left retroareolar region (white arrow) associated with nipple retraction. No calcifications are noted.

Ultrasonography: Ultrasound doppler image of the left breast (Fig. 15.4c) shows diffuse hypoechoic shadowing (white arrows) in the left central retroareolar region located in the mid and posterior third of the breast with hypoechoic tissue extending to the posterior aspect of the nipple causing retraction. No abnormal vascularity demonstrated.

MRI: Axial subtracted DCE T1WI (Fig. 15.4d) shows that the left breast is less pendulous, smaller in size and is completely replaced by diffuse non-mass enhancement (white arrows) indicating locally advanced breast cancer. No involvement of skin or chest wall. There is focal enhancement in the left half of the sternal body (thick white arrow) indicating likely bone metastasis, which would require further confirmation with a whole-body bone scan. Imaging diagnosis is locally advanced invasive mammary carcinoma involving the left breast.

Histopathology: 14G US core biopsy revealed a grade 3, ER+, PR–, HER2– invasive lobular carcinoma.

A2. Axial subtracted DCE T1WI from a post-neoadjuvant re-staging MRI (Fig. 15.4e) shows no change in the appearance of the left breast enhancement (white arrows). Sternal enhancing lesion is also largely unchanged (thick white arrow). This indicates nonresponse to the chemotherapy and indicates worse outcome for the patient. These women will either proceed to palliative surgical or medical management.

A3. Inflammatory carcinoma is a clinical-pathological entity characterized by diffuse erythema and edema (peau d'orange) involving approximately a third or more of the skin of the breast. It is primarily a clinical diagnosis and may or may not have a clinically evident breast mass. Imaging may show a detectable mass with skin thickening. The skin thickening maybe due to metastatic deposits in the dermal lymphatics or metastatic axillary lymphadenopathy. A pathological proof of dermal lymphatic tumor emboli is not necessary to make a diagnosis of inflammatory carcinoma which is primarily a clinical diagnosis. Rapid evolution in 6 months is one of the characteristics of inflammatory carcinoma. A neglected LABC or a cancer invading or ulcerating, skin does not qualify to be labeled as an inflammatory carcinoma.

Notes

Role of Breast MRI in Neoadjuvant Therapy

At the current time, MRI is considered to be the most suitable diagnostic modality to determine response to neoadjuvant chemotherapy. Although it has shown good correlation with pathology size

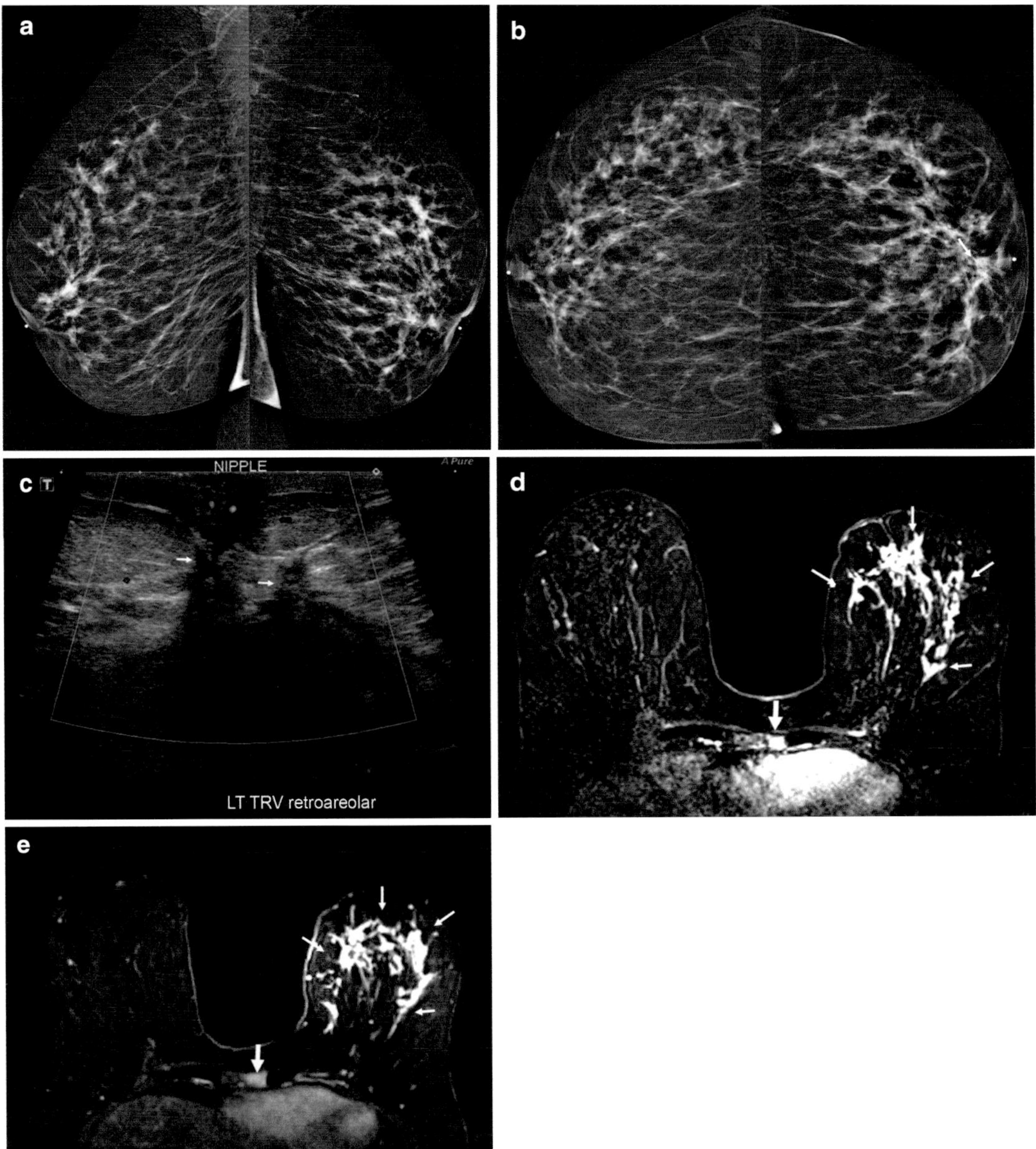

Fig. 15.4 (**a**) Bilateral MLO views. (**b**) Bilateral CC views. (**c**) Targeted left breast ultrasound with doppler. (**d**) Axial DCE T1WI. (**e**) Post-neoadjuvant axial DCE T1WI

estimation, occasionally overestimation as well as underestimation of residual disease have been noted. MRI is the most accurate modality in predicting response in the solid imaging phenotype of TNBC and HER2-enriched breast tumors. In these cases, MRI is highly reliable for surgical planning. On the contrary, cancers that are hormone receptor positive and those demonstrating non-mass enhancement show lower concordance with surgical pathology, making surgical guidance difficult.

It is important to always look for delayed enhancement on post-neoadjuvant MRI as the neoadjuvant chemotherapy can change the vascularization of invasive cancers and may lose the classic early enhancement and washout. T1-weighted images should be assessed for the residual soft tissue component of the residual cancer although sometimes it may be difficult to differentiate residual tumor from the fibrosis in the surgical bed.

ACOSOG Z0011 Trial

Axillary lymph node dissection provides excellent loco-regional control of cancer, but it is associated with significant risk of complications such as lymphedema, numbness, axillary web syndrome, and restricted arm motion.

The American College of Surgeons Oncology Group **Z0011** (ACOSOG Z0011) was a randomized clinical trial to compare the survival outcome in patients with low nodal disease after SLND and ALND in patients undergoing BCS followed by adjuvant radiotherapy and adjuvant systemic therapy. The results of this trial demonstrated that the subgroup of women with T1 or T2 node negative breast cancer and 1 or 2 positive sentinel nodes who were treated with breast-conserving therapy and adjuvant systemic therapy had noninferior overall survival outcomes with those who had ALND with similar adjuvant treatment.

Before the trial, axillary nodal dissection was considered necessary for better cancer control for all preoperative metastatic LN or positive SLNB cases, irrespective of the number of nodes involved. This trial changed the approach to the management of axilla from a complete dissection to a limited axillary intervention. There was a general consensus that axillary dissection was necessary for better cancer control when metastases were identified in sentinel lymph nodes.

Based on more recent trials, (Alliance trial) node-positive invasive breast cancer can also be offered targeted axillary dissection, which includes SLNB along with excision on the biopsy proven (clipped) positive lymph node subsequent to neoadjuvant chemotherapy. This allows for minimally invasive management of low volume axillary metastatic disease.

Suggested Readings

Amin MB, Greene FL, Edge SB, Compton CC, Gershenwald JE, Brookland RK, Meyer L, Gress DM, Byrd DR, Winchester DP. The Eighth Edition AJCC Cancer Staging Manual: Continuing to build a bridge from a population-based to a more "personalized" approach to cancer staging. CA Cancer J Clin. 2017;67(2):93–9.

Aysola K, Desai A, Welch C, Xu J, Qin Y, Reddy V, Matthews R, Owens C, Okoli J, Beech DJ, Piyathilake CJ. Triple negative breast cancer–an overview. Hereditary Genet. 2013;2013(Suppl 2):001.

Boisserie-Lacroix M, MacGrogan G, Debled M, Ferron S, Asad-Syed M, McKelvie-Sebileau P, Mathoulin-Pélissier S, Brouste V, Hurtevent-Labrot G. Triple-negative breast cancers: associations between imaging and pathological findings for triple-negative tumors compared with hormone receptor-positive/human epidermal growth factor receptor-2-negative breast cancers. Oncologist. 2013;18(7):802–11.

Caudle AS, Yang WT, Krishnamurthy S, Mittendorf EA, Black DM, Gilcrease MZ, Bedrosian I, Hobbs BP, DeSnyder SM, Hwang RF, Adrada BE, Shaitelman SF, Chavez-MacGregor M, Smith BD, Candelaria RP, Babiera GV, Dogan BE, Santiago L, Hunt KK, et al. Improved axillary evaluation following neoadjuvant therapy for patients with node-positive breast cancer using selective evaluation of clipped nodes: implementation of targeted axillary dissection. J Clin Oncol. 2016;34(10):1072–8.

Eisenhauer EA, Therasse P, Bogaerts J, Schwartz LH, Sargent D, Ford R, Dancey J, Arbuck S, Gwyther S, Mooney M, Rubinstein L. New response evaluation criteria in solid tumours: revised RECIST guideline (version 1.1). Eur J Cancer. 2009;45(2):228–47.

Giuliano AE, Ballman KV, McCall L, Beitsch PD, Brennan MB, Kelemen PR, Ollila DW, Hansen NM, Whitworth PW, Blumencranz PW, Leitch AM, Saha S, Hunt KK, Morrow M. Effect of axillary dissection vs no axillary dissection on 10-year overall survival among women with invasive breast cancer and sentinel node metastasis: the ACOSOG Z0011 (Alliance) randomized clinical trial. JAMA. 2017;318(10):918–26.

Lobbes MB, Prevos R, Smidt M, Tjan-Heijnen VC, Van Goethem M, Schipper R, Beets-Tan RG, Wildberger JE. The role of magnetic resonance imaging in assessing residual disease and pathologic complete response in breast cancer patients receiving neoadjuvant chemotherapy: a systematic review. Insight Imag. 2013;4(2):163–75.

National Comprehensive Cancer Network. NCCN clinical practice guidelines in oncology: breast cancer version 3. Fort Washington: National Comprehensive Cancer Network; 2014.

Price ER, Wong J, Mukhtar R, Hylton N, Esserman LJ. How to use magnetic resonance imaging following neoadjuvant chemotherapy in locally advanced breast cancer. World J Clin Cases. 2015;3(7):607–13.

Reyal F, Hamy AS, Piccart MJ. Neoadjuvant treatment: the future of patients with breast cancer. ESMO Open. 2018;3(4):e000371.

Simos D, Clemons M, Ginsburg OM, Jacobs C. Definition and consequences of locally advanced breast cancer. Curr Opin Support Palliat Care. 2014;8(1):33–8.

16 Breast Diseases in Pregnancy and Lactation, Inflammation, Infections

16.1 Case 16.1

History: 30-year-old woman presents with a right 12 o'clock palpable painful/tender mass and fever. Currently lactating.

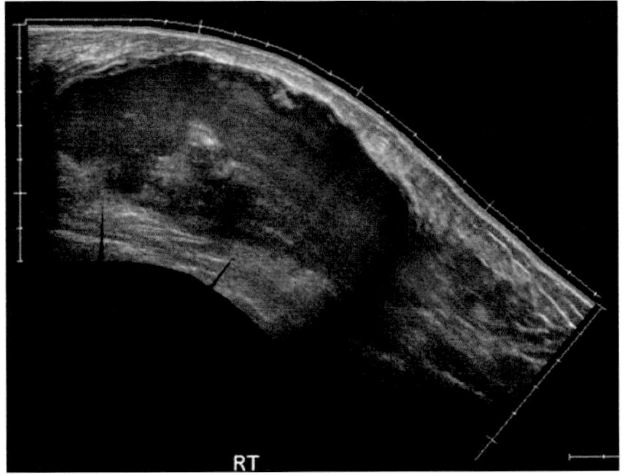

Fig. 16.1 Ultrasound view of the upper right breast (Panoramic)

Questions

Q1. Describe the imaging findings (Fig. 16.1). What would be the next step?
Q2. Provide possible differentials.
Q3. What is the management of the above-described condition?

Answers

A1. Panoramic ultrasound image of the right breast reveals a complex heterogenous collection in the middle third of the breast associated with some posterior enhancement. The surrounding adipose tissue shows increased echogenicity indicating surrounding inflammation. There is mild skin thickening. It is important to assess the remainder breast and axilla.

Given the clinical signs and symptoms, this is likely an inflammatory/infective collection which needs to be aspirated.

A2. Differential Diagnosis:
- Acute puerperal mastitis with abscess formation.
- Infected galactocele.
- Lactational adenoma.
- Infarcted fibroadenoma.

A3. Management includes:
- Aspiration under local anaesthesia with ultrasound guidance.
- Culture and sensitivity of the aspirate.
- Antibiotic coverage.
- Short-term follow-up if patient continues to be symptomatic.

N. Chotai, S. Kulkarni, *Breast Imaging Essentials*, https://doi.org/10.1007/978-981-15-1412-8_16

- Some women may need surgical drainage if the contents are thick along with irrigation of the abscess cavity.
- In cases with nonresolving abscess, a 14 G tissue biopsy may be required to exclude underlying malignancy.

Diagnosis: Puerperal abscess. Gram-positive cocci isolated.

Notes

Inflammation of breast may be focal or diffuse. It may be infectious or noninfectious and may be puerperal or nonpuerperal mastitis. Clinically, patients generally present with breast pain, swelling, redness. On examination, there may be focal or diffuse erythema, tenderness, and warmth. Disruption of skin surface of the nipple-areolar complex may cause breast infection, especially if there is associated milk stasis.

Mammogram may be withheld initially if there are severe inflammatory changes with pain. When done, it may show skin and trabecular thickening, focal asymmetry or increased density of involved part of breast, mass may be seen in abscess formation.

Ultrasound is the best imaging tool and also helps guide aspiration if needed. There may be diffuse or focal increased echogenicity of involved tissue, skin thickening, dilated ducts, irregular hypoechoic mass, or abscess collection with echoes. There may be increased vascularity due to inflammation.

MRI shows T2W hyperintense signal in areas of edema. There may be heterogeneous enhancement in area of inflammation. Abscess may show thick, irregular wall with enhancement.

D/D: Inflammatory carcinoma may be clinically indistinguishable. If the inflammation fails to respond to conservative antibiotic treatment and there is clinical concern, then skin punch biopsy may be needed to differentiate between the two. Another differential to be remembered is granulomatous mastitis which is diagnosed only on histology.

Infectious mastitis secondary to bacterial infection generally are due to *Staphylococcus aureus* or *Streptococcus* bacteria, as in this case. Smoking is shown to increase the risk of subareolar abscess (Zuska's disease) and cause recurrent/nonresponsive mastitis.

Treatment is generally antibiotic therapy and aspiration of abscess, as clinically indicated.

16.2 Case 16.2

History: 37-year-old woman currently lactating presents with a palpable mass.

Questions

Q1. What imaging test would you offer for this woman?

Q2. Describe the ultrasound findings (Fig. 16.2a).

Q3. Describe the mammographic findings (Fig. 16.2b) and give BI-RADS category.

Q4. How would you manage the above condition?

Answers

A1. Sonography is the first line investigation in the assessment of pregnant or lactating women. In lactating women, if required, a single-view mammogram may be performed to aid further diagnosis.

As per the ACR appropriateness criteria, a mammogram may be offered to a nonpregnant woman of age 30 years and above who presents with a palpable finding in addition to an ultrasound exam. In a pregnant woman, ultrasound is the first exam and if suspicious findings are found a limited mammogram can be offered with abdominal shielding if it is thought to impact immediate management. Radiation safety should be discussed with the patient and her referring physician before the mammogram is performed.

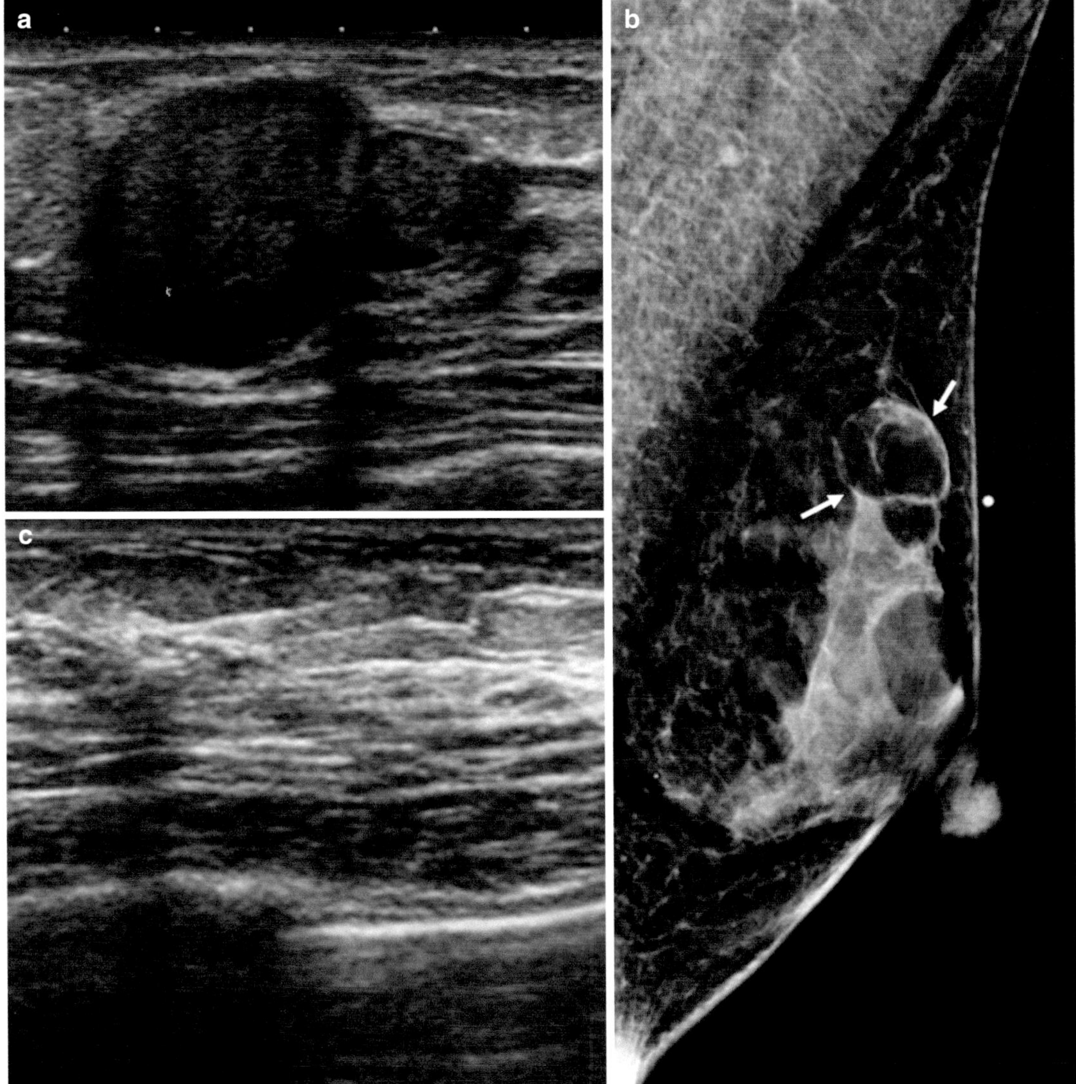

Fig. 16.2 (**a**) Targeted ultrasound image of left breast palpable lump. (**b**) Single-view left mammogram in MLO projection. (**c**) Targeted ultrasound image of left breast lump post aspiration

A2. As the patient presented with a palpable finding, ultrasound was the first exam that was offered to this woman. Single transverse ultrasound image (Fig. 16.2a) of left breast in the area of palpable lump reveals a complex solid cystic mass. It is fairly well circumscribed with mild posterior through transmission. Edge shadows can be appreciated indicating a likely benign etiology. Differentials in the absence of any systemic symptoms (fever, etc.) are galactocele, complex fibroadenoma, fat necrosis, fibroadenolipoma, and lactational adenoma. Given the more solid appearance, a single-view mammogram was offered.

A3. Single-view left MLO (Fig. 16.2b) demonstrates a well circumscribed mass (white arrows) completely fatty in density, which confirms the mass to be a galactocele. Due to the milky contents of a galactocele, it often tends to appear complex on ultrasound but completely fatty on mammography, which is very characteristic.

Diagnosis: Galactocele BI-RADS 2

A4. No further management or follow-up necessary for this essentially benign condition. If the patient is in discomfort, a fine needle aspiration may be offered after obtaining consent for a likely milk fistula or infection. Aspirate will reveal whitish milky fluid and the lesion collapses following aspiration (Fig. 16.2c).

Notes

Galactoceles

Galactoceles, also referred to as **lactoceles**, are the commonest benign breast lesions in young lactating women. Occlusion of a lactiferous duct leads to the formation of a retention cyst. Although termed as galactocele, they commonly occur during pregnancy and on cessation of lactation. Percutaneous aspiration of cyst may reveal fresh milk or thickened white liquid depending on chronicity of the lesion.

Mammographic appearance of galactocele can be varied depending on the fat and protein content and the consistency of the fluid.

Imaging appearances may vary as follows:

1. Pseudolipoma: Predominantly fat content imparts appearance of a radiolucent mass akin to a lipoma on mammogram.
2. Fat-fluid level within cyst: When the milk is in fresh liquid state, a characteristic fat-fluid level is noted due to differential viscosity of fat and fluid. This is well demonstrated in a straight lateral upright mammographic view.
3. Pseudohamartoma: In a long-standing galactocele, high-viscosity contents give a hamartoma-like appearance on the mammogram.

Ultrasound appearances can be widely variable. They could be cystic/multicystic (~50%), mixed solid cystic (~37%), or solid (~13%). Color Doppler interrogation will show lack of blood flow.

Radiation Dose Consideration

The radiation dose from standard 4-view mammogram is less than 3 mGy. This is roughly equivalent to 7 weeks of background radiation. Estimated radiation dose to the uterus following a routine mammogram is less than 0.03 μGy, which far less than the threshold 50 mGy. No known teratogenic fetal effects have been reported below this threshold. Use of lead apron shielding can reduce the radiation dose to the uterus by about 50%, though it should be noted that scatter radiation is the main cause of dose to uterus and shielding has limited effectiveness on scattered radiation. Lead apron shielding should still be offered to all pregnant women. In case of accidental exposure to a mammogram during early pregnancy, the woman should be assured about extremely low risk to fetus during this period. There are no proven theoretical carcinogenic effects of radiation on the lactating breast with active proliferation of breast epithelium.

16.3 Case 16.3

History: 36-year-old woman presents with a palpable mobile mass at the 2:30 location in the left breast. Known saline implant breast augmentation. Currently lactating.

Questions

Q1. Describe the ultrasound findings (Fig. 16.3) and give the BI-RADS category.

Q2. What is the management of the above condition?

Answers

A1. Single transverse ultrasound image reveals a well-circumscribed, oval, heterogeneous

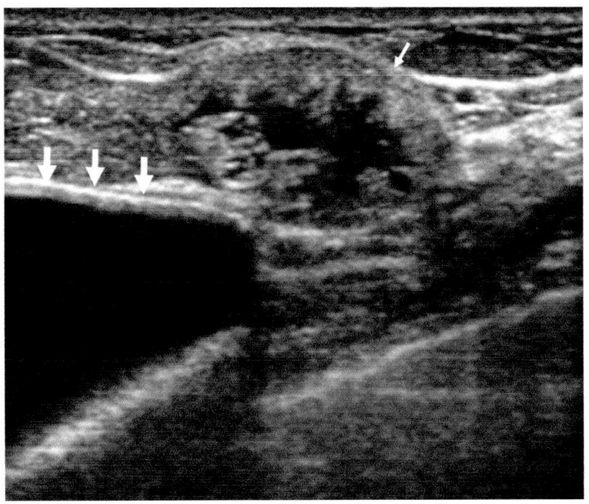

Fig. 16.3 Targeted ultrasound image of left breast palpable lump

echogenicity mass (white arrow) with through transmission situated superficial to the saline implant (thick white arrows) in the left breast.

Differential diagnosis: Fibroadenoma and lactational adenoma.

BI-RADS 4.

Diagnosis: Lactational adenoma.

A2. Typically, lactational adenomas regress following cessation of lactation and no further follow up or intervention is necessary. Occasionally they may infarct in which case they may present as a firm tender mass and in these cases a surgical consultation and close follow-up may be required.

Notes

Lactational Adenoma

Lactational adenoma is a benign breast tumor occurring in pregnancy or lactation. It is thought to be secondary to premature lactational changes occurring in one part of breast tissue out of phase from surrounding breast parenchyma. On pathology it typically shows foamy to vacuolated cytoplasm without any obvious cellular atypia.

On ultrasound, it shows typical benign imaging features like circumscribed hypo to isoechoic mass, parallel orientation, minimal internal vascularity with occasional internal echogenic septum. It may be indistinguishable from fibroadenoma. Imaging is not diagnostic, and biopsy may be suggested to reach diagnosis. The top differentials include fibroadenomata, galactocele, complicated cyst, tubular adenoma, and circumscribed carcinoma.

It has not been shown to have any malignant potential, neither is it shown to increase the risk of breast cancer in the future.

16.4 Case 16.4

History: 36-year-old woman, currently lactating, presents with a swollen left breast and a palpable mass.

Questions

Q1. Describe the imaging findings (Fig. 16.4a–c). What would be the next step?

Q2. What is the definition of a pregnancy-associated breast cancer (PABC)?

Q3. What are the special considerations while performing image-guided biopsies in pregnant and lactating women?

Answers

A1. The left mammogram in MLO projection (Fig. 16.4a) shows diffuse increase in density with poor contrast and thickening of the overlying skin (white arrows). No discreet masses are demonstrated although some distortion is seen in the upper breast (thick white arrow). No calcifications are noted. In such cases, where the breast is clinically swollen, compression is suboptimal, which limits the diagnostic quality of the mammogram.

Ultrasound image of left breast at 12 o'clock (Fig. 16.4b) shows a large underlying mass with irregular and angulated margins. The deeper margin of the mass cannot be discerned due to its size.

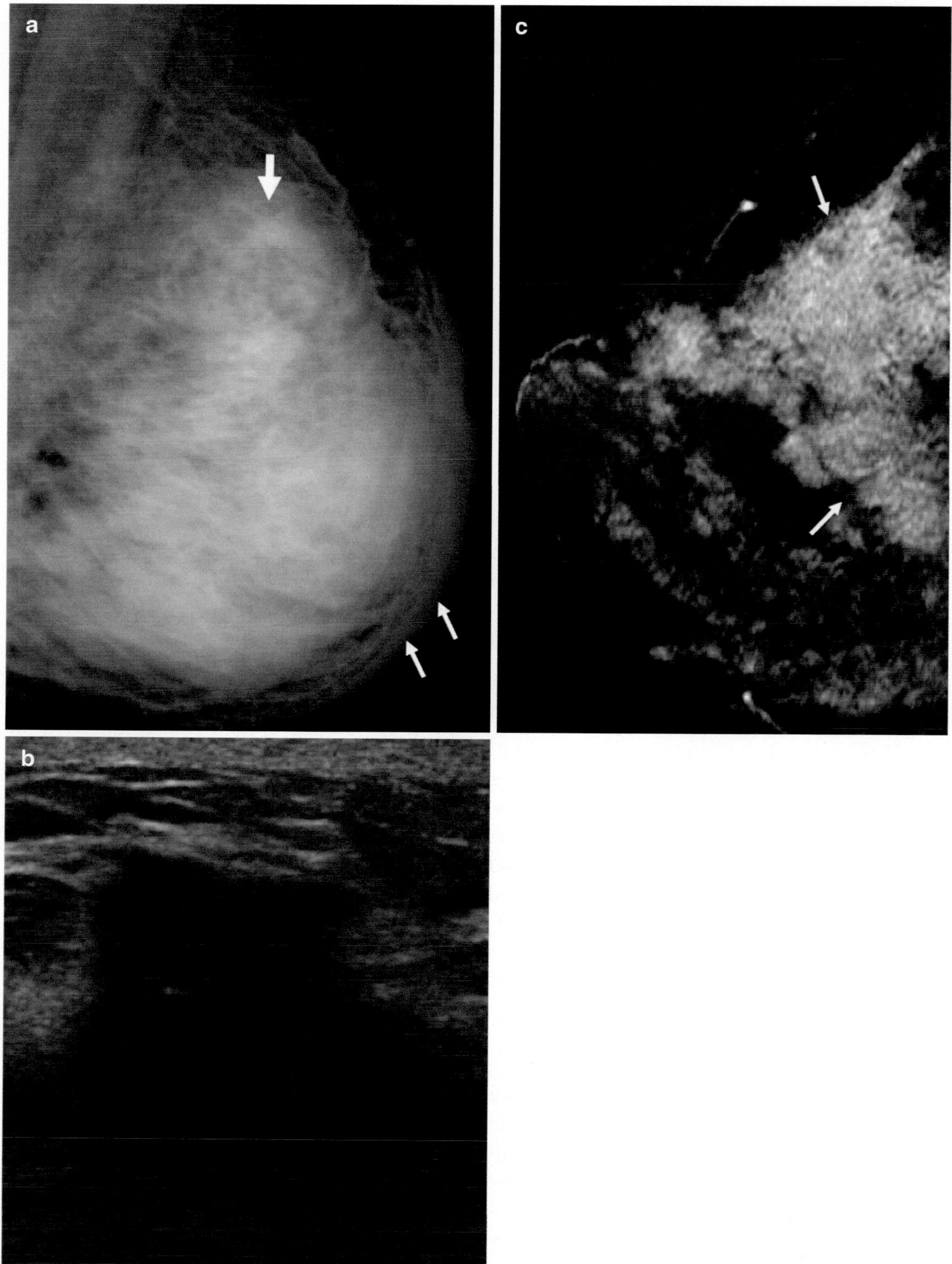

Fig. 16.4 (**a**) Single-view left mammogram in MLO projection. (**b**) Targeted ultrasound image of left breast at the 12 o'clock location. (**c**) Postcontrast T1WI subtracted sagittal MRI left breast

Single sagittal T1W postcontrast subtracted image (Fig. 16.4c) shows replacement of the upper half of the left breast with enhancing masses (white arrows).

Imaging features are suspicious for locally advanced pregnancy-associated breast cancer involving the left breast.

A2. Breast cancer occurring during pregnancy or within 1 year of childbirth is termed as pregnancy-associated breast cancer (PABC). Poor prognosis and advanced stage at diagnosis, likely secondary to a delay in diagnosis, are common in these women. Reported incidence of PABC is 1 in 3000–10,000 pregnancies. It is the commonest cause of cancer-related death in pregnant and lactating women. Presenting symptoms include asymmetrical breast enlargement, a palpable painless lump, skin thickening, focal pain, and bloody nipple discharge.

A3. Pregnant and lactating women have increased breast vascularity and dilated ducts. These increase the risk of procedure-related bleeding and infection. There is a small risk of post-biopsy milk fistula formation in these women, and a written, informed consent with these possibilities should be obtained.

Patients should also be informed about possible presence of blood and lidocaine in the breast milk, post biopsy. Although safe for the infant, the patient can consider pumping and discarding milk from the affected breast for up to 12–24 h after core needle biopsy.

Notes

Pregnancy-Associated Breast Cancer

Pregnancy-associated breast cancer (PABC) is relatively more common in BRCA-1 and -2 gene carriers and are more aggressive than non-pregnancy-related breast cancer. Nearly 85–90% of PABC are high-grade tumors and almost 50% of patients have positive axillary nodes at presentation. Usually the PABC are triple negative (ER/PR/HER2/neu negative) in pregnant patients, while they are more likely HER2/neu positive in lactating patients. Imaging findings are similar to nonpregnancy-related breast cancer, but about 30% of PABC are occult on mammogram due to dense breasts in pregnancy. Ultrasound is the first choice of imaging in pregnancy and lactation period. If the ultrasound features are highly suspicious, supplementary single-view mammogram may be offered with abdominal shield during pregnancy. In lactating woman, mammogram may be done after nursing or pumping. Use of MRI should not be done during pregnancy as gadolinium use should be avoided during the first trimester. Although there is literature endorsing use of MRI in the later part of the pregnancy if the potential advantage outweighs risk to fetus, it is best avoided altogether during pregnancy. Also note should be made of possible increased background enhancement during pregnancy and lactation.

Interruption of pregnancy is not proven beneficial. Modified radical mastectomy with axillary node biopsy/dissection is commonly advised. Chemotherapy and Tamoxifen are generally avoided during the first trimester but can be given in late second and third trimesters. Radiotherapy is given after delivery, when needed.

16.5 Case 16.5

History: 35-year-old woman presents with a tender recurrent right subareolar mass. No history of lactation.

Questions

Q1. Describe the imaging findings (Fig. 16.5a, b).
Q2. What would be the next step?
Q3. What specific history should be asked for?

Answers

A1. Single right CC projection mammogram (Fig. 16.5a) reveals a subareolar irregular density (arrow) with thickening of the periareolar skin.

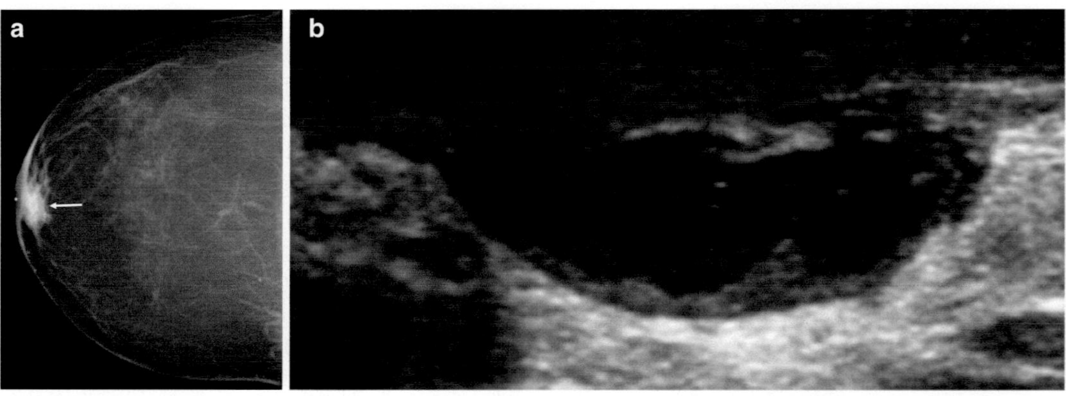

Fig. 16.5 (**a**) Single-view right mammogram in CC projection. (**b**) Targeted ultrasound of right breast areolar region

Ultrasound of right breast image (Fig. 16.5b) reveals the complex subareolar collection associated with skin thickening. Surrounding inflamed mildly echogenic fat is noted.

Imaging features are likely to suggest nonpuerperal subareolar mastitis.

A2. Next step would fine needle aspiration to relieve the symptoms and obtain aspirate for culture sensitivity.

A3. History of chronic smoking should be elicited. A type of recurrent mastitis which is linked to cigarette smoking is called Zuska's disease.

Notes

Zuska's Disease

This being a rare disease, exact pathogenesis is not clear. It is likely related to tobacco use. This is caused by squamous metaplasia and proliferation of lactiferous ducts which causes obstruction and stasis. The obstructed duct ruptures and contents spill into the surrounding stroma, initiating a chronic active granulomatous reaction and abscess formation. The abscess is caused initially by *Staphylococcus* bacteria and subsequently by a mixed flora of bacteria.

Common symptoms are painful, erythematous retroareolar mass with sometime fistula formation. This may be recurrent if the obstructed duct is not removed. Adequate treatment with antibiotics and complete excision of the offending ducts may be needed for complete resolution.

16.6 Case 16.6

History: 70-year-old woman presents with a vague palpable mass in the left upper outer quadrant.

Questions

Q1. Describe the imaging findings (Fig. 16.6a, b) and give the BI-RADS category.

Q2. What is the differential diagnosis?

Q3. Ultrasound core biopsy revealed a histopathology of granulomatous mastitis. What would you recommend next?

Q4. What is granulomatous mastitis?

Answers

A1. Imaging findings are as follows:

The left mammogram in MLO and CC projections (Fig. 16.6a) reveal a dense focal irregular mass in the upper outer quadrant (white arrows). No associated findings noted.

Ultrasound (Fig. 16.6b) shows a hypoechoic irregular solid mass in the left breast at the 2:30 location with a few

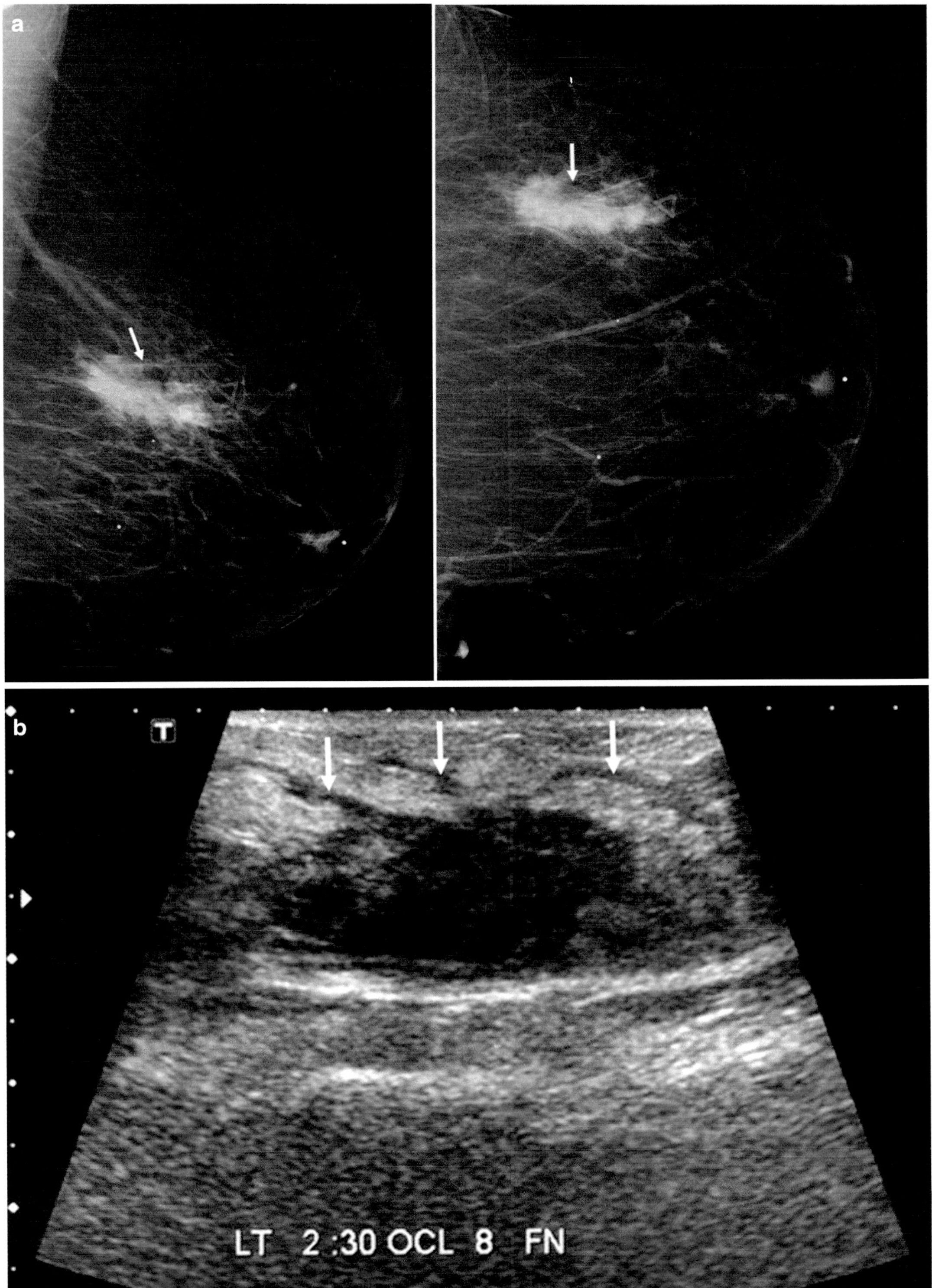

Fig. 16.6 (**a**) Left mammogram in MLO and CC views. (**b**) Targeted ultrasound of left breast

hypoechoic dendritic extensions towards the skin (white arrows). Imaging features are suspicious in a postmenopausal woman and histological correlation is suggested. Category: BI-RADS 4.

Histopathology: Granulomatous mastitis.

A2. Differential diagnosis of this lesion would include invasive mammary carcinoma, granulomatous mastitis, lymphoma, metastatic disease, and atypical fibroepithelial lesion (less likely given the age of patient).

A3. Given the imaging appearance and the histology, it would be deemed as a radio-pathological discordance. These would require a repeat biopsy to ensure that the target lesion was biopsied so that a malignant lesion is not missed.

A4. Granulomatous mastitis is a chronic inflammatory disease of the breast which has a wide differential spectrum, such as the following:

- Infectious causes including organisms such as mycobacterium, fungus, etc.
- Autoimmune process.
- Duct ectasia (plasma cell mastitis).
- Diabetes mellitus, sarcoidosis, etc.
- Idiopathic granulomatous mastitis.

Notes

Idiopathic Granulomatous Mastitis (IGM)

Idiopathic granulomatous mastitis is an idiopathic, noninfective, granulomatous lobular mastitis. Other granulomatous infections including tuberculosis are excluded.

It is typically seen in younger multiparous women presenting with a breast lump. (Our case is seen in a much older woman, which is unusual). There may be recent history of breast feeding in many patients. Common presenting symptoms are tenderness, mass, skin redness, and warmth. Some patients may have discharging sinuses.

On mammography a focal asymmetry, often retroareolar, is seen. There may be associated skin and trabecular thickening in involved part of breast.

Ultrasound shows irregular hypoechoic mass or confluent tubular structures, suggesting dilated ducts. There may be sinus tracts leading to the skin. Sometime there may be abscess collection as well. Increased vascularity in the inflamed breast is a common finding.

MRI: T2WI may show small pockets of abscess. Enhancing irregular mass/non-mass enhancement with tubular structures may be seen on contrast injection. MR is good for evaluating disease extent and monitor treatment response.

Differential diagnosis: Infective mastitis, inflammatory breast carcinoma, tuberculosis of breast. The imaging findings mimic malignancy, which may prompt multiple core biopsies due to perceived radio-pathological discordance.

Treatment of IGM is variable and ranges from surgical excision, steroids, methotrexate, etc.

Suggested Readings

Ayyappan AP, Kulkarni S, Crystal P. Pregnancy-associated breast cancer: spectrum of imaging appearances. Br J Radiol. 2010;83:529–34.

Bakaris S, Yuksel M, Cıragil P, Guven MA, Ezberci F, Bulbuloglu E. Granulomatous mastitis including breast tuberculosis and idiopathic lobular granulomatous mastitis. Can J Surg. 2006;49(6):427.

Darling ML, Smith DN, Rhei E, Denison CM, Lester SC, Meyer JE. Lactating adenoma: sonographic features. Breast J. 2000;6(4):252–6.

Guadagni M, Nazzari G. Zuska's disease. Giornale italiano di dermatologia e venereologia: organo ufficiale, Società italiana di dermatologia e sifilografia. 2008;143(2):157–60.

Leong PW, Chotai NC, Kulkarni S. Imaging features of inflammatory breast disorders: a pictorial essay. Korean J Radiol. 2018;19(1):5–14.

Lepori D. Inflammatory breast disease: the radiologist's role. Diagn Interv Imaging. 2015;96(10):1045–64.

Loibl S, Von Minckwitz G, Gwyn K, Ellis P, Blohmer JU, Schlegelberger B, Keller M, Harder S, Theriault RL, Crivellari D, Klingebiel T. Breast carcinoma during pregnancy: international recommendations from an expert meeting. Cancer. 2006;106(2):237–46.

Sabate JM, Clotet M, Torrubia S, Gomez A, Guerrero R, de Las Heras P, Lerma E. Radiologic evaluation of breast disorders related to pregnancy and lactation. Radiographics. 2007;27(suppl_1):S101–24.

Salvador R, Salvador M, Jimenez JA, Martinez M, Casas L. Galactocele of the breast: radiologic and ultrasonographic findings. Br J Radiol. 1990;63(746):140–2.

Vashi R, Hooley R, Butler R, Geisel J, Philpotts L. Breast imaging of the pregnant and lactating patient: physiologic changes and common benign entities. Am J Roentgenol. 2013a;200(2):329–36.

Vashi R, Hooley R, Butler R, Geisel J, Philpotts L. Breast imaging of the pregnant and lactating patient: imaging modalities and pregnancy-associated breast cancer. Am J Roentgenol. 2013b;200(2):321–8.

17 Post-operative Breast and Implants

17.1 Case 17.1

History: 51-year-old woman with a past history of left lumpectomy 8 years ago for breast cancer. Surveillance mammogram and ultrasound performed.

Questions

Q1. Describe the mammographic findings (Fig. 17.1a, b).

Q2. Describe the findings on ultrasound (Fig. 17.1c) and give appropriate BI-RADS.

Answers

A1. Bilateral MLO (Fig. 17.1a) and CC (Fig. 17.1b) views of both breasts show architectural distortion and contour deformity involving upper central left breast and left axilla (white arrow) in keeping with post-therapeutic changes. Coarse calcifications (thick white arrows) in the operative bed are likely dystrophic in nature. No overtly suspicious features are noted to suggest recurrent tumor. No spiculated mass or suspicious microcalcifications or architectural distortion is noted in the right breast. Bilateral breast skin appears largely unremarkable.

A2. Ultrasound images of the left breast (Fig. 17.1c) are available. Architectural distortion is seen (thick white arrow) in upper outer quadrant of the left breast, in keeping with postsurgical changes. Linear echogenic focus (white arrow) with dense posterior shadowing in the operative bed likely correlates with the dystrophic calcification seen on mammogram. No overtly suspicious imaging features are identified in the given images to suggest recurrence.

Category: BI-RADS 2.

Regular surveillance should be continued.

Notes

On mammography, the surgical scar may show volume reduction, contour deformity and architectural distortion. Skin thickening and trabecular thickening with increased breast density is seen in the initial 2–3 years secondary to postradiotherapy changes (Fig. 17.1d). These changes generally reduce over time and scar may become dense. Postoperative seroma, fat necrosis, and dystrophic calcifications may also be seen in the surgical bed. Calcifications are generally coarse and curvilinear calcifications around a central lucency. When evolving, they can look pleomorphic and therefore if they are newly noted they should undergo workup to exclude recurrence.

N. Chotai, S. Kulkarni, *Breast Imaging Essentials*, https://doi.org/10.1007/978-981-15-1412-8_17

On ultrasound, the surgical scar shows a variable appearance as it evolves. In the initial phase the surgical bed shows a seroma (fluid collection) which can appear quite complex followed by gradual resolution and replacement by fibrous scar tissue, which can show dense shadowing on ultrasound. Most typically the shadowing behind the scar appears wide in one projection and very narrow on the orthogonal plane (Fig. 17.1e). Architectural distortion can also be seen on ultrasound. Imaging of a surgical scar on ultrasound can be difficult at times and correlation with mammography can be helpful.

On MRI, postoperative hematoma may have variable intensity depending on the age of the

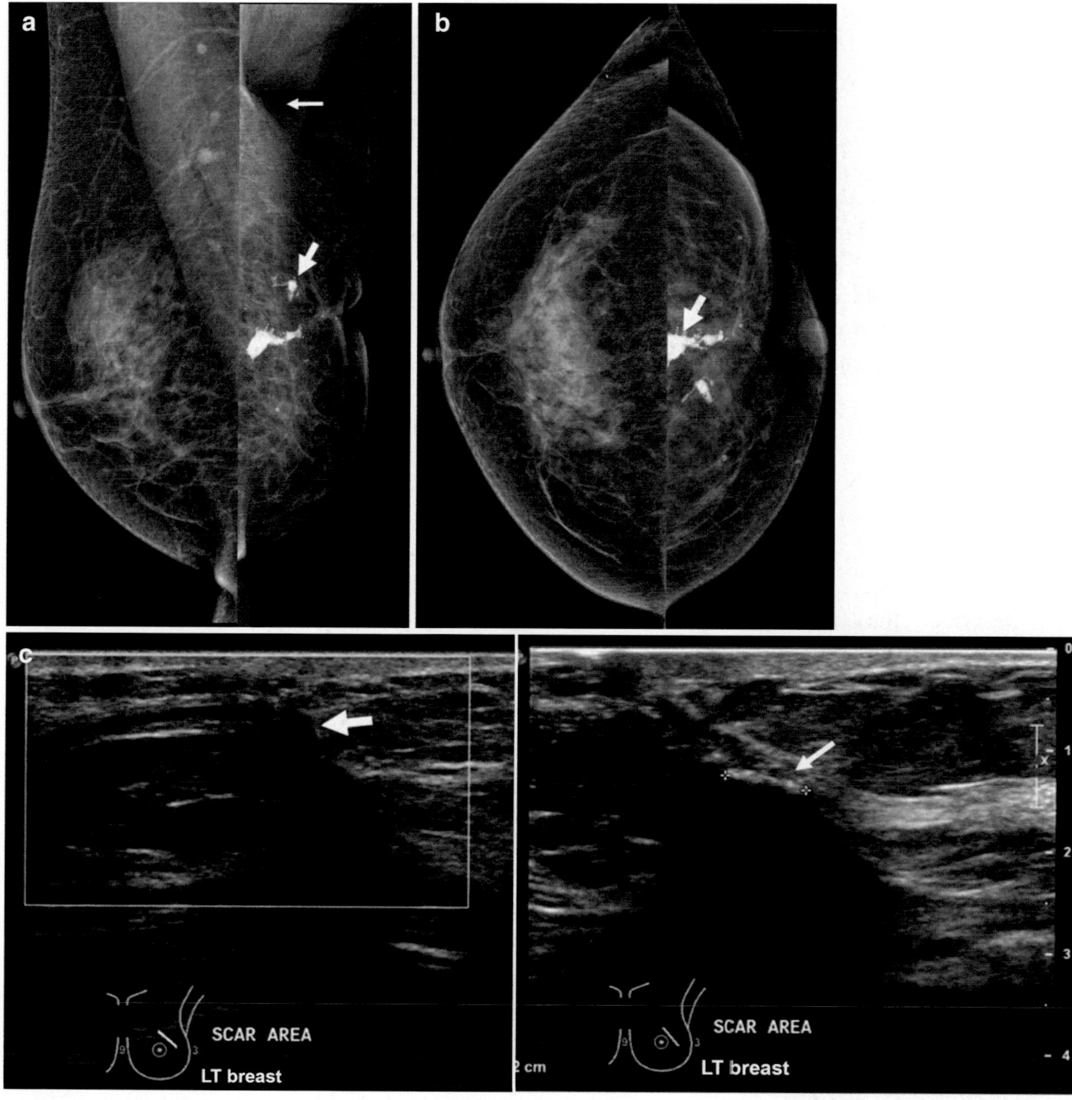

Fig. 17.1 (**a**) Bilateral MLO views. (**b**) Bilateral CC views. (**c**) Targeted left breast ultrasound with color Doppler of the surgical bed. (**d**) Companion case 1: (*a*) Left CC view: Biopsy proved IDC (white arrow) in the outer half. (*b*) Left CC view: Posttherapeutic mammogram shows BCT. Mild architectural distortion, contour deformity, skin and trabecular thickening consistent with postoperative and postradiotherapy change. (**e**) Companion case 2: Appearance of normal surgical scar on ultrasound. Scar is seen as a hypoechoic area with shadowing (white arrow). It appears wide in one plane and narrow and vertically elongated in the orthogonal plane

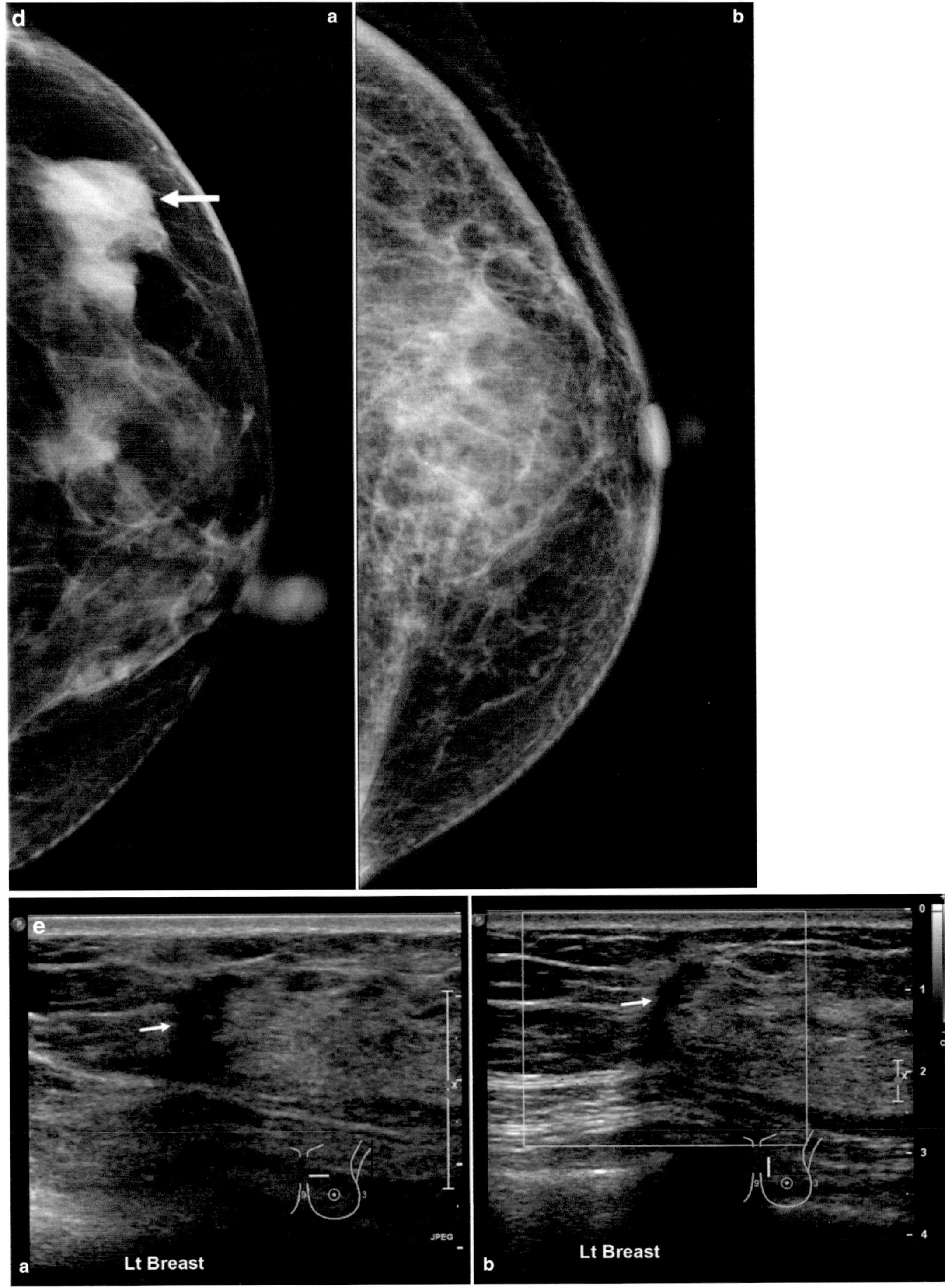

Fig. 17.1 (continued)

blood products. Delayed seroma generally shows a thin, regular wall that may enhance with clear fluid intensity content within the cavity. Enhancement typically resolves by 1.5–2 years. Occasionally, fat necrosis may appear as irregular enhancing mass. Fat intensity signal within the lesion on precontrast images may help differentiate fat necrosis from recurrence. If the findings are not typical, then histology may be needed in some cases to differentiate between the two.

It is important to note that postoperative changes, at times, make it difficult to detect early recurrence. Adjuvant MRI screening may be used for early detection of recurrence in premenopausal women with dense breasts or high-risk status and a personal history of breast cancer (ACR recommendation March 2018). This may not be feasible in many practices with limited resources (access to magnet time and funding) and as an alternative adjuvant ultrasound surveillance may be used.

17.2 Case 17.2

History: 52-year-old woman with previous right lumpectomy for IDC 10 years ago. Now presents with a new palpable lump at the site of surgical scar.

Questions

Q1. Describe the mammogram (Fig. 17.2a) and ultrasound (Fig. 17.2b) findings with the appropriate BI-RADS category.

Q2. Describe the findings on the contrast-enhanced mammogram (Fig. 17.2c).

Q3. Free hand biopsy (without image guidance) of the palpable lesion was performed. The histology was reported as benign post-radiation fibrosis. What would you advise next?

Answers

A1. Right MLO and CC views (Fig. 17.1a) show subtle architectural distortion and skin retraction in central region, mid third of the right breast. This is in keeping with postoperative changes. There is a partially circumscribed, high-density mass (double white arrows) in the right breast in relation to the scar. This correlates with the palpable concern. No associated microcalcifications are seen in this region. Right breast skin, subcutaneous tissue, and nipple are unremarkable. No enlarged axillary nodes are noted.

Ultrasound of the right breast (Fig. 17.2b), in the area of clinical concern, shows a hypoechoic lesion with indistinct margin. Minimal internal vascularity is seen in the mass. The imaging features are concerning for recurrence and histological correlation is suggested.

Category: BI-RADS 4C.

A2. Contrast-enhanced spectral mammography images of the right breast (Fig. 17.2c) in MLO and CC projections show a heterogeneously enhancing mass (thick white arrows) corresponding with the previously documented mass. Enhancement of mass is considered a concerning feature favoring recurrence. No other suspicious enhancement is seen in the right breast.

A3. The imaging features of the mass on all provided imaging are concerning for a malignant mass and a benign biopsy would be considered discordant. A repeat biopsy under image guidance is recommended.

A repeat ultrasound-guided biopsy of the mass was performed.

Histopathology: Grade 2 IDC (recurrence). A completion mastectomy was performed.

Notes

Local Recurrence

Rate of local recurrence is high in younger patients, high-grade tumors, positive surgical margins at lumpectomy, lack of radiotherapy, and triple-negative tumors. Recurrence rate is about 1–2% per year, and about 10–15% over 10 years.

Annual imaging surveillance is recommended for patients for at least 10 years post BCT to detect early recurrence.

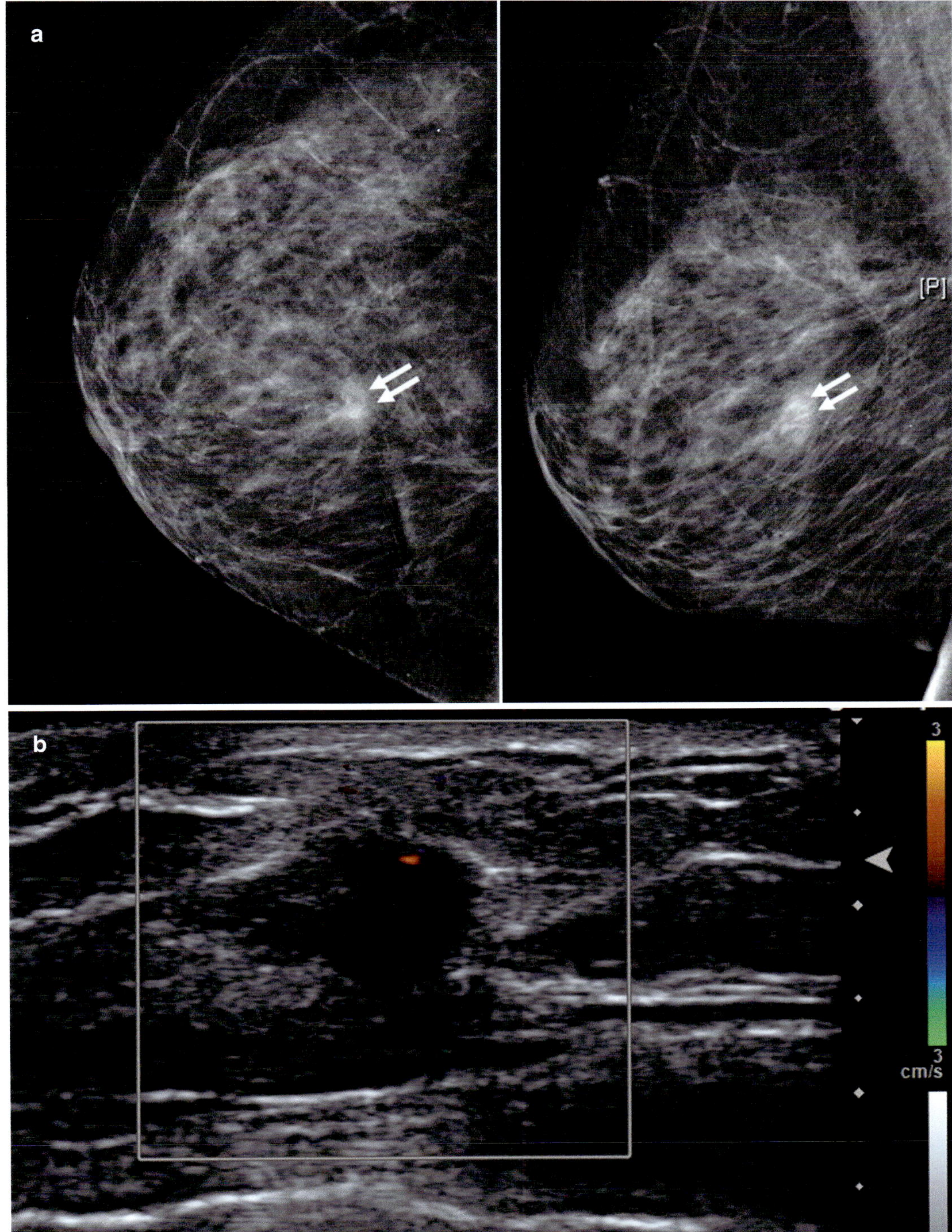

Fig. 17.2 (**a**) Right CC and MLO views. (**b**) Targeted right breast ultrasound. (**c**) Right CESM CC and MLO views

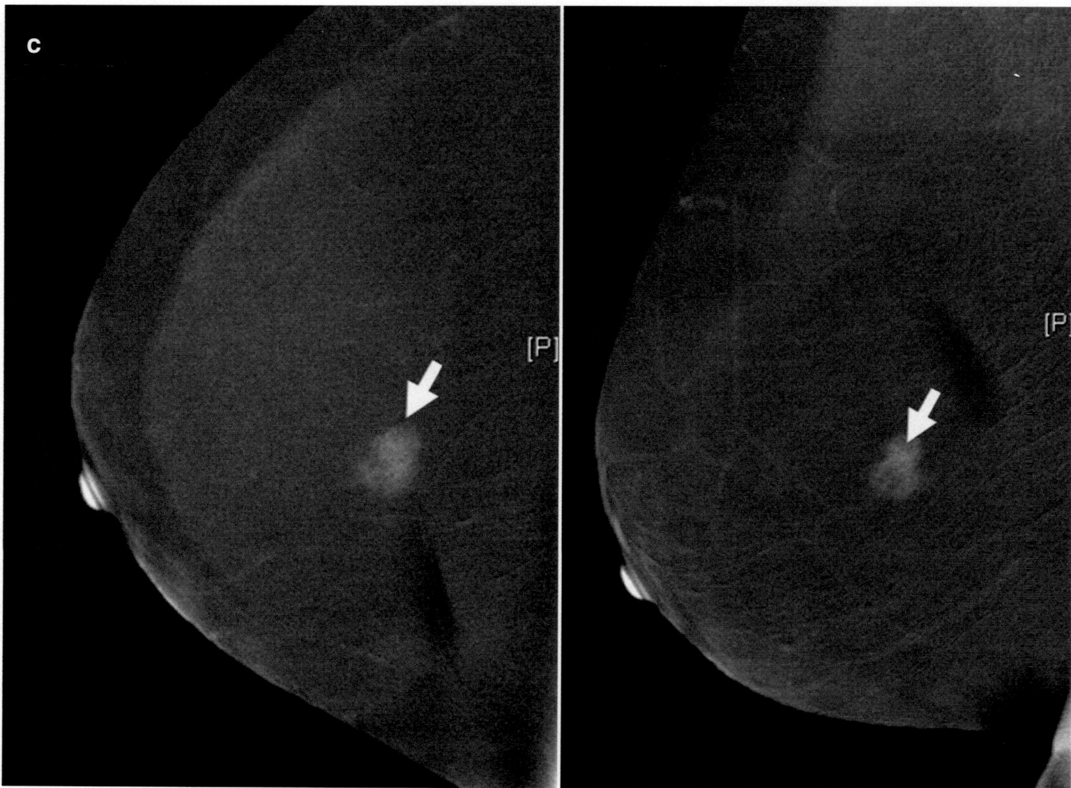

Fig. 17.2 (continued)

Clinically, any new palpable mass at the operative bed, new skin nodules, or new palpable axillary nodes may raise suspicion for recurrence. Occasionally, the recurrence may present with distant metastasis. If recurrence occurs in early postoperative period (within 5 years of treatment), then it reduces the 5-year survival from 70% to 40%.

On mammography, increased density or volume of the scar, new pleomorphic microcalcifications, and a new mass in the operative bed may suggest local recurrence.

On ultrasound, increasing volume of hypoechoic area under the scar, new spiculated or irregular mass separate from the scar may indicate tumor recurrence.

MRI is the most sensitive modality to detect early recurrence after lumpectomy. New enhancement in the operative bed raises suspicion of recurrence.

Management

Local recurrence: Initial treatment of primary breast cancer determines the management of local recurrence. Women developing local recurrence after initial treatment with breast-conserving surgery are usually treated with mastectomy. Women with postmastectomy recurrence are treated by excising the recurrent mass surgically. Subsequent combination of adjuvants like radiation, endocrine therapy, targeted therapy (like trastuzumab), and chemotherapy are used depending on the tumor subtype and patient comorbidity.

Regional recurrence: Regional nodal recurrence is treated by surgical excision of the lymph nodes followed by adjuvant radiotherapy. A combination of adjuvant systemic treatment (such as chemo, targeted therapy, or hormone therapy) may be used.

Distant recurrence: When the breast cancer recurs in other parts of the body, such as the bones, lungs, or brain, the treatment is similar to initial diagnosis of stage 4 disease.

17.3 Case 17.3

History: Multiple images of women with history of breast augmentation.

Questions

Q1. Describe the mammogram findings in Fig. 17.3a, b.
Q2. Describe the ultrasound findings in Fig. 17.3c.
Q3. Describe MRI findings in Fig. 17.3d, e.

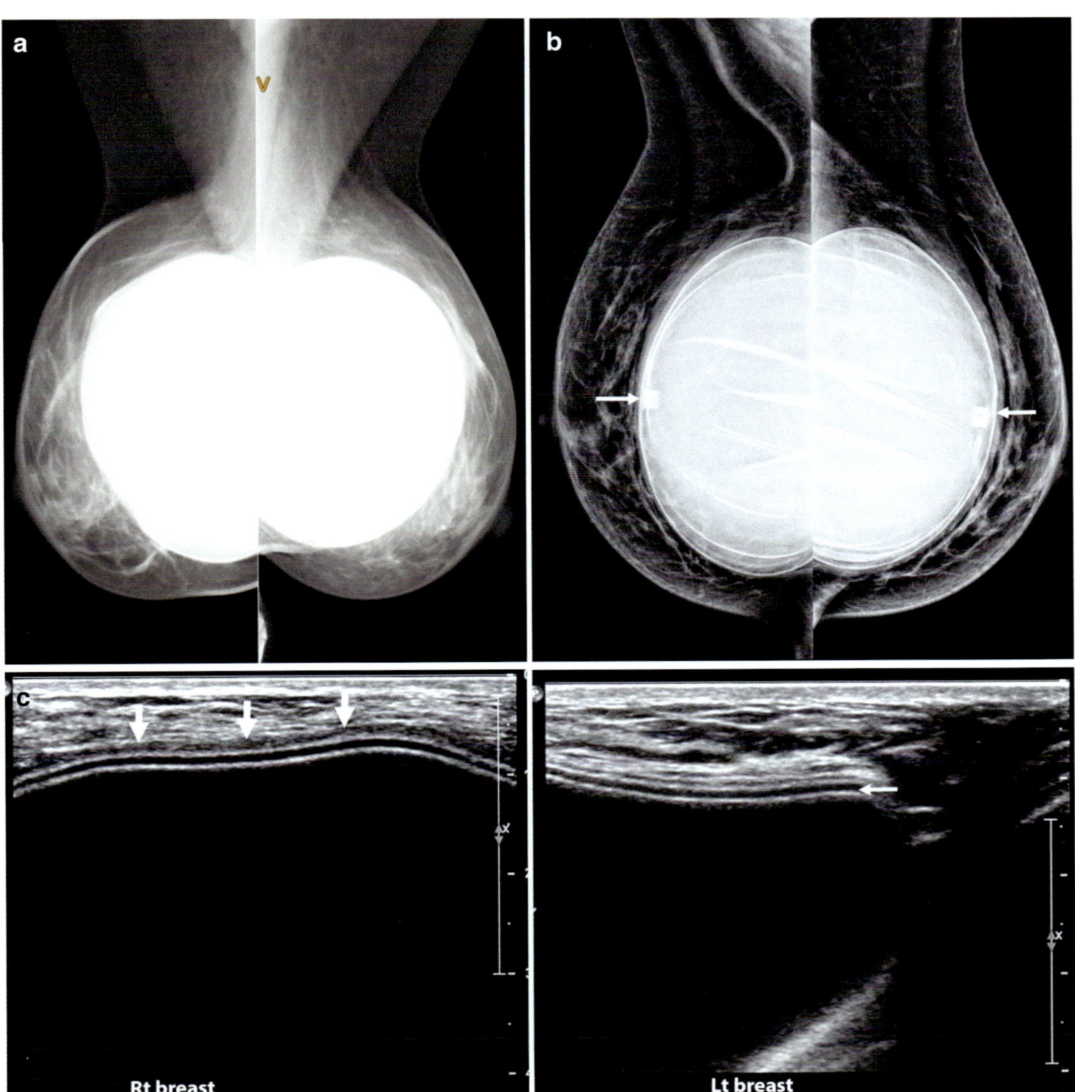

Fig. 17.3 (**a**) Bilateral MLO views. (**b**) Bilateral MLO views. (**c**): Bilateral breast ultrasound. (**d**) (*a–c*): MRI appearance of saline implants. (**e**) (*a–c*): MRI appearance of silicone implants. (**f**) (*a*, *b*): Diagrammatic representation of position of implant with respect to the pectoralis major muscle

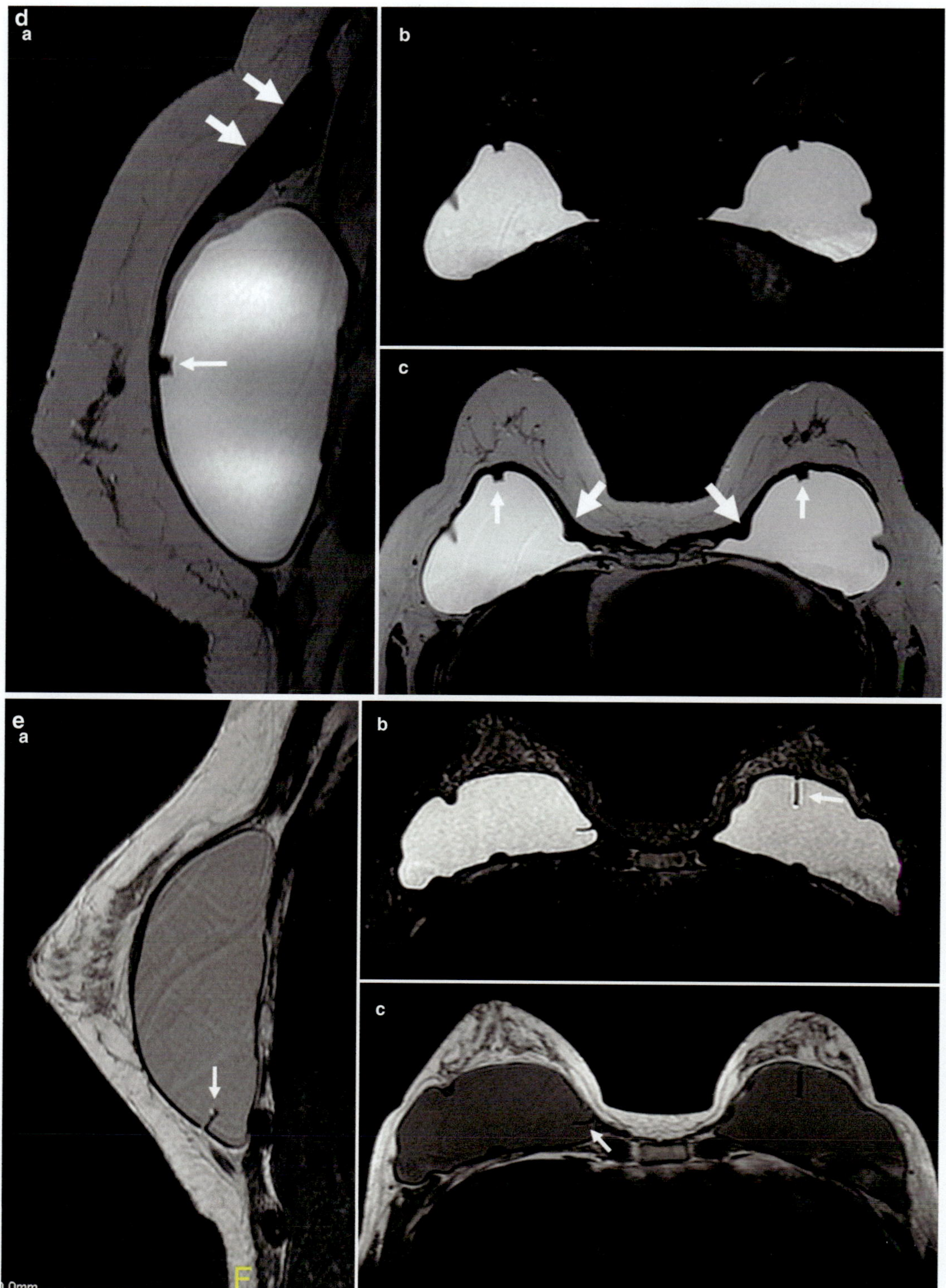

Fig. 17.3 (continued)

f

Augmented RT breast retroglandular implant

Pectoralis major muscle

Gland

Implant

a

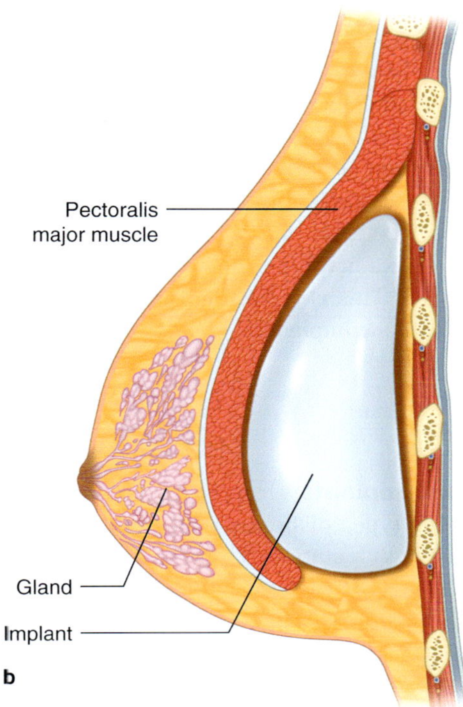

Fig. 17.3 (continued)

Answers

A1. MLO views of two different women are provided.

Figure 17.3a shows heterogeneously dense breast parenchyma. Bilateral homogeneously dense prostheses are noted suggesting silicone implants. The implants are seen anterior to the pectoralis major muscle, suggesting retroglandular location.

Figure 17.3b shows heterogeneously dense breast parenchyma. Bilateral relatively lucent prostheses are noted with a valve (white arrows) in each prosthesis; suggestive of saline implants. The pectoralis major muscle is seen anterior to the implants, suggesting retropectoral location.

The implants in both cases appear symmetrical with smooth and regular outline suggesting mammographically intact implants.

A2. Figure 17.3c shows the ultrasound appearance of a normal intact implant with smooth regular outline. The double/parallel outline of implant represents implant shell (white arrow) and thin outside fibrous capsule (thick white arrows). The implant contents appear anechoic/clear. The thin layer of breast parenchyma anterior to the implants show no suspicious lesion.

A3. MRI images of two different women provided.

In Fig. 17.3d: Sagittal T2WI (a), axial T2WI fat-suppressed (b), and axial T1WI (c).

Bilateral retropectoral implants are noted. The implant outline is smooth, regular, and symmetrical. The pectoralis muscle (thick white arrows) is seen anterior to the prosthesis. Implants appear bright on T2WI and are brighter than fat on T1WI. Symmetrical, nodular hypointense filling defect is seen along the anterior wall of prosthesis (white arrows) suggestive of valves. This is typical of normal saline implants.

In Fig. 17.3e: Sagittal T2WI (a), axial T2WI fat-suppressed (b), and axial T1WI (c).

Bilateral retropectoral implants are noted. The implant outline is smooth, regular, and symmetrical. The pectoralis muscle is seen anterior to the prosthesis. Implants are less bright on T2WI and show hypointense signal on T1WI as compared to the fat. Radial folds (white arrows) are identified. This is typical appearance of normal silicone implants.

Notes

Breast Implants

Various types of breast implants are used for breast augmentation. They are generally categorized by filler type, number of lumen, and surface contour. They can be placed in the retromammary region anterior to the pectoralis muscle (termed as *retroglandular or prepectoral* implants) or behind the pectoralis muscle (termed as *retropectoral* implant) (Fig. 17.3f). The outer layer of the implant is called implant shell and is commonly made of silicone. The content of the implant may be saline or silicone gel giving the name to the implant. The surface of the implant may be smooth or textured. Upon placement in the body, the body responds by developing a fibrous capsule around it.

Most saline implants have valves through which the saline is injected to inflate the implant and reach the desired size for a given patient. The inflation can also be done gradually in multiple sessions. Some saline implants are pre-filled. On mammogram, the implant looks quite lucent and valves are generally seen.

Silicone implant, on the other hand, contains silicone gel within the silicone shell. On mammography, the implants show regular, smooth outline. The capsule may calcify in a quarter of patients. One of the delayed complications of implant is capsular contracture, which leads to a round or a deformed shape of the implant on imaging. Silicone implant rupture can be intracapsular or extracapsular. Another rare possible complication is implant-related anaplastic large B cell lymphoma (ALBCL). This is more common in textured silicone gel implant and may commonly present as peri-implant fluid collection or mass encasing the implant. Assessment of this peri-implant fluid requires a special cytologic assessment for lymphoma cells. Additional imaging with MRI is useful in documenting the extent of the lymphoma.

Many different types of implants with multiple lumens are now available, the common one being double lumen implant with outer saline and inner silicone lumen. Outer saline implant can be filled to varying degrees as per the patient's need. Reverse double lumen implant has an outer silicone and an inner saline compartment. Outer silicone type implant provides a better natural feel. Double lumen implants with silicone in both lumens are also available and are termed as "Gel within gel." It may be hard to diagnose what type of implant the patient has on imaging and at times information from the plastic surgeon may be needed.

Mammography of breast with implants is challenging, and despite performing implant displacement views 30–50% of the overlying breast parenchyma may escape visualization. In women with capsular contracture, implant displacement views may be suboptimal or impossible to perform, further compromising the sensitivity of mammogram. The MLO view best depicts the location of the implant in relation to the pectoralis muscle.

On ultrasound, the intact implant shell appears as a double/parallel echogenic line with anechoic contents. Anterior reverberation artefact is more pronounced in silicone implants compared to saline implants. A small amount of peri-implant fluid is commonly seen and is normal.

17.4 Case 17.4

History: 44-year-woman with bilateral breast implants done 12 years ago presents with complaint of asymmetric right breast contour.

Questions

Q1. Describe the mammogram (Fig. 17.4a, b) and ultrasound (Fig. 17.4c) findings.

Q2. Describe the MRI findings (Fig. 17.4d).

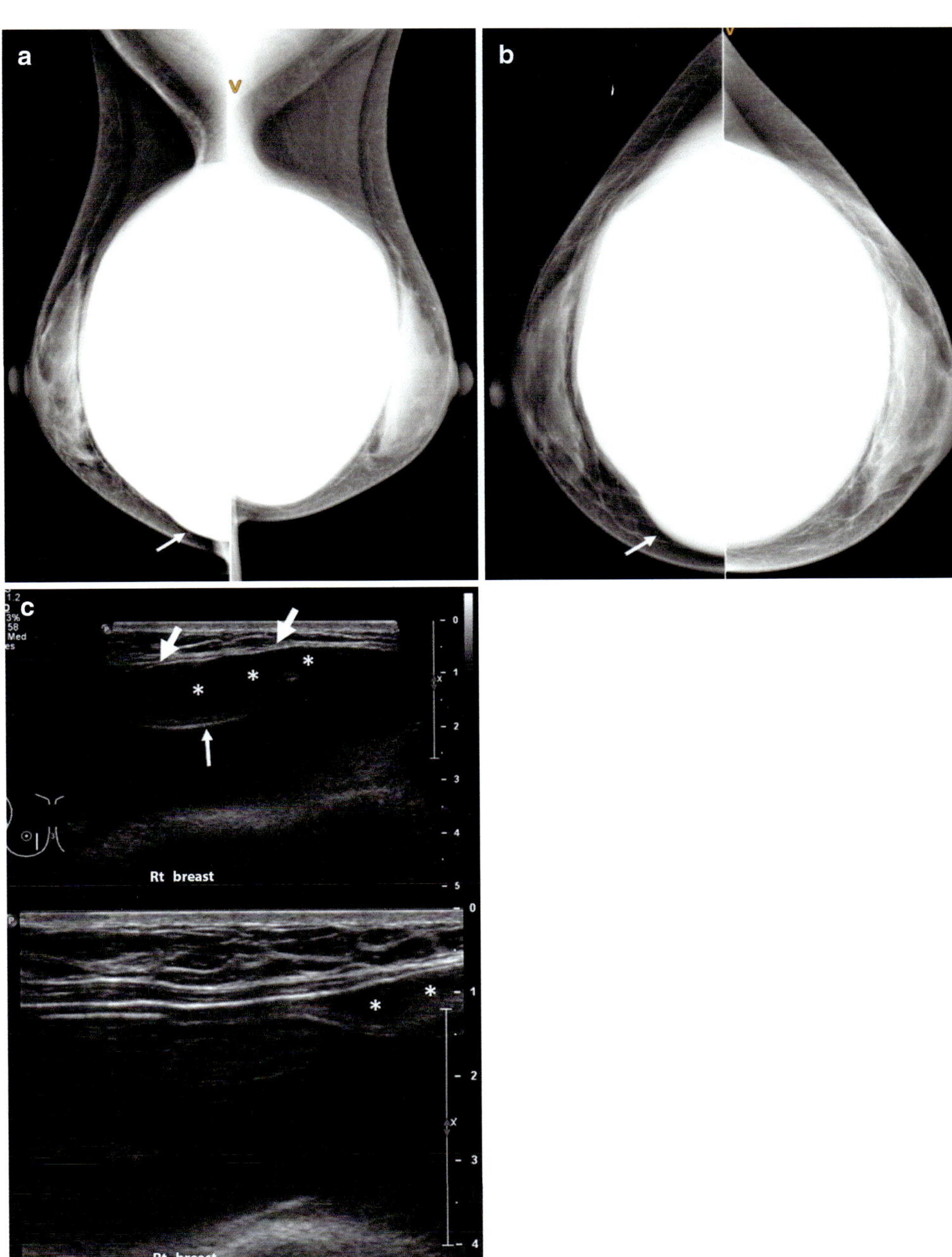

Fig. 17.4 (**a**) Bilateral MLO views. (**b**):Bilateral CC views. (**c**) Right breast ultrasound. (**d**) (*a–c*): MRI: Axial T1WI (*a*), axial T2WI fat-suppressed (*b*), and Sagittal T2WI (*c*). (**e**) Sagittal T2WI showing collapsed implant shell—“Linguine sign” suggesting intracapsular rupture

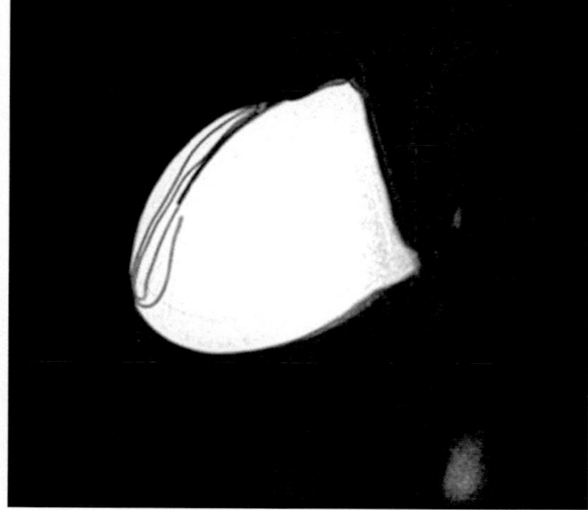

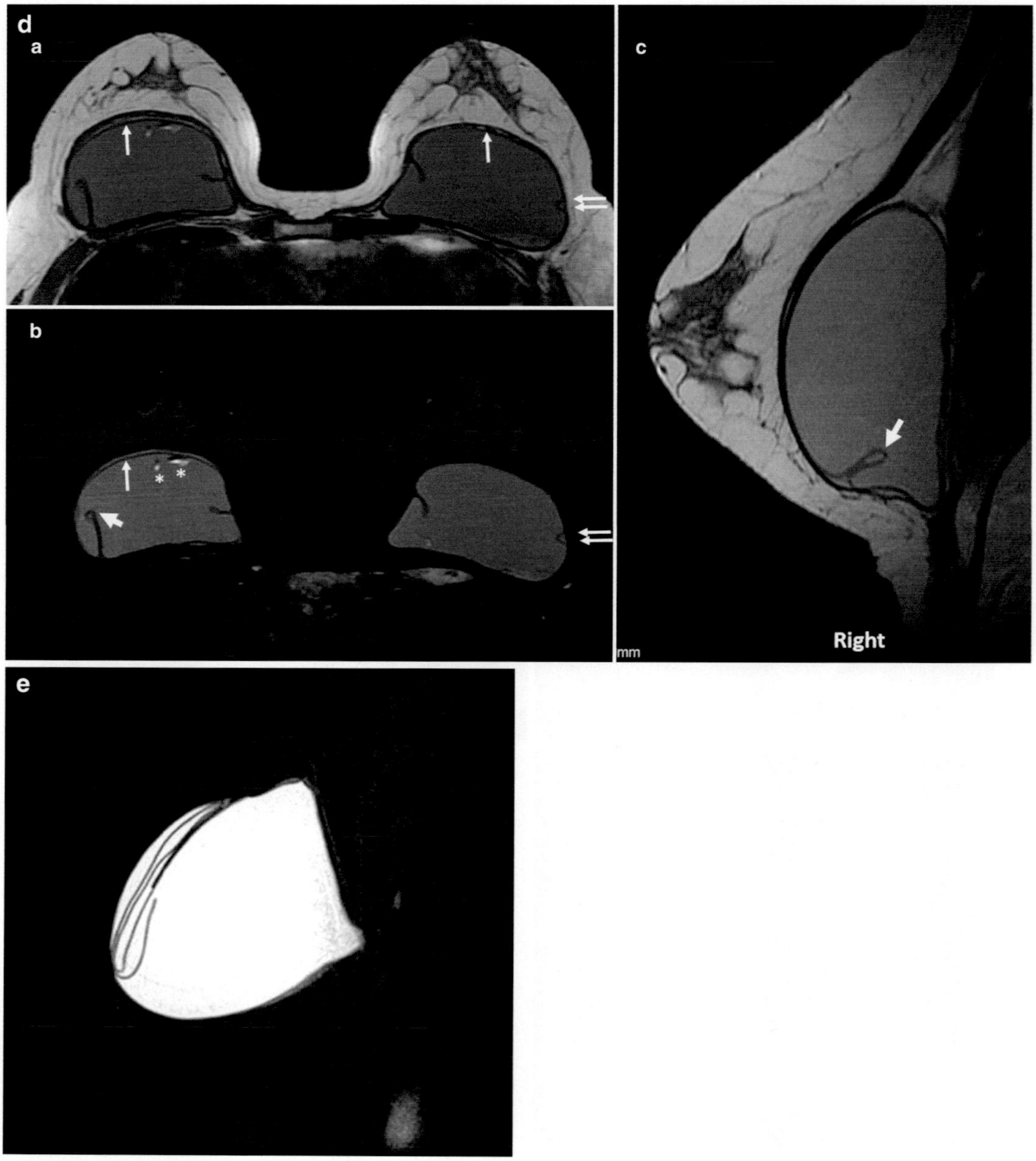

Fig. 17.4 (continued)

Answers

A1. MLO (Fig. 17.4a) and CC (Fig. 17.4b) views of both breasts are available to review. Both the breasts show heterogeneously dense breast parenchyma. Bilateral retro pectoral silicone implants are noted in situ. There is minimal irregularity noted involving right implant outline with a focal bulge noted in the lower inner quadrant (white arrow). No suspicious feature is noted in the overlying breast parenchyma; though implant displacement views should also be done for better assessment of the overlying breast parenchyma. Ultrasound (Fig. 17.4c) shows separation of implant shell (white arrow) from the capsule (thick white arrows) with leaking of silicone gel between them (asterisks), producing subcapsular line/step ladder sign. There is isoechoic gel (asterisks) noted in other image that is also suggestive of intracapsular implant rupture. Overall, the imaging findings are suggestive of right intracapsular implant rupture.

A2. Fig. 17.4d Axial T1WI (a), axial T2WI fat-suppressed (b), and Sagittal T2WI (c).

Bilateral retropectoral silicone implants are noted in situ. Right implant shows subcapsular lines (white arrows), teardrop sign (thick white arrows), and salad-oil sign (asterisks). Left implant shows subcapsular line (white arrow) and noose sign (double white arrows). Findings indicate bilateral intracapsular rupture.

In some women with intracapsular rupture, the ruptured implant shell is seen freely floating within the prosthesis. This is called the Linguine sign (Fig. 17.4e).

17.5 Case 17.5

History: 51-year-woman with history of breast implants. Now new palpable concern in upper outer quadrant of left breast.

Questions

Q1. Describe the findings on mammogram (Fig. 17.5a, b).

Q2. Describe the findings on ultrasound (Fig. 17.5c).

Q3. What history should be elicited? What is the appropriate BI-RADS?

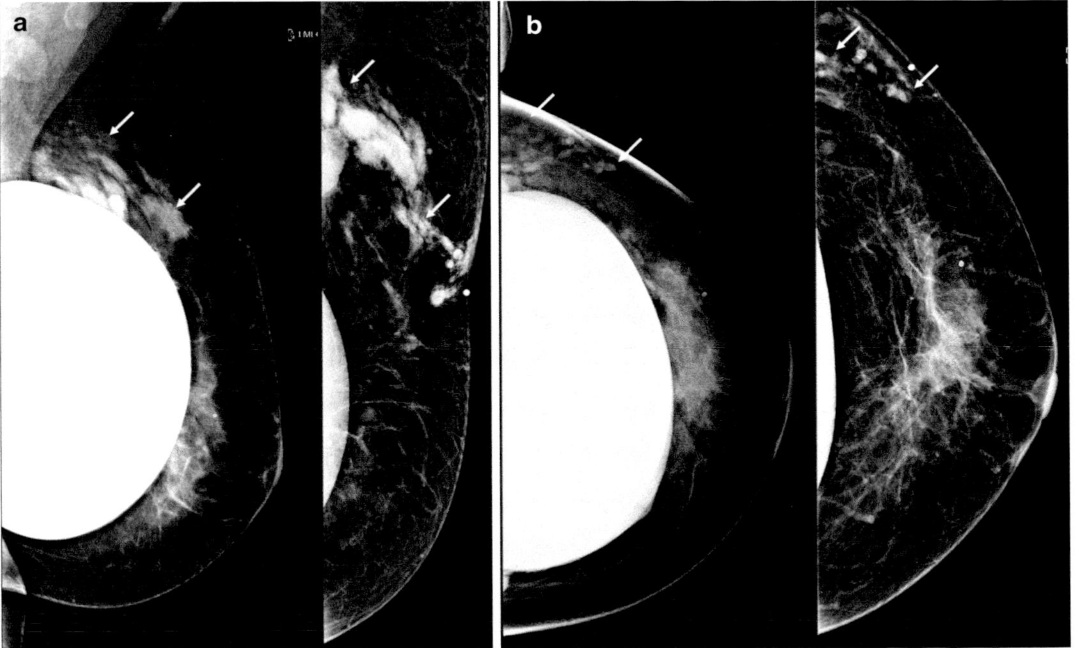

Fig. 17.5 (**a**) Left MLO standard and implant displacement views. (**b**) Left CC standard and implant displacement views. (**c**) Targeted left breast ultrasound. (**d**) Companion case (*a*, *b*): Bilateral MLO (*a*) and CC (*b*) views. Partially collapsed left retroglandular saline implant. Implant is reduced in volume and is folded on itself. Intact right saline implant. (**e**) (*a*, *b*): Bilateral breast ultrasound. (*a*) Left retroareolar image shows collapsed implant shell (white arrow) with anechoic fluid between shell and capsule (asterisks). (*b*) The right breast implant is intact

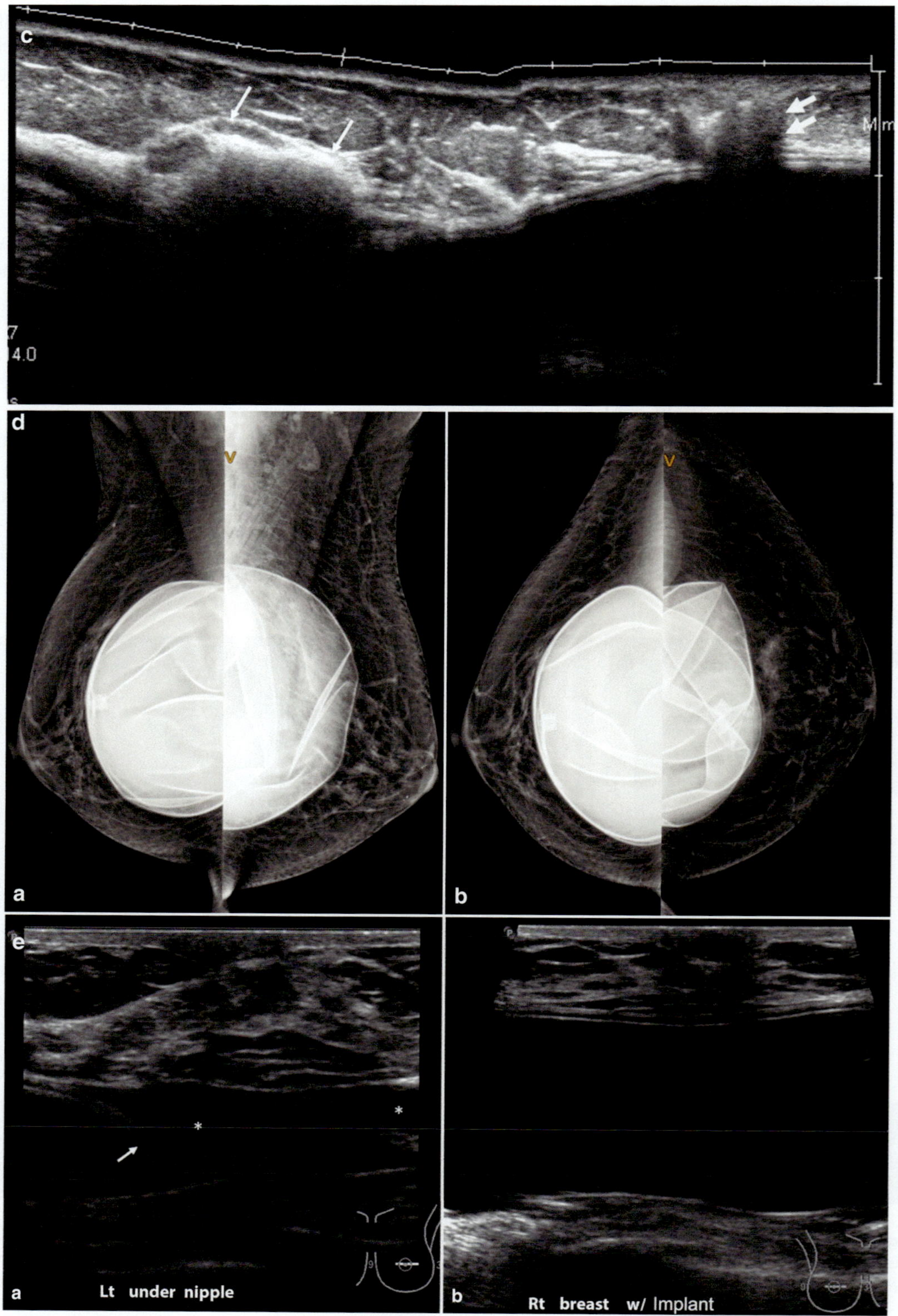

Fig. 17.5 (continued)

Answers

A1. Fig. 17.5a Left MLO standard and implant displaced views. Figure 17.5b: Left CC standard and implant displaced views. Retroglandular silicone implant shows smooth contour. A metallic bead marker annotates the area of palpable lump in the upper outer quadrant of the left breast. Underneath the marker are seen several, round to oval, high-density lesions (white arrows) with density similar to silicone. The breast parenchyma is otherwise unremarkable.

A2. Fig. 17.5c Panoramic ultrasound image of the left breast shows a retroglandular implant with echogenic areas along the outer surface of the implant with dirty shadowing. This is called the "snow-storm" appearance (white arrows). These appearances represent extracapsular free silicone in the breast parenchyma.

A3. History of implant revision surgery must be elicited. This woman shows findings consistent with extracapsular silicone implant rupture. However, the implant seen on the mammogram is smooth and appears intact. This is seen in women who undergo explantation (removal) of a previously ruptured silicone gel implant and exchanged with a new implant. In these women an intact new implant is seen along with the older residual calcified capsule and silicone granulomas that could confuse the reader. History of implant replacement on the patient history form or technologist notes can help clinch the diagnosis as in this case.

Category: BI-RADS 2.

Notes

Implant Rupture

Breast implant rupture is a recognized complication of a breast implant that occurs due to the aging of the implant. It generally becomes apparent about 10–15 years after implant insertion. Other causes of rupture include manufacturing defect, under filling that results in more folds, incompetent valve and rarely blunt trauma.

Saline Implant Rupture: Rupture of saline implant is a clinical diagnosis as it immediately deflates and is termed as "flat tire." Imaging is generally not required to make the diagnosis of ruptured saline implants. The saline soon gets absorbed by the body. On conventional imaging, the collapsed implant shell can be well seen on mammogram (Fig. 17.5d) and ultrasound (Fig. 17.5e). About a fifth of saline implants need revision surgery.

Silicone Implant Rupture: Silicone implant rupture can be intracapsular (85%), when confined by the surrounding fibrous capsule, or extracapsular (15%), when silicone freely extravasates.

An *intracapsular* rupture occurs when the implant shell ruptures within the intact fibrous capsule formed by the body. The intact fibrous capsule prevents free silicone extravasation which precludes its clinical or mammographic diagnosis. This makes it difficult to detect on clinical exam or mammography. On imaging, the intracapsular rupture may be seen as a focal bulge or contour deformity on mammogram. On ultrasound, a "step-ladder" sign or isoechoic silicone between shell and capsule may suggest intracapsular implant rupture.

Breast MRI is by far the best modality for the assessment of implant integrity and does not require contrast injection. A collapsed implant shell within the fibrous capsule, seen on MRI, is diagnostic of intracapsular rupture. A minimally collapsed shell may appear as a parallel line to the capsule, termed as the "subcapsular line sign." A ruptured implant shell allows the free silicone to seep onto the outer surface of the shell, thereby producing classic signs like the "keyhole sign," "noose sign" or "teardrop sign." A significantly collapsed shell appears as a group of wavy lines, termed the "linguine sign." In these signs, silicone is demonstrated on both sides of the radial fold. A normal radial fold will not demonstrate such an appearance.

An *extracapsular* rupture involves breakage of the fibrous capsule in addition to the implant shell. This can lead to altered implant contour, which can be detected on clinical examination and mammography. An extracapsular rupture implies associated intracapsular rupture. Extracapsular rupture on mammogram is seen as the macroscopic silicone density seen outside of implant confines, within breast tissue or the pectoralis muscle, or axillary nodes. On ultrasound, extracapsular silicone is seen as echogenic masses with "snowstorm" appearance seen outside the implant outline. Occasionally, silicone is also seen within the axillary nodes giving a "snowstorm" appearance in the axillary nodes. Ultrasound overall performs poorly, with sensitivity and specificity rates ranging between 59–85% and 55–79%, respectively.

On MRI, free silicone appears hypointense on T1WI images with no enhancement and demonstrates increased signal T2WI (STIR) images. Mixing of silicone with saline in a ruptured double lumen implant may produce a nonspecific "salad oil sign."

Occasionally, free silicone show enhancement on postcontrast images due to surrounding inflammation and granuloma formation, thereby mimicking an enhancing breast cancer (Fig. 17.5f) and may require a biopsy for differentiation.

17.6 Case 17.6

History: 63-year woman with implants for 14 years. Now new palpable lump in right lower inner breast at about 5 o'clock.

Questions

Q1. Describe the imaging findings on MRI (Fig. 17.6a).

Q2. Describe the imaging features on ultrasound (Fig. 17.6b) and give the appropriate BI-RADS.

Answers

A1. Axial MRI images in T2WI fat-suppressed (a and b), silicone bright sequence (c), postcontrast T1W fat-suppressed (d), sagittal T2WI right breast. Bilateral retropectoral silicone implants are noted in situ. Right breast prosthesis shows subcapsular line (white arrow), teardrop sign (double white arrows), and silicone signal in right axillary nodes (asterisks), suggesting implant rupture. In the lower inner quadrant of the right breast at about the 5 o'clock location, an oval mass with silicone signal intensity is seen (thick white arrows), correlating with the palpable concern. This mass shows enhancement on DCE.

The above finding may represent an enhancing silicone granuloma or a T2 bright, enhancing tumor.

A2. Corresponding ultrasound images show a thick isoechoic layer in the anterior third of the right implant (a) separating the implant shell and capsule (asterisks). Typical snowstorm appearance of right axillary node is suggestive of silicone in node (b). At the 5 o'clock location in the right breast there is an oval, partially circumscribed echogenic lesion outside the implant (white arrow), corresponding to the enhancing mass on MRI. Snowstorm appearance is suggesting this to represent extracapsular silicone rather than a real breast tumor.

Diagnosis: Right enhancing silicone granuloma and silicone axillary adenopathy due to extracapsular rupture of the silicone implant.

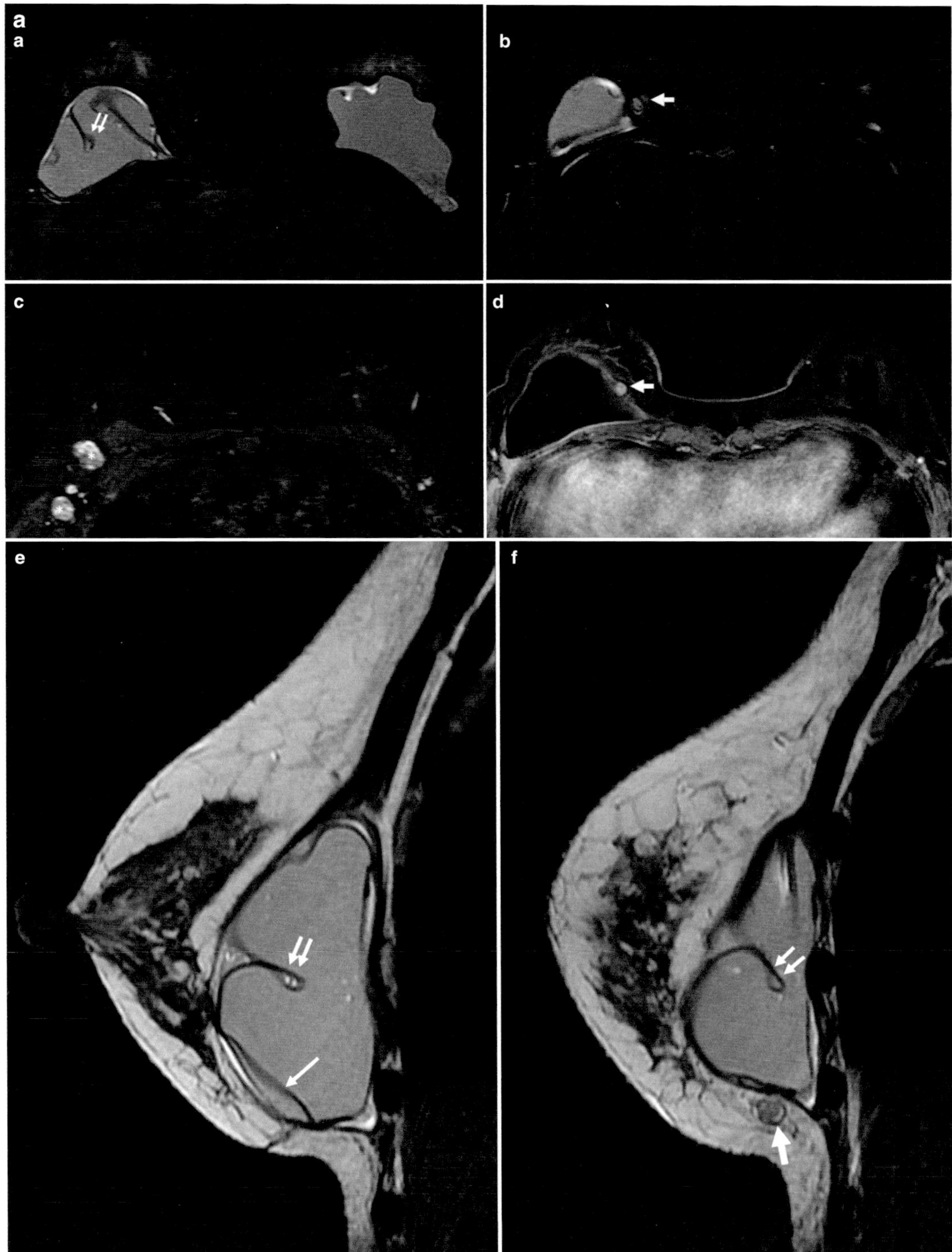

Fig. 17.6 (**a**) MRI (*a*): Axial T2WI (*a*, *b*), silicone bright (*c*), post contrast T1WI fat-suppressed (*d*), sagittal T2WI (*e*, *f*). (**b**) Ultrasound images of right breast and axilla

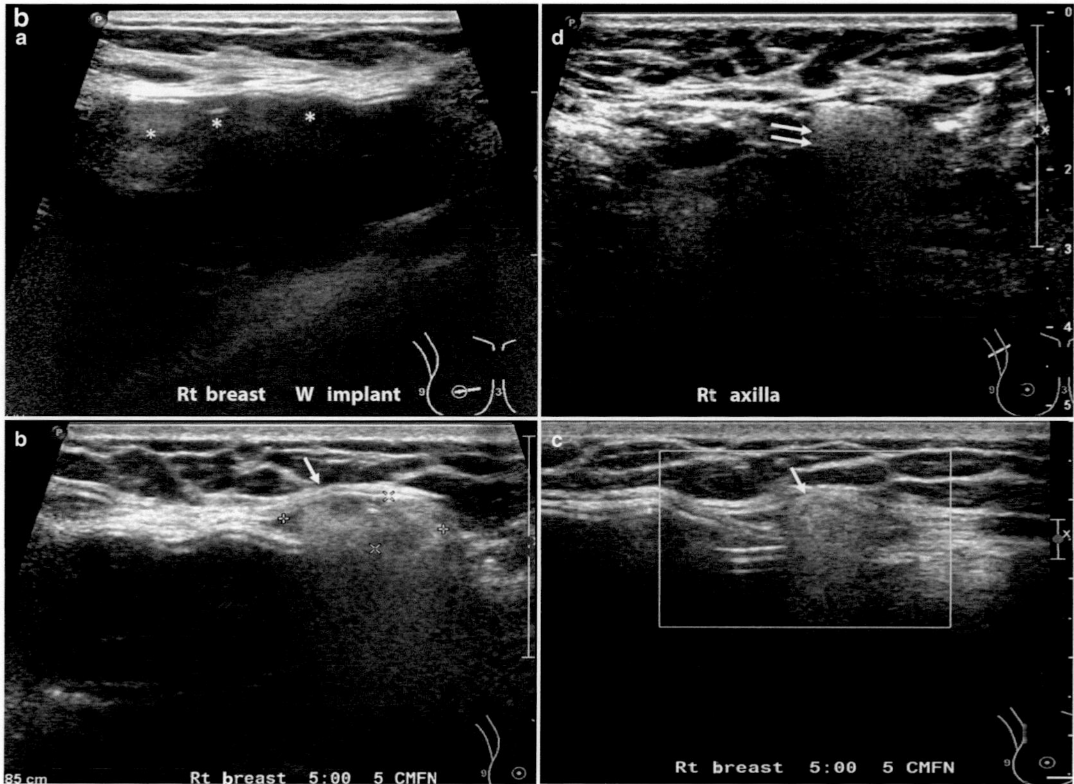

Fig. 17.6 (continued)

Suggested Readings

Berg WA, Caskey CI, Hamper UM, et al. Diagnosing breast implant rupture with MR imaging, US, and mammography. Radiographics. 1993;13(6):1323–36.

Brenner RJ, Pfaff JM. Mammographic features after conservation therapy for malignant breast disease: serial findings standardized by regression analysis. Am J Roentgenol. 1996;167(1):171–8.

Di Benedetto G, Cecchini S, Grassetti L, Baldassarre S, Valeri G, Leva L, Giuseppetti GM, Bertani A. Comparative study of breast implant rupture using mammography, sonography, and magnetic resonance imaging: correlation with surgical findings. Breast J. 2008;14(6):532–7.

Huston TL, Simmons RM. Locally recurrent breast cancer after conservation therapy. Am J Surg. 2005;189(2):229–35.

Immonen-Räihä P, Kauhava L, Parvinen I, Holli K, Kronqvist P, Pylkkänen L, Helenius H, Kaljonen A, Räsänen O, Klemi PJ. Mammographic screening reduces risk of breast carcinoma recurrence. Cancer. 2005;103(3):474–82.

Juanpere S, Perez E, Huc O, et al. Imaging of breast implants-a pictorial review. Insights Imaging. 2011;2(6):653–70.

Mendelson EB. Evaluation of the postoperative breast. Radiol Clin N Am. 1992;30(1):107–38.

Monticciolo DL, Newell MS, Moy L, Niell B, Monsees B, Sickles EA. Breast cancer screening in women at higher-than-average risk: recommendations from the ACR. J Am Coll Radiol. 2018;15(3):408–14.

Paredes ES. Atlas of mammography. In: Lippincott Williams & Wilkins. Philadelphia; 2007. isbn:0781764335.

Raj SD, Karimova EJ, Fishman MD, Fein-Zachary V, Phillips J, Dialani V, Slanetz PJ. Imaging of breast implant–associated complications and pathologic conditions: breast imaging. Radiographics. 2017;37(5):1603–4.

Safvi A. Linguine sign. Radiology. 2000;216(3):838–9.

Saslow D, Boetes C, Burke W, Harms S, Leach MO, Lehman CD, Morris E, Pisano E, Schnall M, Sener S, Smith RA. American Cancer Society guidelines for breast screening with MRI as an adjunct to mammography. CA Cancer J Clin. 2007;57(2):75–89.

Shah AT, Jankharia BB. Imaging of common breast implants and implant-related complications: a pictorial essay. Ind J Radiol Imag. 2016;26(2):216.

Yang N, Muradali D. The augmented breast: a pictorial review of the abnormal and unusual. Am J Roentgenol. 2011;196(4):W451–60.

18 Augmentation and Reconstruction

18.1 Case 18.1

History: 53-year-old woman with history of breast augmentation 10 years ago presents for a routine mammogram. Family history of breast cancer in mother.

Questions

Q1. Describe the findings on the provided mammogram (Fig. 18.1a, b) and ultrasound (Fig. 18.1c).

Q2. Describe the findings on MRI (Fig. 18.1d).

Q3. Provide possible differentials in this case.

Answers

A1. Bilateral MLO (Fig. 18.1a) and CC views (Fig. 18.1b) show numerous 5–10 mm, round, circumscribed, dense masses diffusely scattered in both breasts. Some of them show rim calcifications (white arrow). Some of these are seen in the pectoralis muscle (asterisks). Ultrasound images (Fig. 18.1c) show bilateral, symmetrical, highly echogenic noise with dense shadowing and "snowstorm" appearance in both breasts. This obscures visualization of the breast parenchyma. There are a couple of clear cystic lesions (white arrows) seen with posterior enhancement. The skin is thickened.

Imaging features are highly suggestive of free silicone gel injection for breast augmentation. Conventional imaging is not useful as screening modalities in these patients, as the silicone granuloma can obscure a tumor. In such patients, MRI should be used for breast cancer screening.

A2. MRI image (Fig. 18.1d) shows multiple variable sized, round to oval, masses scattered in both breasts; predominantly in the retroglandular region, in the subcutaneous region, and also some in the intraparenchymal region (white arrow). They are isointense on T1W images (a) and hyper to mixed intensity on T2W images (b). No enhancement is seen in these masses (c). Bilateral breast skin thickening is noted. MIP image does not show any abnormality (d).

Diagnosis: Free silicone injections breast augmentation.

A3. This appearance is highly typical of free silicone injection and no other differential is considered especially if there is history of breast augmentation available. Rarely, widespread dystrophic calcifications in scleroderma, post radiotherapy calcifications may give similar appearance to a lesser degree.

N. Chotai, S. Kulkarni, *Breast Imaging Essentials*, https://doi.org/10.1007/978-981-15-1412-8_18

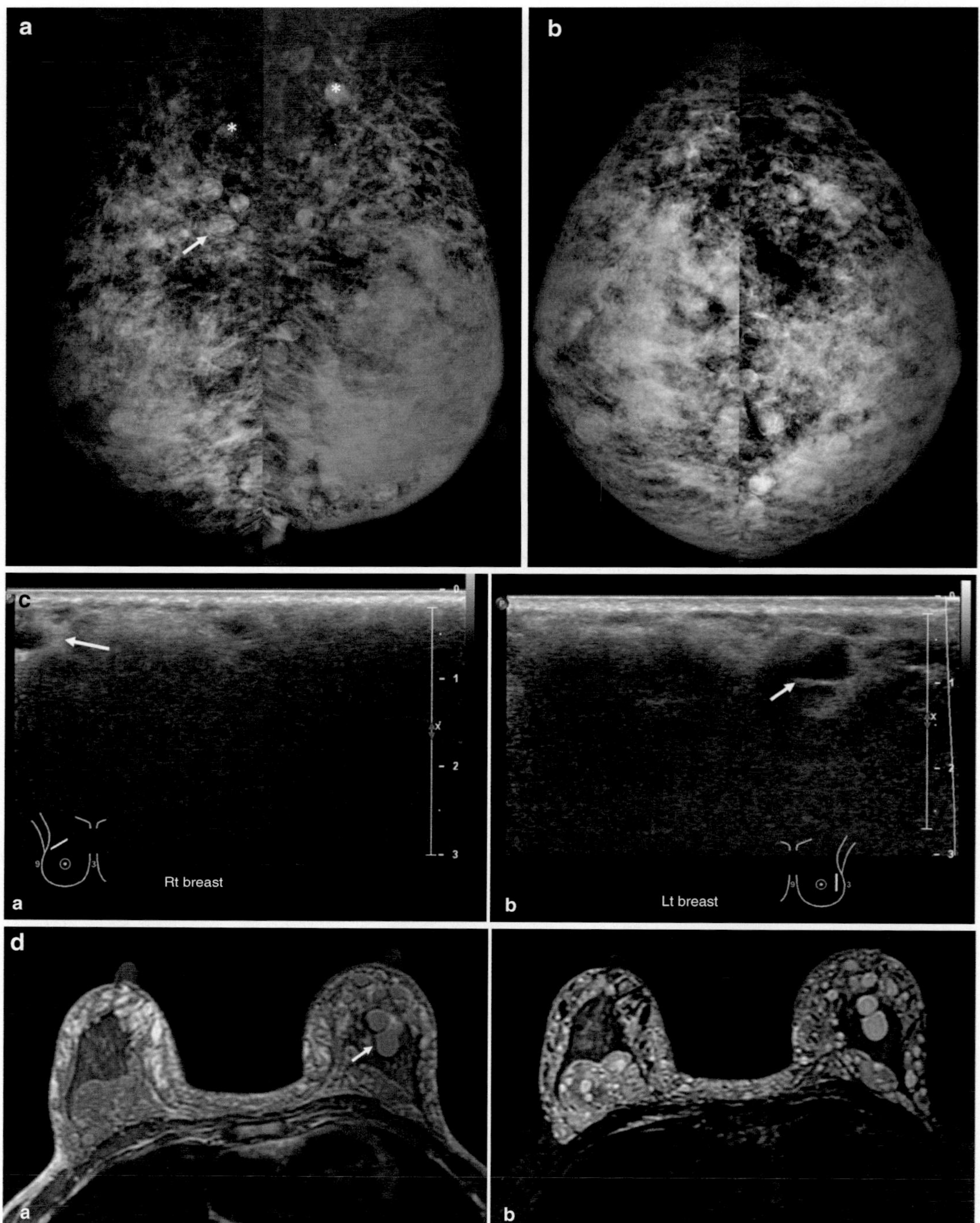

Fig. 18.1 (**a**) Bilateral MLO views. (**b**) Bilateral CC views. (**c**) Bilateral breast ultrasound. (**d**) Axial TIWI (*a*), T2WI (*b*), DCE Subtracted image (*c*), and Axial MIP (*d*)

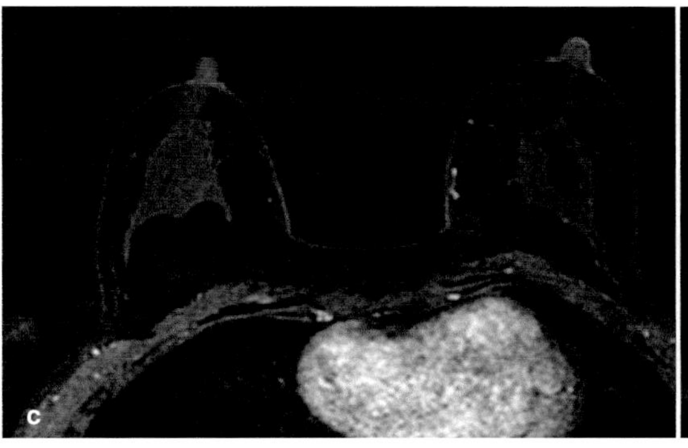

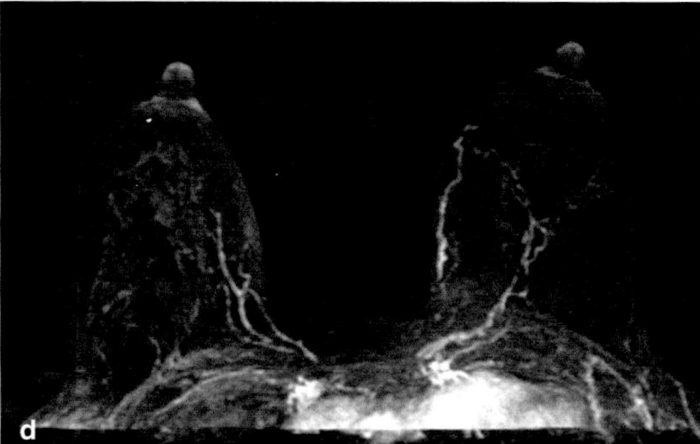

Fig. 18.1 (continued)

18.2 Case 18.2

History: 39-year-old woman with palpable lump in the 1 o'clock position of the right breast. No family history of breast cancer.

Questions

Q1. Describe the findings on mammogram (Fig. 18.2a, b) and ultrasound (Fig. 18.2c).

Q2. What history would you like to elicit from the patient?

Answers

A1. Bilateral MLO (Fig. 18.2a) and CC (Fig. 18.2b) views show heterogeneously dense breast parenchyma. There are a few, round, circumscribed lucent lesions with rim calcifications seen in the right breast (white arrows). The dominant lesion is seen in the upper half of right breast in posterior third depth, correlating with the palpable lump. Multiple bilateral benign round calcifications are noted. Ultrasound image (Fig. 18.2c) shows a palpable, complicated cystic lesion with internal echoes at 1 o'clock in the right breast, with no significant internal vascularity, to correlate with the mammographic lucent fatty lesion. Another smaller cystic lesion is seen at 9 o'clock, which also correlates with the fat density lesion seen on mammogram. Findings are likely to represent fat necrosis/oil cysts with calcifications.

A2. History of breast augmentation procedure with free fat injections should be elicited. This appearance on mammogram is typical of free fat injection followed by necrosis and calcifications seen bilaterally.

18.3 Case 18.3

History: 47-year-old average-risk woman for a mammogram. Previous history of breast augmentation done.

Questions

Q1. Describe the findings on mammogram (Fig. 18.3a) and ultrasound (Fig. 18.3b).

Q2. Describe the findings on MRI (Fig. 18.3c).

Q3. State known complications of this augmentation material.

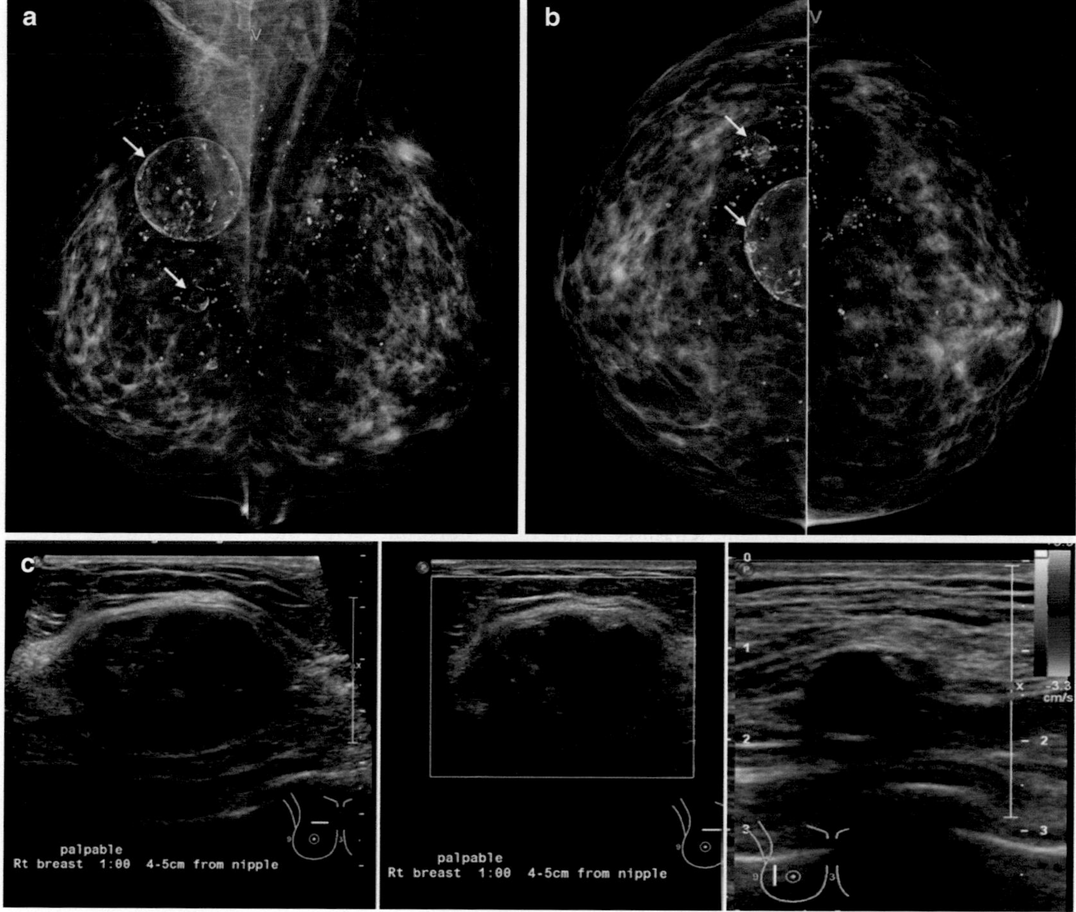

Fig. 18.2 (**a**) Bilateral MLO views. (**b**) Bilateral CC views. (**c**) Right breast ultrasound and color Doppler

Answers

A1. Bilateral MLO views (Fig. 18.3a) show large, symmetrical, homogeneously isodense opacities in both breasts (white arrows), predominantly in the retroglandular space. No suspicious mammographic feature is identified. Ultrasound images of both breasts (Fig. 18.3b) show large, unilocular, anechoic fluid collection (thick white arrows) in both breasts with few floating internal echoes. Findings are suggestive of breast augmentation with free polyacrylamide gel (PAAG) injections.

A2. MRI (Fig. 18.3c) show bilateral nearly symmetrical retroglandular space collections (white arrows) that are predominantly hyperintense on T2w image (a), isointense on T1w image (b), shows mild peripheral enhancement on DCE T1W subtracted image (c). No suspicious lesion is seen on MIP image to suggest malignancy (d).

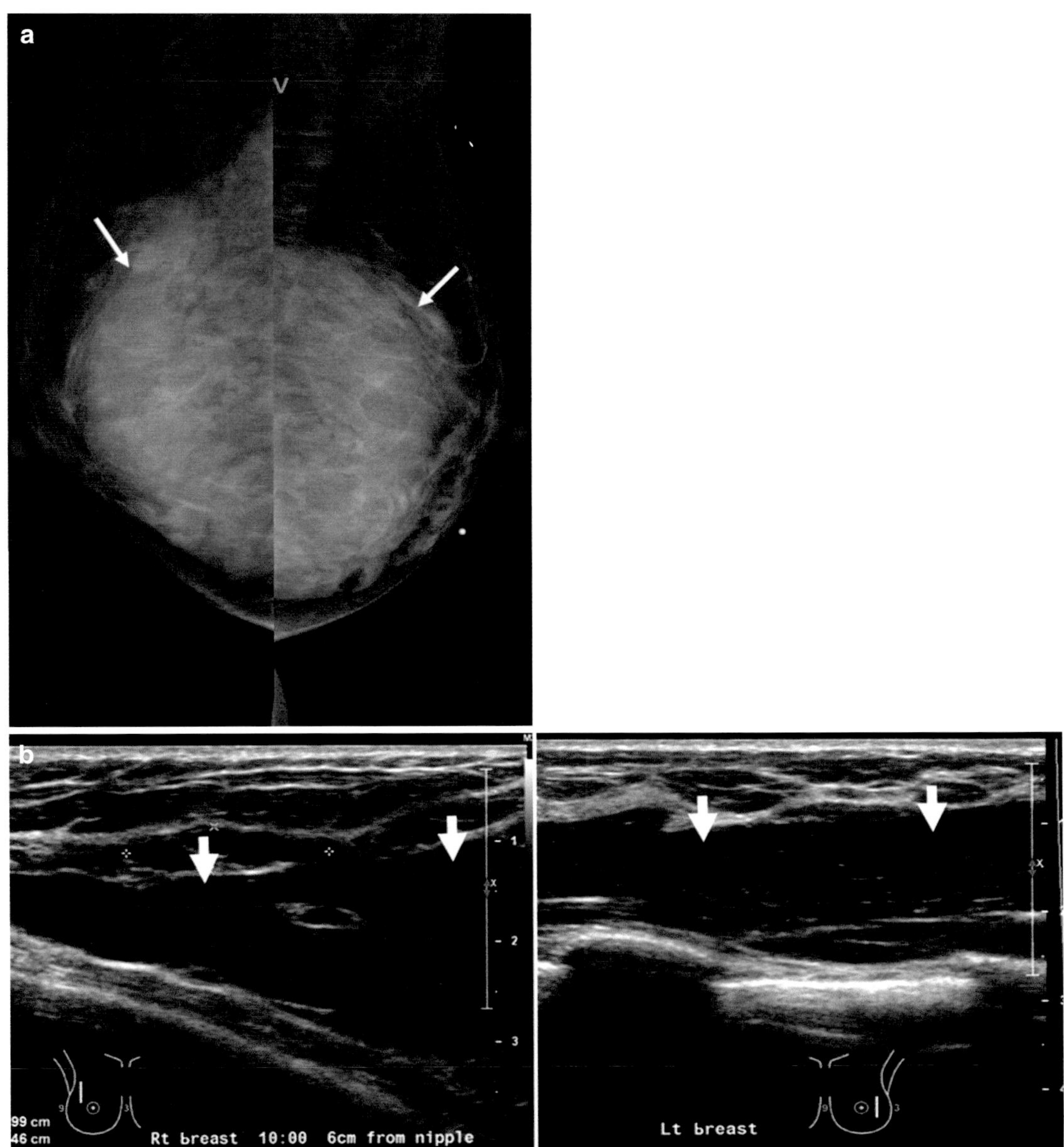

Fig. 18.3 (**a**) Bilateral MLO views. (**b**) Bilateral breast ultrascund. (**C**) MRI: Axial T2WI (*a*), T1WI (*b*), DCE subtracted image, (*c*) and Axial MIP (*d*)

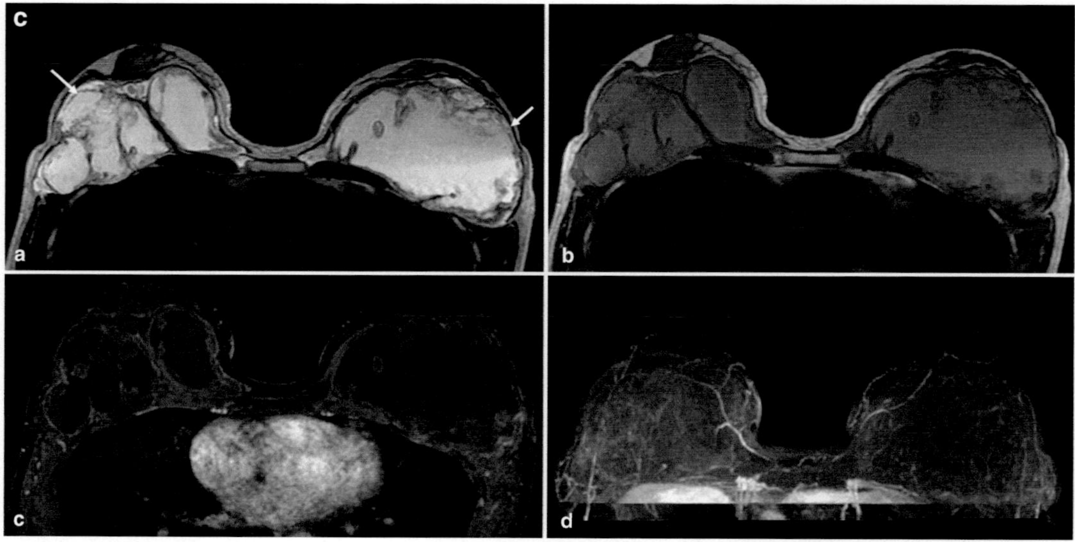

Fig. 18.3 (continued)

A3. PAAG was initially considered as a nontoxic, nonbiodegradable, safe material that was introduced in the 1980s as a type of minimally invasive cheap breast augmentation material as an alternate to implants. Generally, it was thought to lack severe tissue reaction and hence does not result in capsule formation, contracture, pain, or fibrosis. But some impure polymers in PAAG may cause neurotoxicity and are teratogenic. It can also lead to embolism and portal hypertension, if it enters circulation. Repeated infection/inflammation and muscle necrosis are also known with PAAG injections. Being hydrophilic, it absorbs water and increases risk of infection. Migration beyond breast into axilla, chest, and abdominal wall are also well known complications, with formation of granulomas.

Notes

Breast Augmentation with Injectable Fillers

Free cosmetic material injection for breast augmentation is now illegal in some countries, but is still used in some parts of Asia. The common materials used for injections are free silicone, autologous fat, polyacrylamide hydrogel (PAAG), and paraffin.

Free silicone gel injections (Case 18.1) are typically seen on a mammogram as multiple, variable-sized, round, dense masses scattered diffusely in breast parenchyma, retromammary fat, the subcutaneous layer, and many times even within the pectoralis muscles. Some of them show rim calcifications. Skin may be thickened in many patients. Occasionally, silicone may be seen in nodes that appear dense on mammogram. On ultrasound, they may appear as cystic lesions or in the form of a "snowstorm." On DCE-MRI, these silicone granulomas may show variable enhancement, mimicking malignancy.

Autologous fat may be used as a free fat injection material in many cases (Case 18.2). Mammogram typically shows multiple, circumscribed, fat density lesions in both breasts; some of them may be calcified. The injected fat frequently undergoes necrosis and calcification at a later date. The calcification is generally seen as bilateral, symmetrical, diffusely scattered benign calcifications. Ultrasound may show circumscribed, cystic lesions with internal echoes and occasional calcified walls. MRI may show typical fat intensity lesions in both breasts. Sometimes, fat necrosis may show bizarre postcontrast enhancement raising concern, but central fat intensity may help in differentiation between fat necrosis and real tumor.

Paraffin is generally seen as a localized, globular material, isodense to breast parenchyma on mammogram, forming paraffinomas. It is generally injected in retromammary fat.

Polyacrylamide gel (PAAG) is another commonly used free injection material (Case 18.3). It has almost 95% water content and hence is seen as a bilateral, nearly symmetrical, large isodense opacity on mammogram and as large fluid collections with echoes on ultrasound. PAAG is commonly injected to be in the retroglandular space. On MRI, PAAG injections are generally seen as large, homogeneous, and single to multiple variable-sized T1W hypointense and T2W hyperintense collections in the retroglandular region. It produces less foreign body response and hence lacks fibrous capsule, increasing the chances of migration and asymmetry in breasts. No significant enhancement is noted with PAAG injection. Complications such as chronic infection, deformity, etc., are known with PAAG injection.

MRI is the best modality for screening women with injectable filler augmentation.

18.4 Case 18.4

History: 67-year-old woman with free silicone injection 20 years ago. Had left mastectomy with reconstruction 5 years ago for breast cancer.

Questions

Q1. Describe the mammogram (Fig. 18.4a) and ultrasound (Fig. 18.4b) findings.

Q2. Describe MRI findings (Fig. 18.4c) and give possible diagnosis. What would you advise next?

Answers

A1. Right MLO and CC views (Fig. 18.4a) show a large spiculated high-density mass in upper outer quadrant of the right breast in posterior third depth of the breast (white arrows). There are multiple variable-sized, round, circumscribed calcified opacities seen diffusely scattered in the right breast as well as the axillary region (thick white arrows). There is reticulation with thickening of subcutaneous tissue as well as breast parenchyma (asterisks). No enlarged axillary nodes are noted. The findings are concerning for a breast mass with free silicone granulomas in the right breast. Ultrasound image (Fig. 18.4b) of the right breast at 6 o'clock (a) shows diffuse dense echogenicity in the subdermal layer with intense posterior snowstorm shadowing obscuring the breast parenchyma. This is due to free silicone injection. At 12 o'clock (b), 5 cm from nipple, an irregular hypoechoic lesion is seen with dense posterior shadowing (white arrow), correlating with the spiculated mass seen on mammogram. The features are indeterminate and biopsy should be considered to establish histology. No prior study was available for comparison. Category: BI-RADS 4.

Histopathology: Ultrasound-guided biopsy: Stromal fibrosis. This was thought to be discordant hence repeat biopsy and a bilateral breast MRI was suggested.

A2. MRI images (Fig. 18.4c) of the same patient is available in T1W axial image (a), T2W axial of right breast (b), postcontrast axial T1W fat saturated image (c), and postcontrast T1w subtracted image of right breast (d). MRI shows left mastectomy with autologous flap reconstruction. There is fat necrosis seen in the medial aspect of left reconstructed breast (white arrow) that shows no enhancement on post contrast images. There is spiculated mass seen in the right breast (asterisk). It is isointense on T1W image, slightly hyperintense on T2W image and lacks post contrast enhancement.

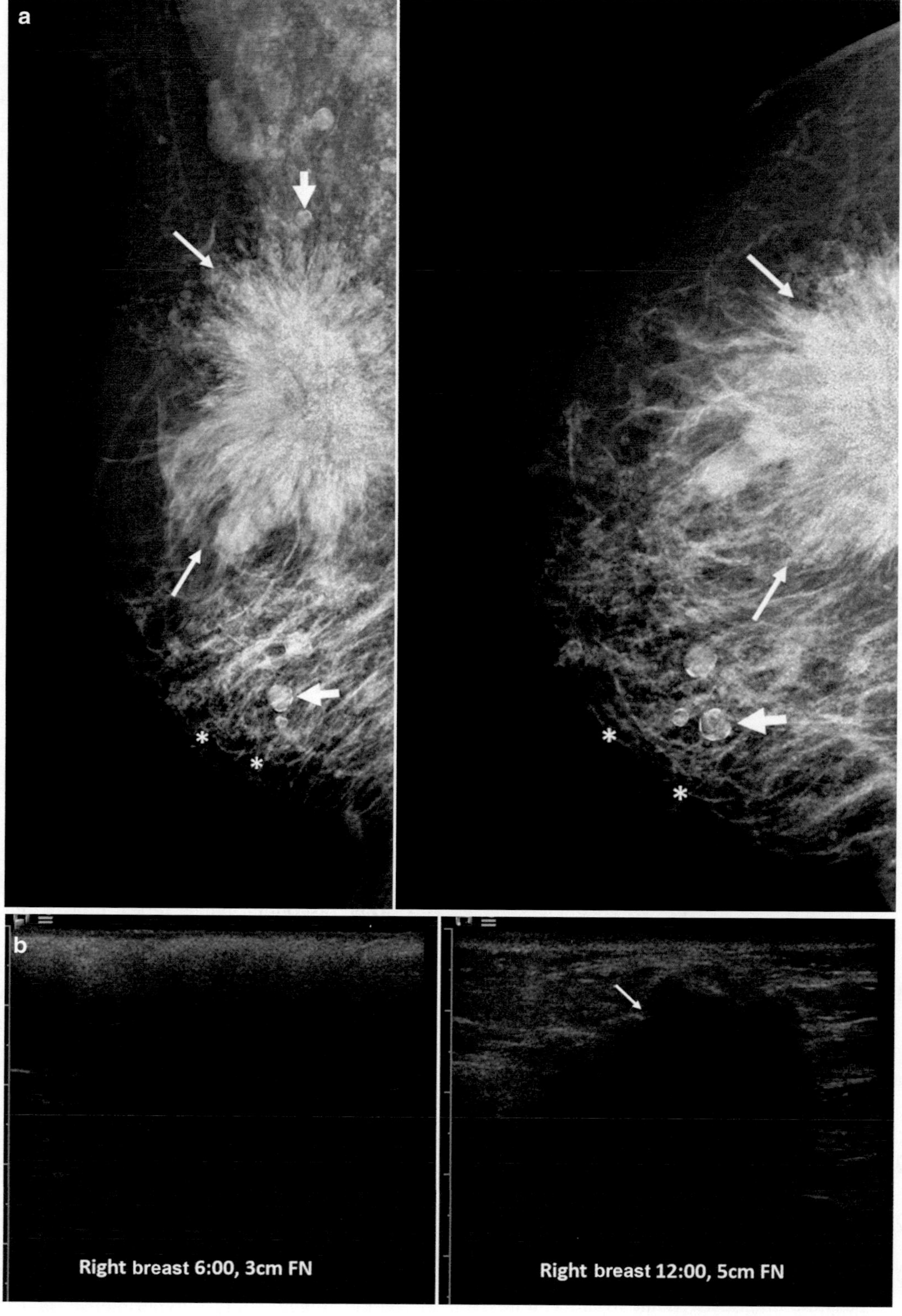

Fig. 18.4 (**a**) Right MLO and CC views. (**b**) Right breast ultrasound. (**c**) MRI: Axial T1WI, T2WI, DCE T1WI fat-suppressed, and DCE subtracted

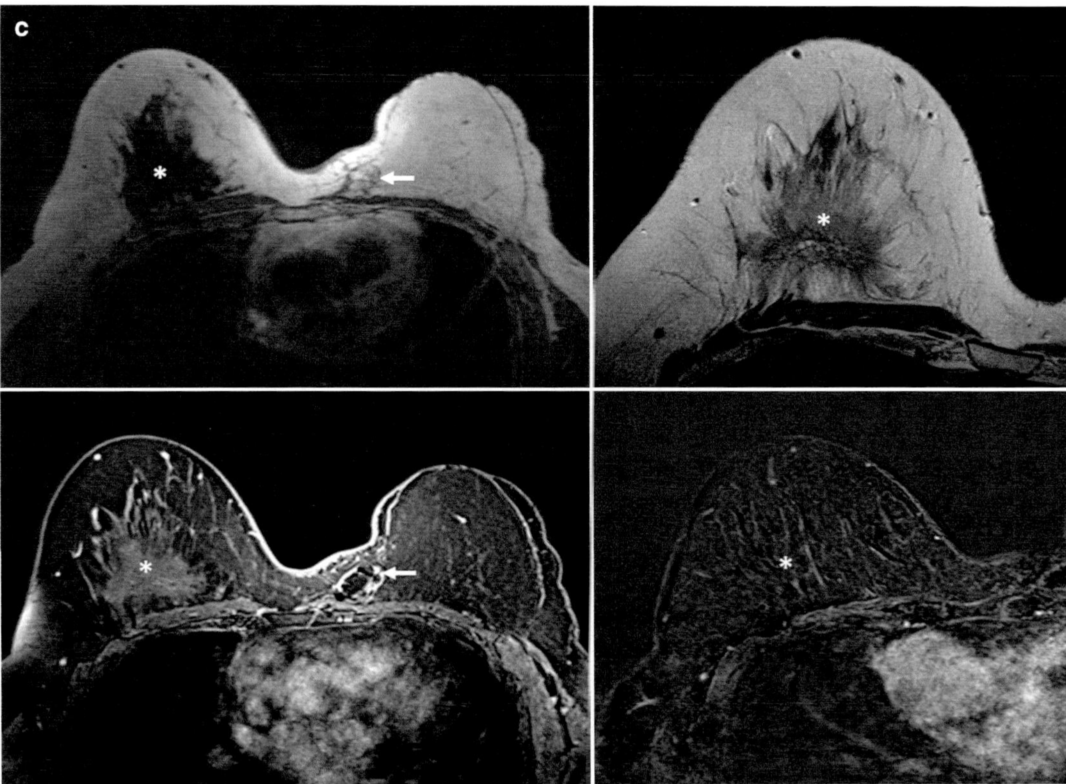

Fig. 18.4 (continued)

In the absence of enhancement, the diagnosis of stromal fibrosis was considered concordant and follow-up was suggested.

Two-year stability was established. The large area of fibrosis was thought to be secondary to free silicone injection. Patient returned to routine surveillance.

Notes

Free Silicone Injections

Free silicone injection for breast augmentation was used commonly in the 1960s. Various complications are identified in patients who undergo free silicone injection for breast augmentation. The common complications reported are silicone mastitis, silicone granuloma formation, and silicone migration. No definite relation between silicone injection and breast cancer risk has been established. It is also well established that in patients with free silicone injections, the routine breast cancer screening modalities including clinical breast examination, mammography, and ultrasound may not be adequate tools. The dense silicone obscures a large amount of breast tissue and underlying breast cancer can easily be hidden. MRI is the most effective method to detect breast cancer in these patients. Migration of silicone into liver, chest wall, abdomen, and neck region is also a reported complication. A few cases of pulmonary embolism and death due to respiratory failure are also reported. Rarely, the silicone granuloma may incite severe foreign body reaction and result in extensive fibrosis, as seen in this case. It mimics breast cancer due to its irregular shape and spiculated margins. Histology would be needed in such cases to differentiate between benign and malignant causes.

18.5 Case 18.5

History: 55-year-old woman with known BRCA 2 gene mutation diagnosed with left breast cancer underwent bilateral mastectomy with reconstruction.

Questions

Q1. Describe the findings on MRI (Fig. 18.5).

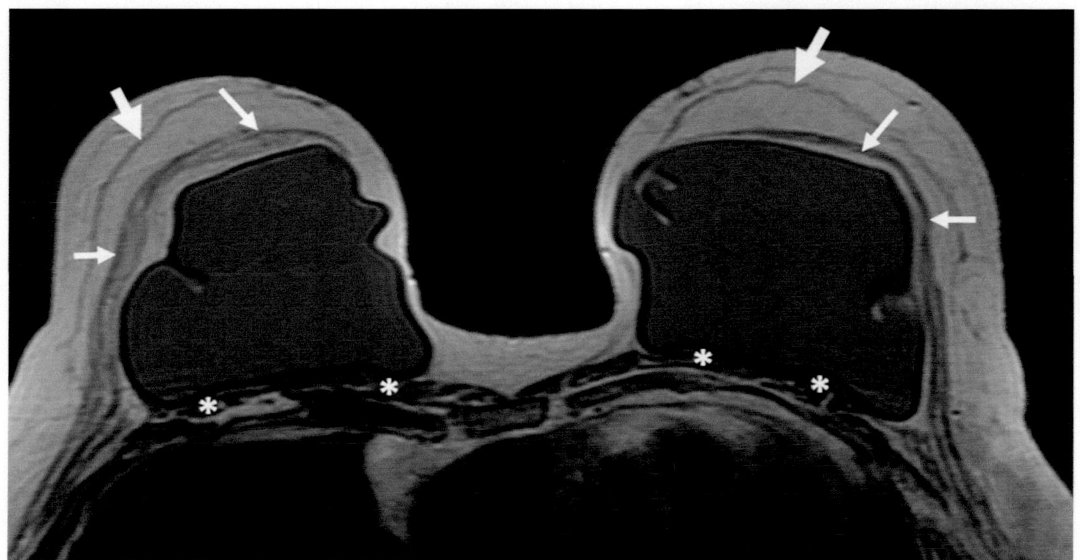

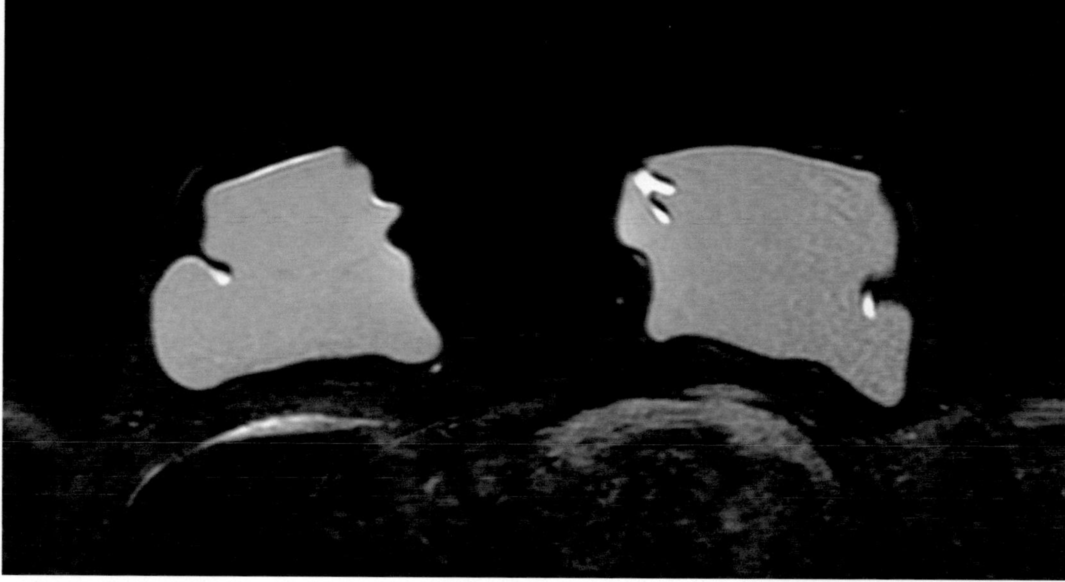

Fig. 18.5 MRI breast images in T1W (top) and T2W fat-suppressed (bottom) sequences. Silicone gel implant reconstruction with LD flap. Thin muscle fibers seen draping the anterolateral surface of the implants (white arrows). The contact zone between the native adipose tissue and transplanted tissue seen anteriorly on T1WI as a thin line (thick white arrows). Pectoralis major seen posterior to implant (asterisks)

Answers

A1. T1W (top) and T2W fat-suppressed (bottom) axial non-contrast-enhanced MRI images are provided. Note is made of bilateral mastectomy with reconstructed breasts. There are bilateral silicone implants noted in situ. The implants appear intact with normal radial folds. The implants are seen placed anterior to the pectoralis major muscle (asterisks). The myocutaneous Latissumus Dorsi myocutaneous flap (LDMF) flap is seen anterior to the implant (white arrows). A few LD muscle bundles are seen laterally and anteriorly. The adipose tissue is seen subcutaneously along with the junction line (thick white arrows) between native tissue and transposed tissue.

Notes

Mastectomies are performed either as part of breast cancer treatment or as a risk-reduction strategy in high-risk women. The different surgical types of mastectomies seen are radical mastectomy (palliative), modified radical mastectomy, skin sparing mastectomy, and nipple sparing mastectomy.

Post mastectomy, implant reconstruction can be done immediately (at the same time as mastectomy) if there is adequate skin available to cover the implant after mastectomy and if is known that the patient would not be requiring adjuvant radiotherapy. Otherwise, staged reconstruction (delayed) using tissue expander may be done to allow the skin to be stretched adequately in stages and make adequate room. Once ready, the expander is exchanged with the prosthesis as second stage of surgery.

18.6 Case 18.6

History: 44-year-old woman with previous right mastectomy and TRAM reconstruction 5 years ago. Now returns with skin nodules over the right reconstructed breast.

Questions

Q1. Describe the findings of the CT scan in Fig. 18.6a.
Q2. Describe the findings of the PET scan in Fig. 18.6b.

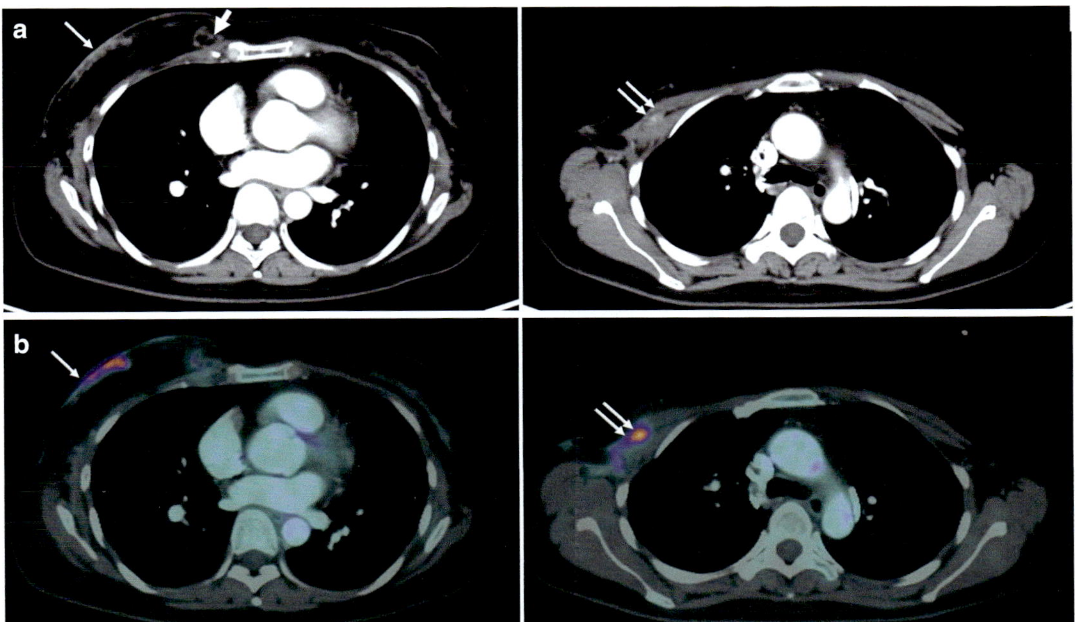

Fig. 18.6 (**a**) Postcontrast CT scan images of thorax. (**b**) PET scan images of thorax

Answers

A1. Contrast-enhanced CT scan images of thorax (Fig. 18.6a) show status post right mastectomy with transverse rectus abdominis myocutaneous flap (TRAM) reconstruction. The reconstructed breast is mainly seen to contain fat tissue. Anteriorly, at the junction line between the flap and native breast tissue, there is thickening with nodularity noted (white arrow). The skin in this region is also thickened. A soft tissue density with internal fat is noted along the medial aspect of the flap in the parasternal region (thick white arrow) suggestive of fat necrosis. No other abnormalities noted.

An image at a higher level shows an enhancing lymph node in the interpectoral region (Rotter's node) (double white arrows). The findings are concerning for locoregional TRAM flap recurrence. Fibrotic strands in the right axillary region are due to prior surgery.

A2. PET study of the same patient (Fig. 18.6b) show FDG avid activity anteriorly in the thickened skin and skin nodules of TRAM flap (white arrow), suggestive of tumor recurrence in the skin overlying the flap. There is increased FDG uptake also seen in the Rotter's node (double white arrows), suggesting nodal metastasis.

Histopathology: The reconstructed right breast nodule punch biopsy proved recurrent grade 3 invasive ductal carcinoma. Patient underwent chemotherapy and mastectomy.

18.7 Case 18.7

History: 62-year-old BRCA-gene-mutation-positive women with bilateral risk-reduction mastectomy and reconstruction.

Questions

Q1. Describe findings on mammogram (Fig. 18.7a, b).

Q2. Describe findings on MRI of the same patient with appropriate BI-RADS (Fig. 18.7c).

Answers

A1. Bilateral mammogram in MLO (Fig. 18.7a) and CC (Fig. 18.7b) views show bilateral mastectomy with fatty autologous deep inferior epigastric perforator (DIEP) flap reconstruction. Fat necrosis with calcification is seen in the upper outer quadrant of the left breast (thick white arrow), which is a common complication in autologous reconstruction. A thin, distinct contact line is seen anteriorly in the reconstructed breast that represents the junction between grafted flap and native skin/subcutaneous layer.

A2. MRI of the same patient (Fig. 18.7c) in T1W non-fat-suppressed image (a) and postcontrast T1W subtracted image (b) is available. In the left reconstructed breast an irregular, peripherally enhancing mass (thick white arrow) is seen that shows fat intensity signal in the center. This is a typical appearance of fat necrosis and biopsy is not required in such cases. Category: BI-RADS 2.

18.8 Case 18.8

History: 49-year-old woman with left mastectomy and DIEP flap reconstruction done 5 years ago. Now presents with new palpable lump in upper outer quadrant of the left reconstructed breast.

Questions

Q1. Describe the findings on the provided mammogram (Fig. 18.8a) and ultrasound (Fig. 18.8b).

Q2. Describe the findings on MRI (Fig. 18.8c).

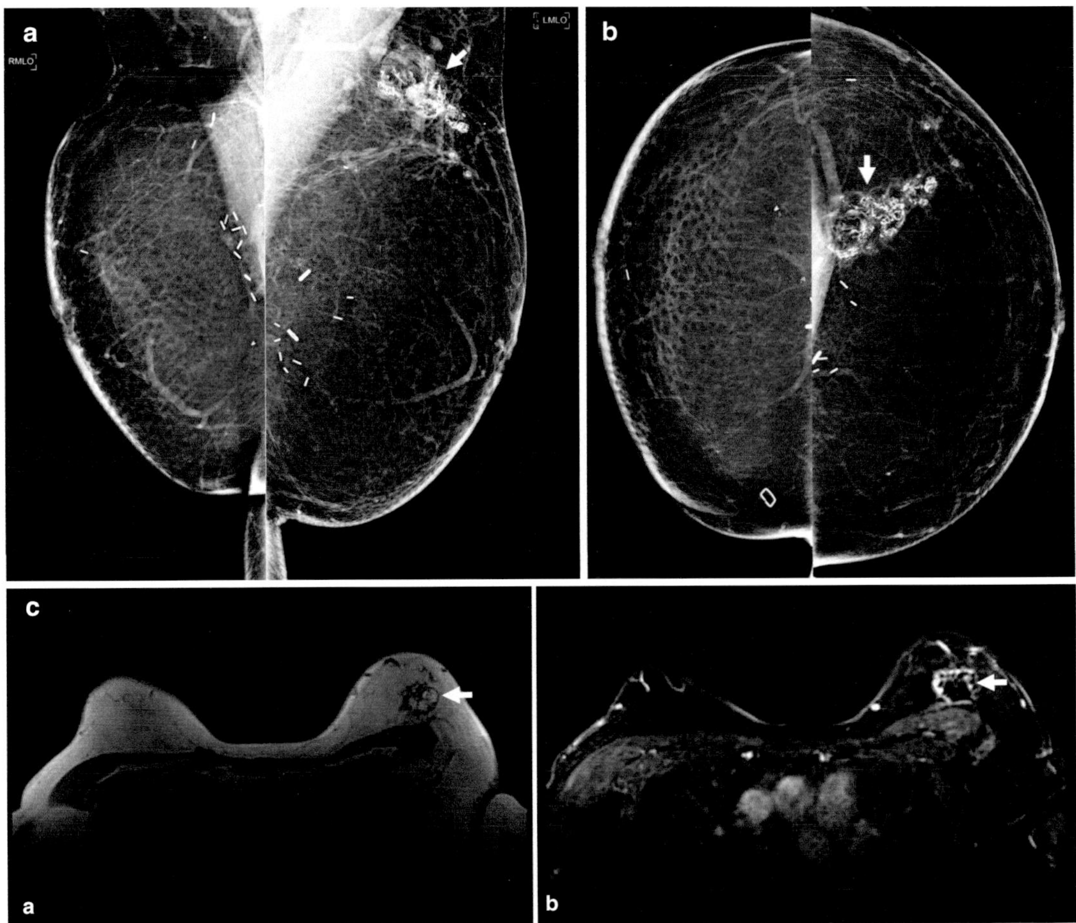

Fig. 18.7 (**a**) Bilateral MLO views. (**b**) Bilateral CC views. (**c**) MRI: T1WI non-fat-suppressed (*a*) and DCE subtracted T1WI

Answers

A1. Left mammogram in MLO and CC views (Fig. 18.8a) show left post-mastectomy autologous flap reconstruction status. The flap is predominantly fatty. A metallic BB marker annotates the site of palpable concern. Underneath the marker is seen an isodense mass (white arrows). Ultrasound image (Fig. 18.8b) of area of concern at the 2 o'clock location shows a heterogenous echogenicity mass in the anterior aspect of the reconstructed breast (white arrows) along the junction line, raising concern of a recurrent tumor.

A2. MRI of the same patient (Fig. 18.8c) shows an isointense mass (white arrow) in the left reconstructed breast that shows intense post-contrast enhancement. The rest of the junction line is thin and clear (thick white arrows). This was biopsy-proven DIEP flap recurrence.

Notes

Autologus Breast Reconstuction

The main advantage of breast reconstruction using autologous tissue transfer is perceived naturalness. The flaps may be conventional pedicled

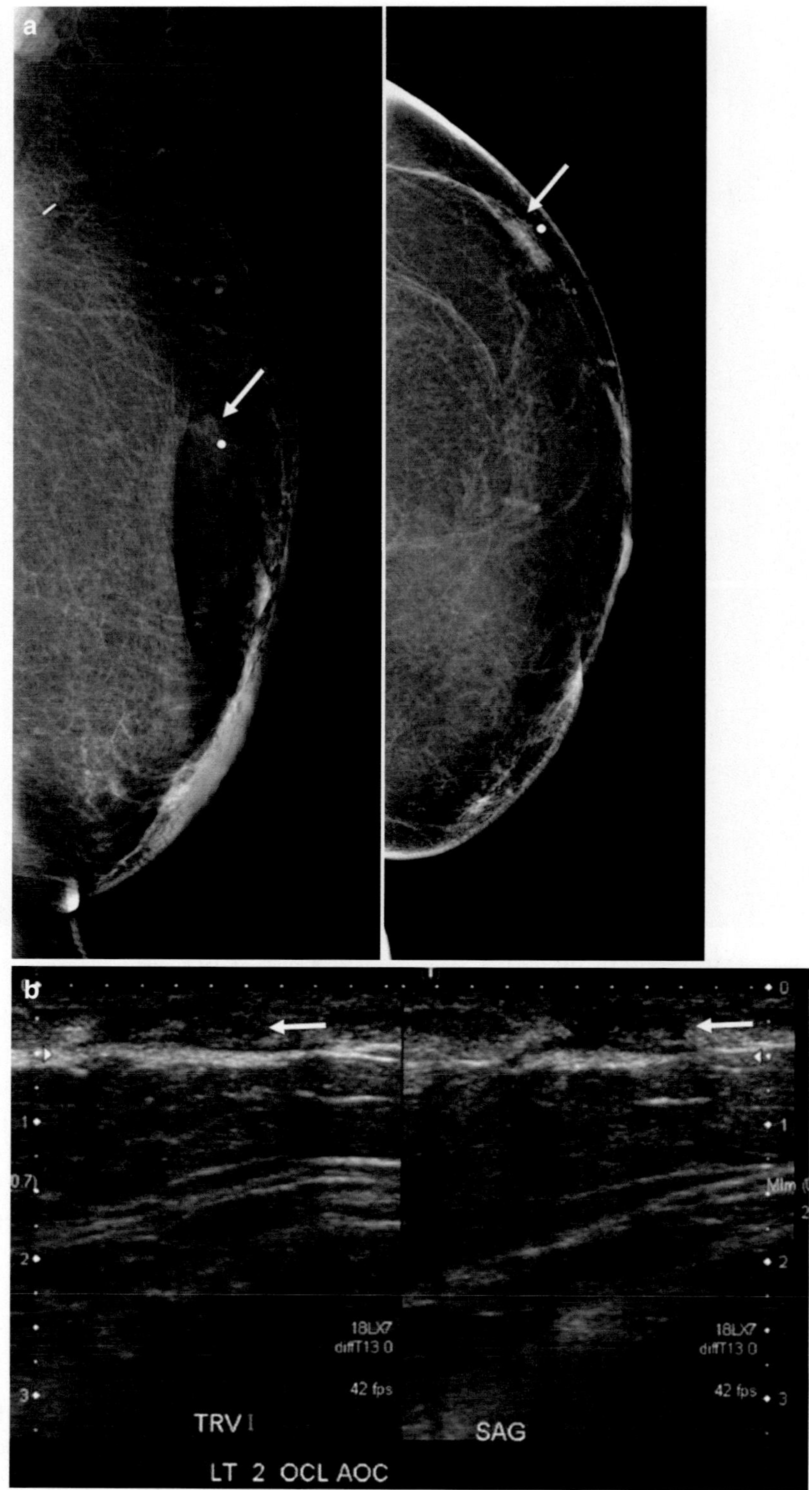

Fig. 18.8 (**a**) Left MLO and CC views. (**b**) Left breast ultrasound. (**c**) MRI: T1WI non-fat-suppressed (*a*) and DCE TIWI subtracted (*b*)

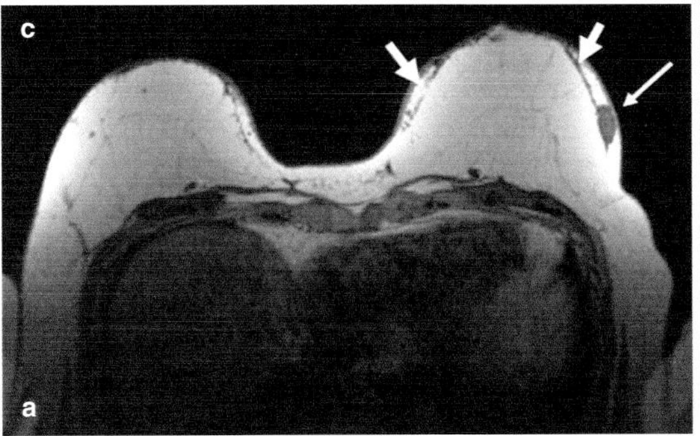

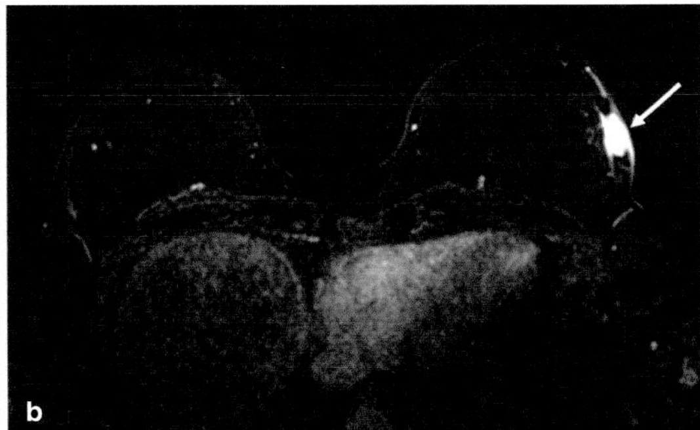

Fig. 18.8 (continued)

flaps like TRAM (transverse rectus abdominis muscle) or LDMF (latissimus dorsi muscle flap). These are myocutaneous flaps that contain muscle, overlying fat, and skin. The flap maintains its blood supply from original vessel and is tunneled to reconstruct the mastectomy bed.

Newer flaps are free flaps where the donor tissue is completely separated from its original blood supply and then re-anastomosed with recipient vessels (most commonly internal mammary vessels). This requires microsurgery. TRAM flap can also be performed as a free flap. Other, more common free flaps are perforator flaps like DIEP (deep inferior epigastric perforator), SIEP (superficial inferior epigastric perforator), or superior or inferior gluteal artery perforator flaps. The DIEP and SIEP flaps do not include muscle. Free flaps offer advantage over pedicled flaps by providing increased skin volume for harvesting, better skin contouring, improved blood flow, and preservation of abdominal wall integrity.

Most recurrence occurs in the skin envelop that may contain the remnant native breast tissue. This lies superficial to the autologous flap and would be easily diagnosed clinically on physical examination. Mammographic screening of flap reconstructed breast is controversial and not commonly done. On imaging, the myocutaneous flaps may have small muscle posteriorly, which may atrophy due to denervation. The flaps are predominantly fatty. In DIEP flaps (Fig. 18.6c), a thin soft tissue curvilinear band is seen underneath the skin that represents de-epithelialized abdominal skin. Extensive fat necrosis is commonly seen in the flaps and may be associated with lacey calcifications and enhancement on MR (Fig. 18.6d). Radiolucent appearance on mammogram and typical fat intensity on T1WI help the diagnosis of fat necrosis. Fat necrosis is commonly seen at periphery of the reconstructed breast. Rarely, it may mimic malignancy and biopsy may be needed for final differentiation. It is important for the radiologist to check for the contact zone between the flap and native breast tissue on imaging, which should be seen as a clear, thin line. The recurrence would generally occur at this site (Fig. 18.8c).

Suggested Readings

Adrada BE, Whitman GJ, Crosby MA, Carkaci S, Dryden MJ, Dogan BE. Multimodality imaging of the reconstructed breast. Curr Probl Diagn Radiol. 2015;44(6):487–95.

Leibman AJ, Misra M. Spectrum of imaging findings in the silicone-injected breast. Plast Reconstr Surg. 2011;128(1):28e–9e.

Liu S, Lim AA. Evaluation and treatment of surgical management of silicone mastitis. J Cutan Aesthet Surg. 2012;5(3):193.

Margolis NE, Morley C, Lotfi P, Shaylor SD, Palestrant S, Moy L, Melsaether AN. Update on imaging of the post-surgical breast. Radiographics. 2014;34(3):642–60.

Peters W, Fornasier V. Complications from injectable materials used for breast augmentation. Can J Plast Surg. 2009;17(3):89–96.

Schmauss D, Machens HG, Harder Y. Breast reconstruction after mastectomy. Front Surg. 2016;2:71.

Wong T, Lo LW, Fung PY, Lai HY, She HL, Ng WK, Kwok KM, Lee CM. Magnetic resonance imaging of breast augmentation: a pictorial review. Insight Imag. 2016;7(3):399–410.

19 Interventional Procedures

19.1 Interventional Breast Procedures

Percutaneous image-guided biopsies are becoming more common to obtain a diagnosis prior to any surgical intervention. They enable reduction of unnecessary surgical procedures in women. Image-guided biopsies, when performed in a prescribed manner, are extremely safe with minimal harm, side effects, and complications and ensure appropriate management of women with breast diseases.

Image-guided biopsies can be performed under mammographic (stereotactic), ultrasound, or MRI guidance. Many different spring-loaded core needle biopsy (CNB) [14-18G] and vacuum assisted biopsy (VAB) devices [7-12G] are commercially available.

Other interventional procedures of the breast that are commonly performed are preoperative localization, fine needle aspirations (FNA), and clip placements.

All biopsy procedures require verbal and written consent with clear information regarding the procedure, clips, post biopsy mammograms, possible complications, and follow up discussed with the patient in a language that the patient understands.

Discussion about failure of procedure or cancellation due to technical reasons should also be discussed where relevant.

Patient should be made aware as to how the patient will receive the pathology results and who she should contact in case of complications or emergencies. Typically the referring physician's office should be responsible for this process.

Women with implants should always be consented for possible implant rupture. This should be included in the written consent.

Women who are pregnant or lactating should be consented for possible nonhealing fistula that drains milk. Although a rare complication, it must be included in the consent.

Some women may be on anticoagulants for other medical conditions or may have coexisting thrombocytopenia, etc. Specific instructions should be given regarding discontinuation of anticoagulants especially for vacuum-assisted biopsies given the use of larger bore needles. Generally, anticoagulants should not impact small needle gauge procedures like CNB and FNA. All centers/institutions should have their standard guidelines for managing such patients.

For example, standard guidelines for some of the commonly used anticoagulants are as follows:

1. Warfarin: A recent international normalised ratio (INR) should be provided by the referring physician. A pre-procedure INR is obtained only if the patient is currently on warfarin or there is a high suspicion for vitamin K deficiency or liver disease. Proceed to biopsy if INR

N. Chotai, S. Kulkarni, *Breast Imaging Essentials*, https://doi.org/10.1007/978-981-15-1412-8_19

is less than or equal to 2.5. Consider using a smaller gauge needle if clinically appropriate.

2. Low-molecular-weight heparin (LMWH) therapeutic doses/Intravenous (IV) Heparin: Recommend stopping medication approximately 12 h prior to the procedure for LMWH and 1–2 h prior to the procedure for IV Heparin. Consider using a smaller gauge needle if clinically appropriate.
3. Thrombocytopenia: The platelet count should be greater 30 × 10^9/L. Consider using a smaller gauge needle if clinically appropriate.
4. Aspirin and Plavix: May proceed if clinically indicated. Consider using a smaller gauge needle if clinically appropriate.
5. New oral anticoagulants: These include Dabigatran, Rivaroxaban, etc., and should be held for 24–48 h (if normal renal clearance) prior to procedure. None of these medications have an antidote or reversal agent; hence it's important to stop them prior to the procedures.

All transcutaneous procedures are comfortably performed under local anesthesia. Lidocaine 1% is utilized for superficial anesthetic instilled subcutaneously. Lidocaine with epinephrine (1:100000) is utilized for deeper anesthesia, especially for VAB. The epinephrine helps in prolonging the anesthetic effect and helps in hemostasis.

Standard post-biopsy care includes firm compression of the biopsy site till the bleeding stops. Steristrips are utilized to close the skin nick allowing the edges to grow back together and keep the wound clean and protected while it heals. These usually fall off in 5–7 days. These are covered with a clean folded piece of gauze and held down by regular tape or a compression surgical tape. An icepack can be provided if available.

At discharge, printed instructions for post-biopsy care should be given to the patient.

*If a clip has been placed during biopsy, a post-biopsy mammogram should be performed.

Proper process of specimen handling, labeling, and delivering it to pathology labs must be established.

19.2 Stereotactic Core Biopsy

A stereotactic core biopsy is performed to assess suspicious lesions (BI-RADS 4 or 5) that are visualized on mammography. This is performed primarily for suspicious calcifications and also for masses, asymmetries, and architectural distortion that are not visualized on ultrasonography.

A stereotactic core biopsy can be either performed on prone table where the patient lies in the prone position or on an upright table where the patient is positioned sitting up or lying on her side. DBT-guided biopsies can also be performed using a prone or upright unit.

Stereotactic core biopsies can be performed using CNB (14G); however, there is increasing shift to using VAB (9-12G). VAB allows retrieval of larger biopsy tissue thereby decreasing the likelihood of upgrade at surgery.

Breast is positioned so as to get the shortest distance to the target. After obtaining a scout view to confirm appropriate positioning of the target, a stereotactic pair of images is acquired (+15 and −15 degree angle from the midline) in the X and Y axes. This allows the calculation of the Z axis (depth) coordinates using the parallax shift of the target on the stereotactic image pair. The key to appropriate positioning is to ensure that you have enough stroke margin (distance between the lesion and the receptor plate) so as to prevent puncturing the other side of the breast and hitting the receptor plate. After obtaining the target, the needle is placed through the skin incision at the depth using the correct coordinates. Pre- and post-fire image pairs can be acquired to ensure appropriate positioning of the tip of the needle prior to sampling (Fig. 19.1).

When the biopsy is being performed for suspicious microcalcifications, it is essential to confirm the presence of adequate calcifications in the retrieved biopsy sample by performing a specimen radiograph (Fig. 19.2). A clip can be placed in the biopsy cavity (Fig. 19.3). Institutional practices may vary. It is a good rule of thumb to always leave a clip at the site of biopsy when the group of microcalcifications is very small and there is a risk of them being completely removed during the biopsy or in cases where there are multiple groups of microcalcifications and you need to mark the group biopsied. The clip placement is always followed by an ipsilateral mammogram to document the position of the clip. Multiple varieties and shapes of clips are available commercially and it is important to choose an MRI-compatible clip that produces a mild artifact should the patient proceed to an MRI examination. When multiple sites are biopsied, different clip shapes are used so at to be able to identify different biopsy sites accurately.

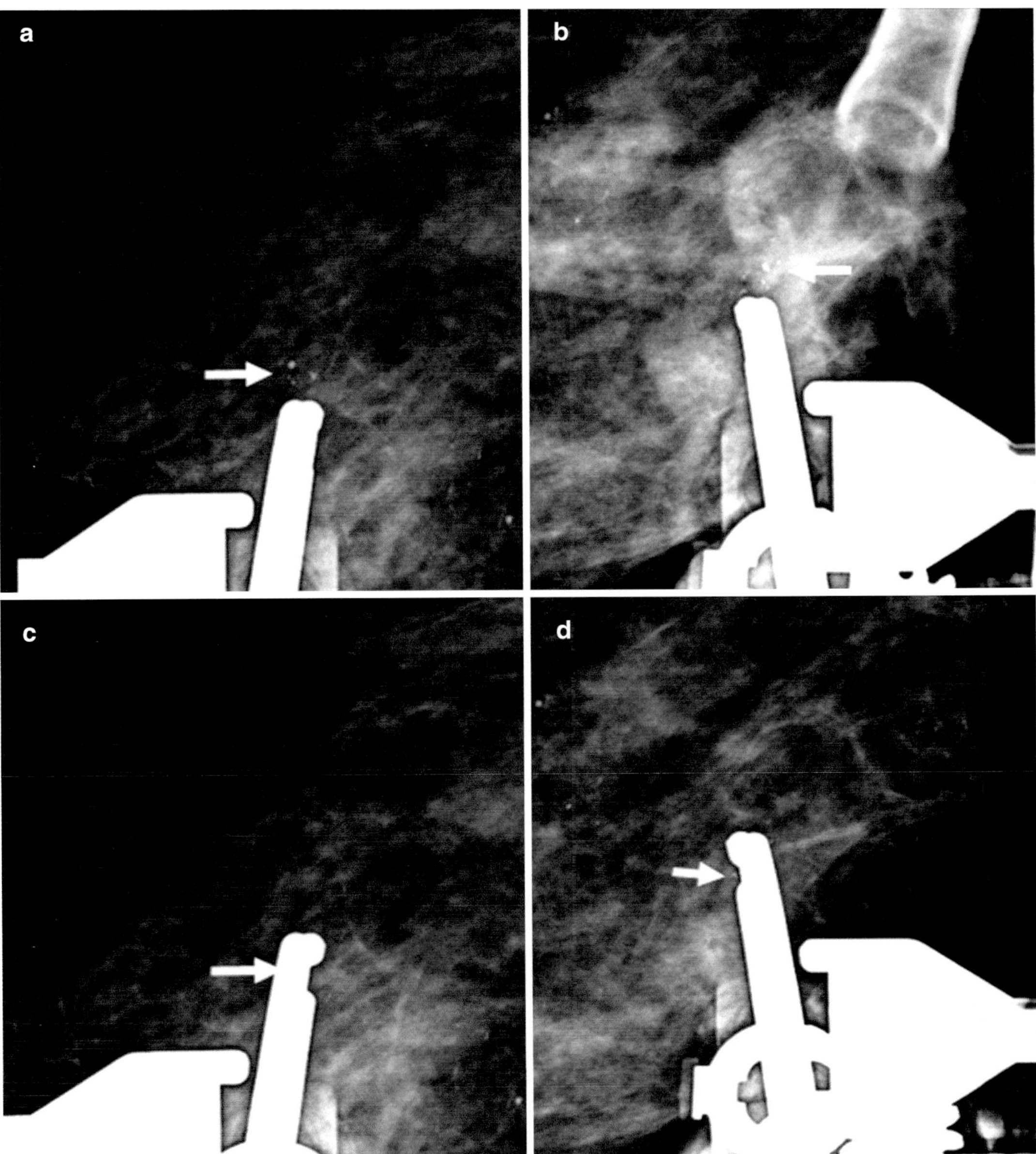

Fig. 19.1 Stereotactic biopsy of a small group of microcalcifications seen in right breast. Pre-fire stereotactic image pair shows the tip of the needle close to the target (**a**, **b**). Post-fire stereotactic image pair shows needle in post-fired position with the needle through the target (**c**, **d**)

Technical Challenges

1. Stereotactic biopsy may be technically challenging in women with small breasts (inadequate stroke margin), lesions close to the chest wall or high up in the axilla. In these cases, it is important to make the patient understand the possibility of failed/cancelled biopsy due to technical factors before embarking on the procedure.
2. Patient movement can lead to X, Y, or Z axis errors in position of the tip of the needle on post-fire views, which need to be corrected in order to succeed in the retrieval of microcalcifications. The vendor of the biopsy equipment will usually provide a chart to help with these corrections. It is important to have a trained technologist who can help you identify and rectify these errors.

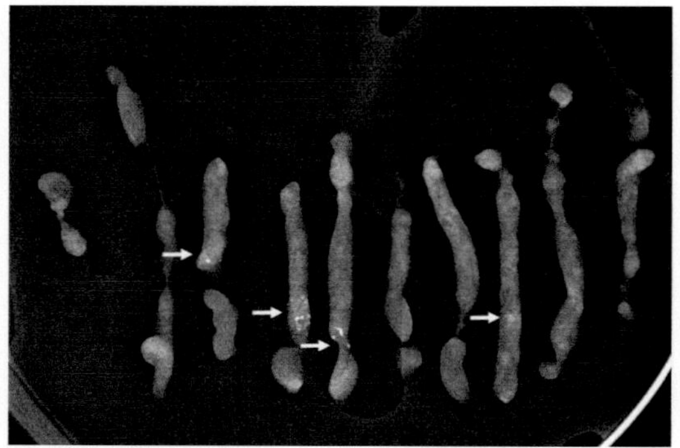

Fig. 19.2 Radiograph of the biopsy core tissue is done to check adequate retrieval of the microcalcifications (white arrows)

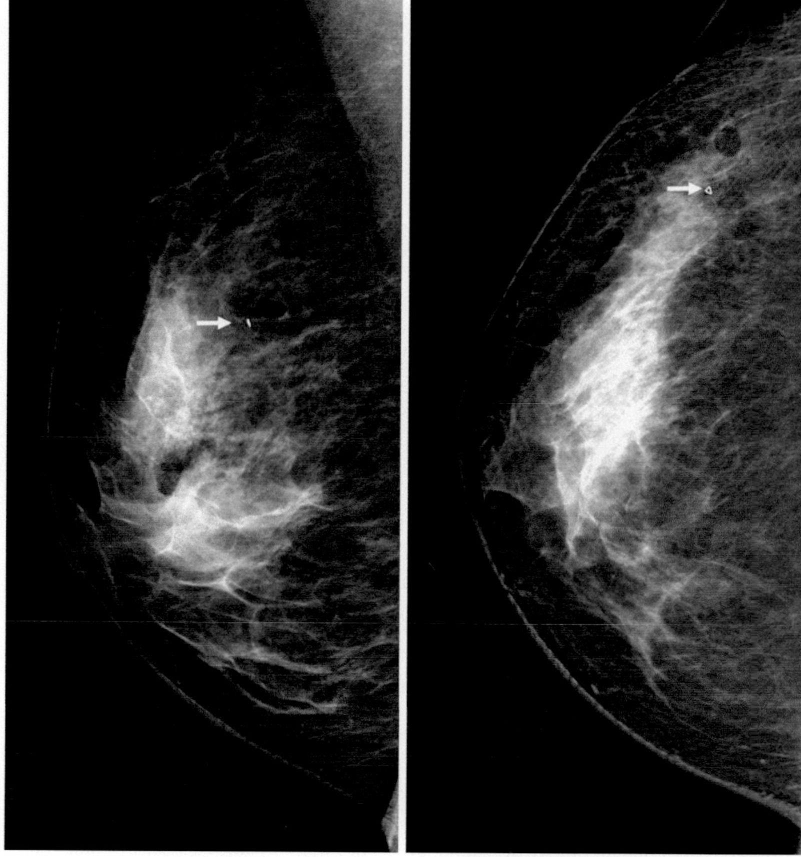

Fig. 19.3 Post-procedure mammogram is done to document the position of marker (white arrow). Migration of the marker clip, if any, should be documented

Complications

1. Bruising and hematoma.
2. Infection.
3. Clip migration: This may occur during the sudden release of compression from the biopsy unit upon completion of the biopsy. This causes the clip to move in the direction of the compression and is called the *accordion effect*. This can be avoided by careful and slow release of the compression. The clip may sometimes move distal to the biopsy cavity due to hematoma or needle movement. If this occurs, one needs to document residual microcalcifications in the biopsy cavity, in an event that all microcalcifications have been removed, a second clip may have to be placed in the biopsy cavity.
4. No retrieval of microcalcifications. This may occur due to technical challenges or in an uncooperative patient. Sometimes, despite several attempts microcalcifications may not be retrieved and the patient may have to be booked for a repeat appointment.

19.3 Ultrasound-Guided Core Biopsy

Ultrasound-guided core needle biopsy (CNB) is a real-time procedure where the target is directly visualized as a needle is being placed in it. This allows for more accuracy, is faster, and is technically much easier for the patient. It does not require breast compression, ionizing radiation, or contrast. Ultrasound-guided biopsy is usually performed for BI-RADS 4 or 5 ultrasound nonpalpable masses. Some women that present with extensive microcalcifications which can be visualized by high-resolution ultrasound probes can also undergo biopsy of these microcalcifications under ultrasound guidance. In these cases the sampling should be more extensive (6–8 passes) than the standard sampling for masses (2–3 passes) to avoid undersampling error. The biopsy samples should undergo a specimen radiograph to document retrieval of target microcalcifications just as in stereotactic core biopsies.

Ultrasound-guided biopsies are also easier for axillary masses and lymph nodes and allow safe biopsy, avoiding critical structures like blood vessels.

Generally, for a routine CNB, 14-18G needles are used. Some institutions also perform ultrasound-guided VAB. VAB is generally performed to completely remove the benign appearing lesions such as solitary papillomas and small fibroadenomata.

Just as in stereotactic biopsies, clips can be placed following ultrasound-guided biopsies especially in subcentimeter solid masses, complex cysts, axillary lymph nodes, etc., always followed by a post-clip unilateral mammogram.

Positioning of the patient and breast is critically important. For lateral lesions a supine oblique position works best and for medial lesions a supine position is used. The underlying principle is to spread out the breast evenly so as to have easy access to the lesion and achieving the shortest distance from the site of skin entry of the needle to the lesion. It is important to support the patients arm and shoulder and provide the most comfortable position. You may also tip the bed of the patient depending on where the lesion is in the breast to allow gravity to assist positioning. Cleaning and draping of breast is performed to prevent fluids/blood from running down on the patient's body and neck. A longitudinal approach to the lesion may be the easiest to perform; however, a radiologist may prefer medial or lateral approach to the lesion based on their comfort level and expertise. It is important to fix the hand holding the probe on the patient in order to stabilize the lesion and keeping it visible throughout the procedure. After instillation of local anesthesia, a generous skin nick is made to allow easy entry of the needle tip into the breast. Once the needle tip is introduced, the needle should be made parallel to the skin and transducer. This allows visualization of the needle as it travels in the breast and prevents inadvertent pneumothorax while sampling deep lesions. Once the needle tip reaches the target lesion, the device should be fired so that the needle traverses the solid mass. Pre- and post-fire images must be documented for every pass of the needle (Fig. 19.4). Check

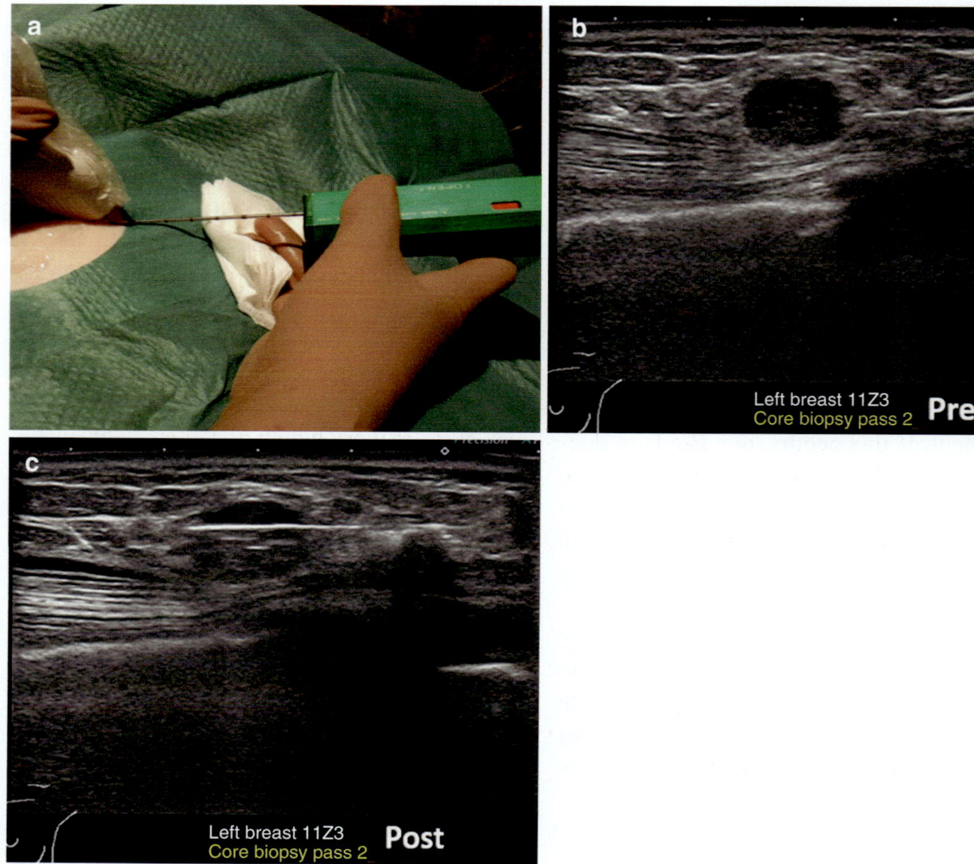

Fig. 19.4 Ultrasound-guided core needle biopsy of a breast lesion is demonstrated. The region is cleaned and draped (**a**). The probe covered with a sterile cover is held in an immobilized position to show the target. Under vision, the needle is advanced close to the edge of the target (**b**) and then fired (**c**) so that it passes through the target to retrieve a sample

that the retrieved samples are not fragmented. Good samples generally sink to the bottom of the specimen jar while fatty fragmented ones float. Additional cores should be acquired if sample quality is not adequate. Biopsy of hard masses could be challenging, leading to the bending of core biopsy needles. In these cases you may need to change the biopsy needle between samplings. When sampling multiple lesions or bilateral lesions, the biopsy needle should be changed for each new lesion biopsied to prevent specimen contamination.

For biopsy of deep breast lesions and lymph nodes, single-use needles that do not fire beyond the lesion (no throw needles) can be used such as the Temno/Quikcore needles. These needles sample at the depth that they are placed in the lesion (Fig. 19.5). Coaxial systems are also available that allow multiple core specimens through a single insertion of the needle.

Technical Challenges

1. Hematoma created by the first needle fire may obscure a small target making further sampling difficult or impossible.

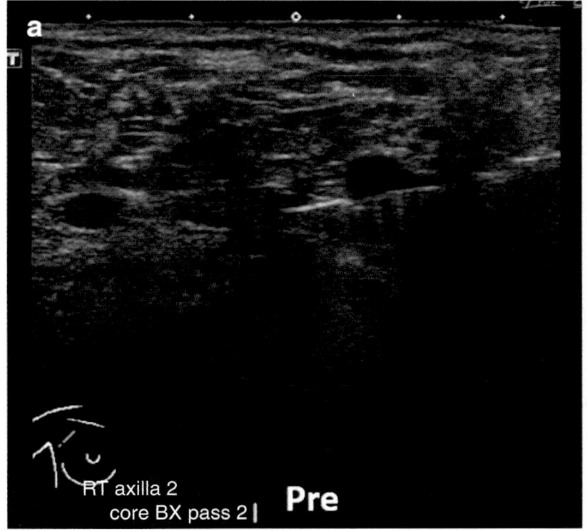

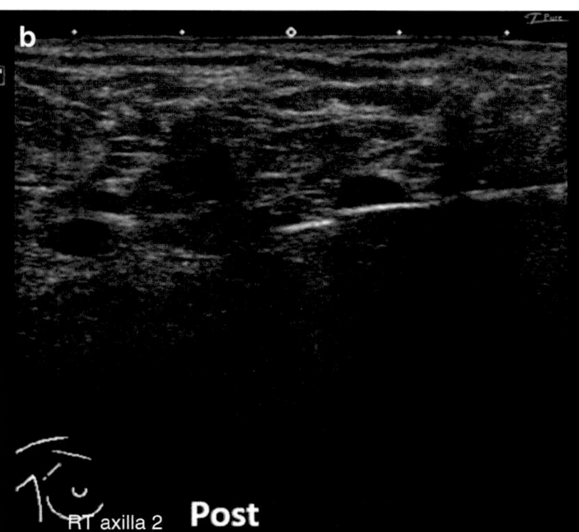

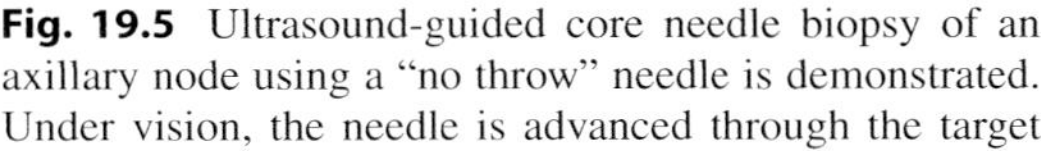

Fig. 19.5 Ultrasound-guided core needle biopsy of an axillary node using a "no throw" needle is demonstrated. Under vision, the needle is advanced through the target lesion till the desired level (**a**) and then fired (**b**) to avoid inadvertent damage to important structures, like axillary vessels distal to the target

2. Patient may not be cooperative and patient anxiety may deter adequate biopsy of a target lesion.
3. Biopsy of wrong lesion due to triangulation errors.
4. Deep lesions may be difficult to access.
5. Superficial lesions located on implant surfaces.

Complications

1. Bruising and hematoma.
2. Infection.
3. Clip migration: The clip may sometimes move distal to the biopsy cavity due to hematoma or needle movement. If this occurs, a second clip may have to be placed in the biopsy cavity under ultrasound guidance.

19.4 Fine Needle Aspiration Biopsy (Fig. 19.6)

This is a simple, fast, cost-effective, and easy procedure using thin 21G–25G needle to obtain sample of tissue/fluid from a solid/cystic lesion as well as for cyst drainage. Under ultrasound guidance, the needle can be precisely passed into the desired part of the lesion to sample, e.g., an intracystic mural mass. Superficial local anesthesia should be used as needed.

It may be a procedure of choice at centers with lack of facility of core biopsy or an experienced practitioner. FNA may be preferred in women with coagulopathy or those who cannot discontinue their anticoagulant therapy for the biopsy.

However, as far as possible an FNA should be avoided for masses to prevent undersampling errors. Small complex cystic lesions may disappear on FNA, making it very difficult to locate them in the case of a malignant diagnosis. Some centers have a practice of placing clips after FNA.

1. Difficulty in differentiation between invasive and in situ carcinoma and papillary masses.
2. High rate (25%) of nondiagnostic aspiration needing repeat procedure.
3. Requires an experienced breast cytopathologist for accuracy for, e.g., to be able to differentiate true atypical cells from lactational change, etc.

Localization procedures are typically performed preoperatively to assist the surgeons to excise the target lesions.

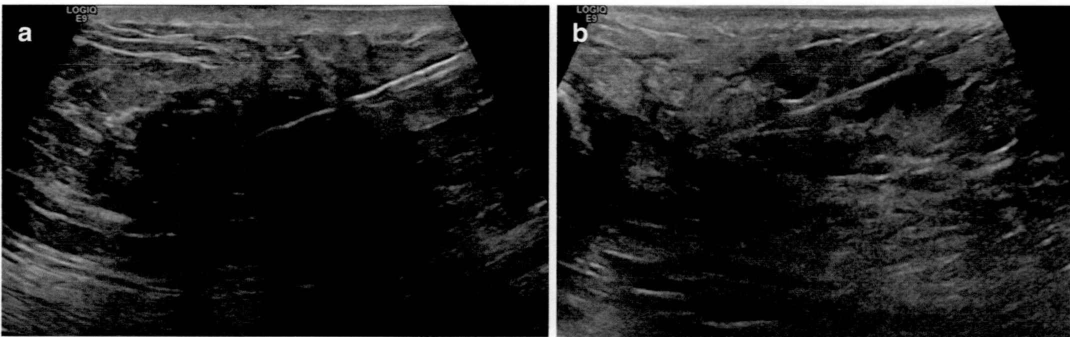

Fig. 19.6 34-year-old lactating woman with right breast abscess. A large-size needle is inserted under ultrasound guidance (**a**) in the collection to drain the liquefied abscess. Post aspiration, collapsed abscess cavity is noted (**b**)

19.5 Mammographic Wire Localization and Bracketing

Preoperatively (hook) wire localization is performed under mammographic alphanumeric grid-based approach (Fig. 19.7a, b) or stereotactic or DBT guidance in order to localize the microcalcifications/clips to be excised. The reinforced portion of the wire is usually placed through the center of the target with the hook beyond the target. If the area of microcalcifications is larger, then two or more wires can be placed along the edges to ensure complete excision of the area. This is termed as bracketing (Fig. 19.8).

One has to watch for vasovagal reaction in patients who are usually fasting for their surgery, are anxious, and are sitting up with their breast in a compression grid. These complications are less frequent when using a prone table.

Mammographic wire localization is also performed for localizing post-MRI biopsy clips for lesions that need excision, particularly in clips that are not visualized by ultrasound. Clipped masses that are no longer visible on ultrasound following neoadjuvant treatment or because they have collapsed can also be localized under mammographic guidance.

Hook wire is placed under superficial local anesthesia.

The skin entry point selected is the shortest possible distance to approach the lesion, which is targeted using either with an alphanumerical grid, DBT, or stereotactic guidance. The hook wire system is introduced such that the tip of the needle is beyond the target (1 cm). The wire is gently deployed and the needle is gently withdrawn taking care not to withdraw the wire.

Post-procedure mammogram is performed to demonstrate the position of the wire in relation to the target. These need to be appropriately annotated and sent to the PACS server so that they can be visualized in the operating room by the surgeon. The site of skin entry is marked with a radiopaque bead/marker so that the surgeon can calculate the length of the wire that is in the patient as well as decide the site of incision.

Once the lesion is excised, the specimen is sent for radiography to ensure that there has been adequate excision, that the clips are retrieved, and that there are no microcalcifications at the margins (Fig. 19.7b-*d*). This information is relayed to the surgeon in the operating rooms with recommendations of revision of margins, if necessary.

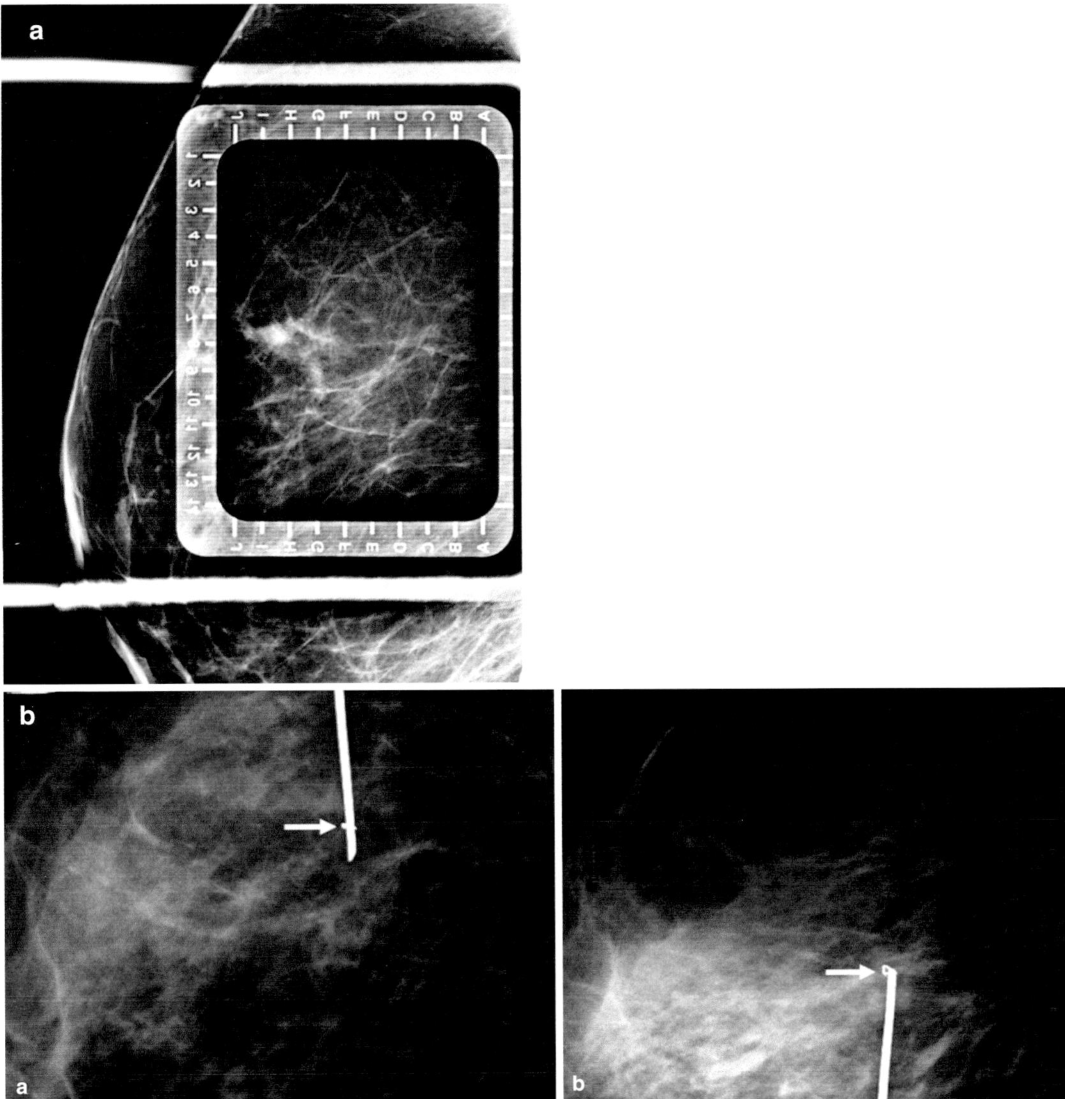

Fig. 19.7 45-year-old woman with microcalcifications that are biopsy-proven ADH. (**a**) Mammographic wire localization of the biopsy site (marked with clip) performed using an alphanumeric grid. (**b**) (*a*, *b*) Hook-wire needle system is advanced with the tip just beyond the target (white arrow) under stereotactic guidance. After confirming the correct position in orthogonal views, the wire is deployed. The needle is withdrawn holding the wire in place. (*c*) Post procedure mammogram shows proper placement of the hook wire in relation to the target (marker clip). (*d*) Post-excision specimen radiograph confirms excision of target lesion and clip

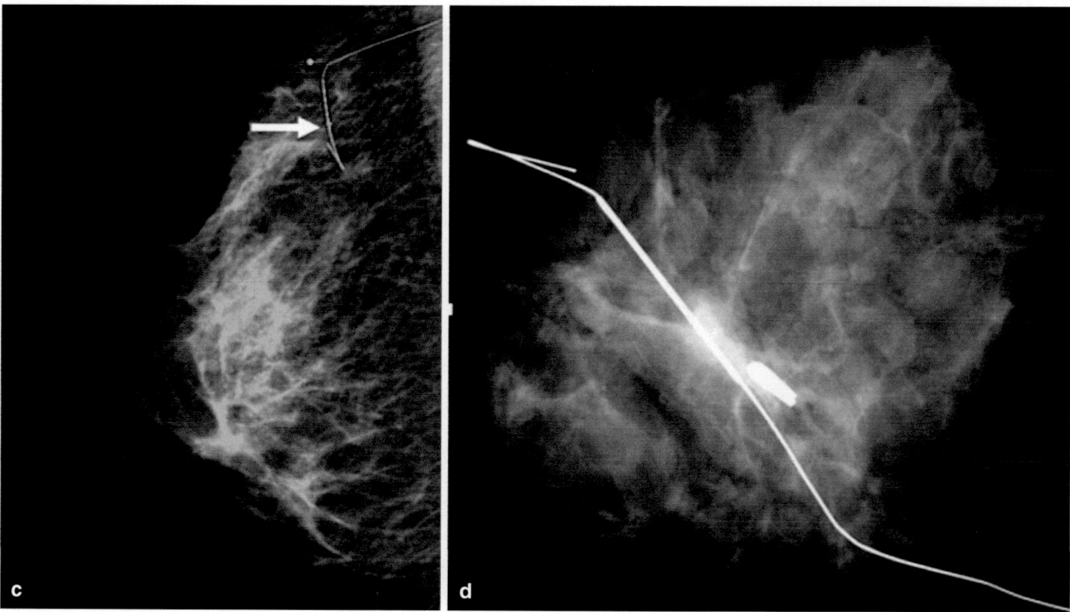

Fig. 19.7 (continued)

Complications: Though rare, some possible complications with wire localization include migration of wire; fragmentation of wire; bleeding, which is generally self-limiting; and pneumothorax.

19.6 Ultrasound-Guided Lesion Localization

Preoperative hook wire procedure under ultrasound guidance is relatively simple to perform. The patient is lying down and there is real-time evaluation of the position of the tip of the localizing wire. Some post-biopsy clips can be visualized under ultrasound and these can be localized under ultrasound guidance as well.

The correct target lesion needs to be properly visualized. Under superficial local anesthesia, the hook wire is inserted just past the lesion, wire is deployed, and needle withdrawn gently over the wire (Fig. 19.9a, b). Post-procedure ultrasound and mammogram are performed to document the position of the wire in relation to the target. The site of skin entry is marked with a radiopaque bead/marker so that the surgeon can calculate the length of the wire that is in the patient as well as decide the site of incision.

Postoperative specimen radiography is performed to confirm excision of the intended lesion satisfactorily, complete removal of the wire, and to document location of the lesion within the specimen to assist the pathologist for targeted sampling. Additionally, ultrasound of the specimen (Fig. 19.9c) is also performed when the wire localization is done under ultrasound guidance. This helps to assess the anterior and posterior margins of the specimen. This information is relayed to the surgeon in the operating room with recommendations of revision of margins, if necessary.

Complications: Though rare, some possible complications with wire localization include migration of wire; fragmentation of wire; bleeding, which is generally self-limiting; and pneumothorax.

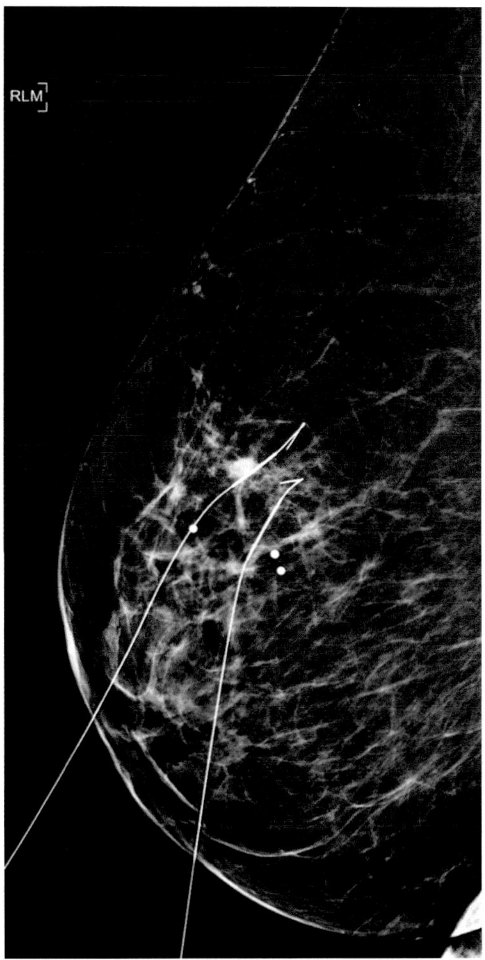

Fig. 19.8 Lateral radiograph showing "bracketing" technique for a larger area of microcalcifications. Two localizing wires bracket the extent of the microcalcifications, allowing complete excision with clear margins

More recently there have been newer techniques of localization that are replacing the traditional wire localization. The benefit of these techniques it to decouple the localization procedures from the day of surgery, thereby making workflow more efficient.

RSL is a relatively effective and cheap technique wherein a radioactive seed akin to a prostate seed is placed in the target lesion several days prior to the patient's surgery. The downside however is the associated radiation risk to all personnel and the patient (Fig. 19.10).

Magnetic seed localization is quite easy akin to any clip placement procedure but is at the current time fairly expensive and requires specialized nonmagnetic surgical instruments, which prevent signal noise at the time of locating the magnetic seed with a special probe.

Radiofrequency localization is also similar to other techniques using an RF tag for localization and is gaining wide acceptance as a localizing procedure. This requires its own handheld probe to localize the RF tag and does not require any changes in surgical equipment.

Occasionally, localization with a fine needle may also be performed by a radiologist as a method of triangulation. In this procedure a fine needle is placed in a lesion documented on ultrasound and taped to the skin. A mammogram with gentle compression is performed to show that the lesion seen on ultrasound indeed corresponds to the lesion seen on mammography. Once this is proven, the fine needle is removed and if required further sampling and clip placement is performed.

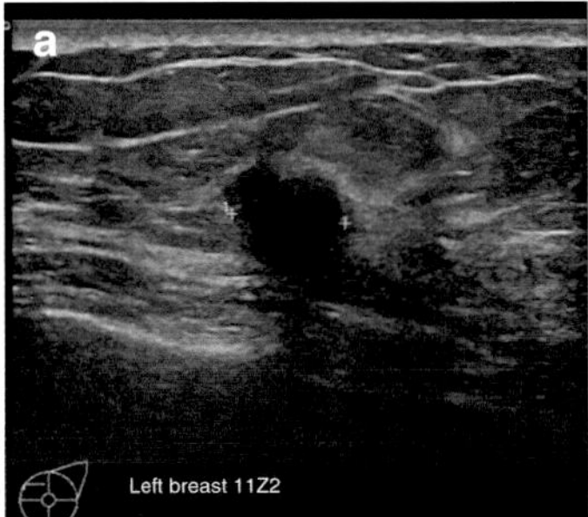

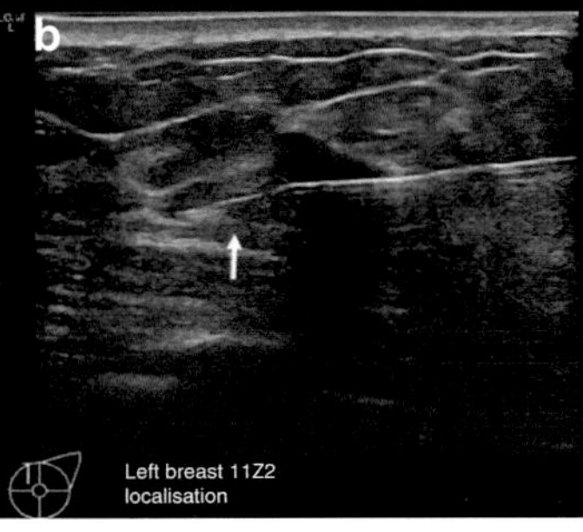

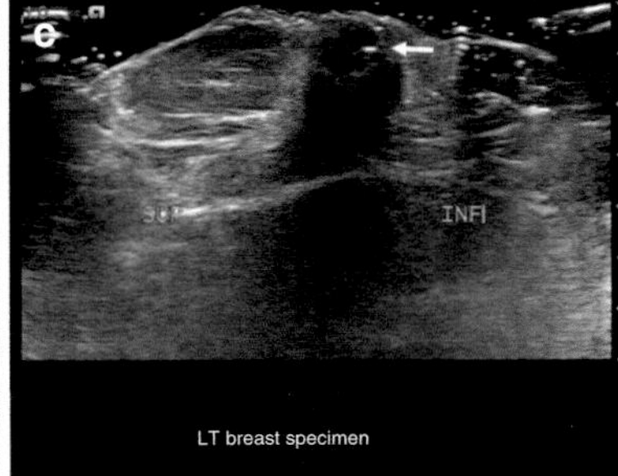

Fig. 19.9 43-year-old woman with biopsy-proven left breast invasive ductal carcinoma at the 11 o'clock location. (**a**) Shows biopsy proven left breast cancer. (**b**) Shows hook wire through the mass with the hook portion of the wire just beyond the lesion (white arrow). Post-lumpectomy specimen ultrasound (**c**) shows the lesion to be completely excised with close anterior margins at the specimen surface. The hook wire is seen through the lesion (white arrow)

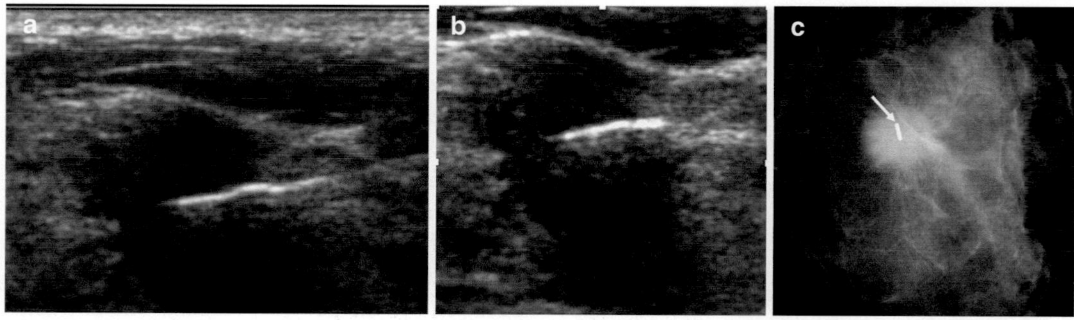

Fig. 19.10 (**a**) Image reveals an ultrasound-guided radioactive seed localization of a biopsy proven cancer. (**b**) Echogenic seed seen deployed in the mass. (**c**) Post excision radiograph shows the excised mass along with the seed (white arrow)

19.7 Clip Insertion (Fig. 19.11a, b)

As described above, metallic clip markers are placed in the biopsy cavity following the biopsies. Numerous varieties of clips (materials and shapes) are available commercially.

All commercially available clips (titanium or steel) come loaded in their coaxial system and are very easy to deploy under any modality. These clips are tiny and will not set off any airport security metal detector, will not be palpable to the patient, and will not elicit any kind of allergic reaction. Some clips with a small amount of nickel can be avoided in the rare occurrence of nickel allergy in a patient.

The biopsy clip serves as a marker documenting where the tissue was sampled in the breast. If in the event that the lesion is no longer visible by imaging after the biopsy, the marker is the only guide to know where the tissue was sampled. This can then be used for localization or for follow-up. The most important indication of the clip is in the neoadjuvant setting and its role has been discussed in the chapter on neoadjuvant treatment.

19.8 MRI-Guided Biopsy

MRI is a very sensitive test but lower in specificity, indicating detection of many findings not all of which will be malignant. Often in the setting of staging or high-risk screening, such findings can pose a dilemma. Not all of them show corresponding mammographic or ultrasound correlate. When relevant, these lesions require MRI-guided biopsy. Diligent assessment of the patients' mammogram (microcalcifications) and second look ultrasound can help in locating the MRI finding, allowing a biopsy to be performed using much cheaper and easier modalities. Every MRI lesion that is biopsied using either ultrasound or mammographic guidance should have a post-biopsy clip placed in the biopsy cavity so that a follow-up MRI can demonstrate that the correct area was sampled. (Clip will be seen in the MRI lesion). In the scenario where the significant MRI lesion is occult on conventional imaging, an MRI biopsy is arranged. All pre-biopsy discussions with patient, anticoagulation guidelines, consent process, and post-biopsy care are similar to other biopsies discussed before. Occasionally, the target lesion may not be visualized on the day of MRI-guided biopsy. The cause is not known, but it may be due to factors like breast compression, background parenchymal enhancement, or timing of biopsy in relation to the menstrual cycle. About 10% of cancelled MRI-guided biopsies due to nonvisualization develop ipsilateral breast cancer on follow-up. This exceeds BI-RADS 2 likelihood (>2%) and hence all such cancelled cases warrant a 6-month follow-up MRI (BI-RADS 3).

Team work between the breast MRI technologist and the radiologist is necessary for optimum positioning and localization of the target lesion.

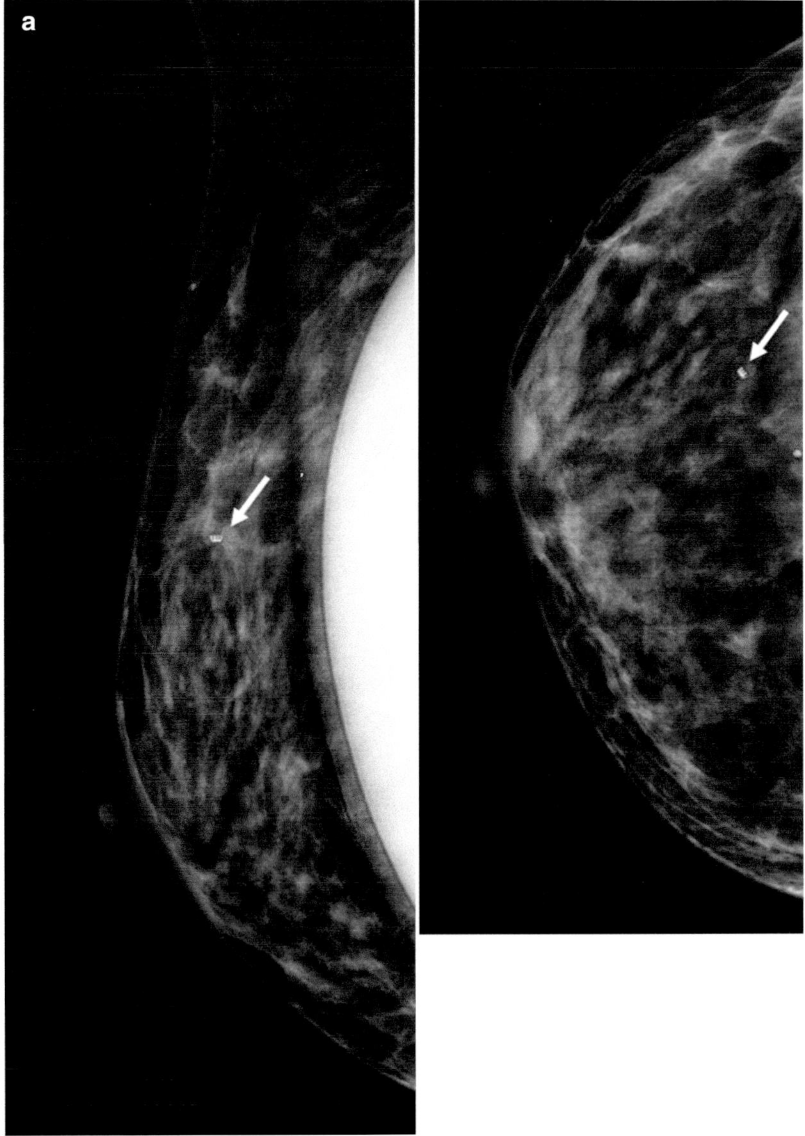

Fig. 19.11 49-year-old woman with history of previous benign breast biopsy with clip insertion. Right mammogram (**a**) in implant displaced MLO and CC projections show retropectoral implant. A metallic clip marker (white arrow) is seen in the upper outer quadrant of the right breast. (**b**) Ultrasound image of right breast at the 12 o'clock location shows an echogenic area with surrounding hypoechoic rim. This represents a metallic marker embedded in collagen (Hydromark clip) that improves ultrasound visibility of the clip for a longer duration

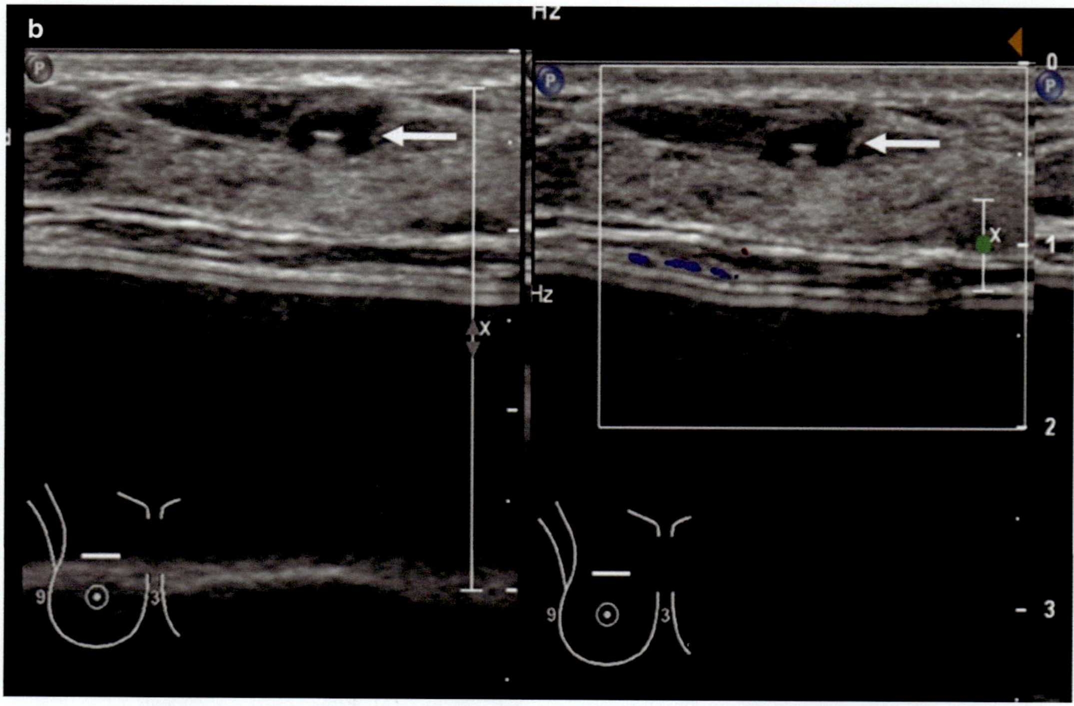

Fig. 19.11 (continued)

Positioning of the patient for the MRI-guided biopsy is very critical as is the familiarity with the biopsy equipment, and therefore a trained MRI technologist is an important team member who needs to be involved in all steps of the procedure starting with the initial discussion with patient and consent.

The biopsy is performed in the prone position with the area of biopsy adequately covered in the biopsy grid. A disposable sterile grid not only helps triangulation but also acts as a compression plate for the breast. Optimal compression is necessary to immobilize the breast and prevent tenting during needle placement. Excessive compression can impede blood flow and prevent lesion visualization. Lesions may be approached through the lateral or medial direction depending upon where they are located in the breast to allow safe biopsy without puncturing the distal surface akin to stroke margin on stereotactic biopsy.

A fiducial is placed in one of the grid openings. This acts as a reference point to determine the positional coordinates of the target lesion. Precontrast images are obtained and used to ensure that the lesion lies in the confines of the biopsy grid, and if required the breast can be readjusted.

Multiple dynamic sequences are then obtained to demonstrate the target. Once confidently identified, the coordinates can be determined either by manual calculations or vendor-specific biopsy software, which will guide one to the appropriate grid opening through which the target lesion can be assessed.

After instilling superficial and deep local anesthesia, a small nick is made on the skin and a sharp metal trocar with a plastic sheath is introduced into the breast at the appropriate calculated depth. The trocar is then withdrawn and replaced with an obturator to allow scanning. The tip of the obturator is easily visualized on MRI and corresponds to the center of the sampling notch and should lie at the center of the lesion on the prebiopsy images (Fig. 19.12).

The position of the trocar is confirmed on axial (which shows the obturator in full length) as well as sagittal images (that shows the obturator in cross sections). Once adequate obturator position is achieved, the obturator is exchanged with the

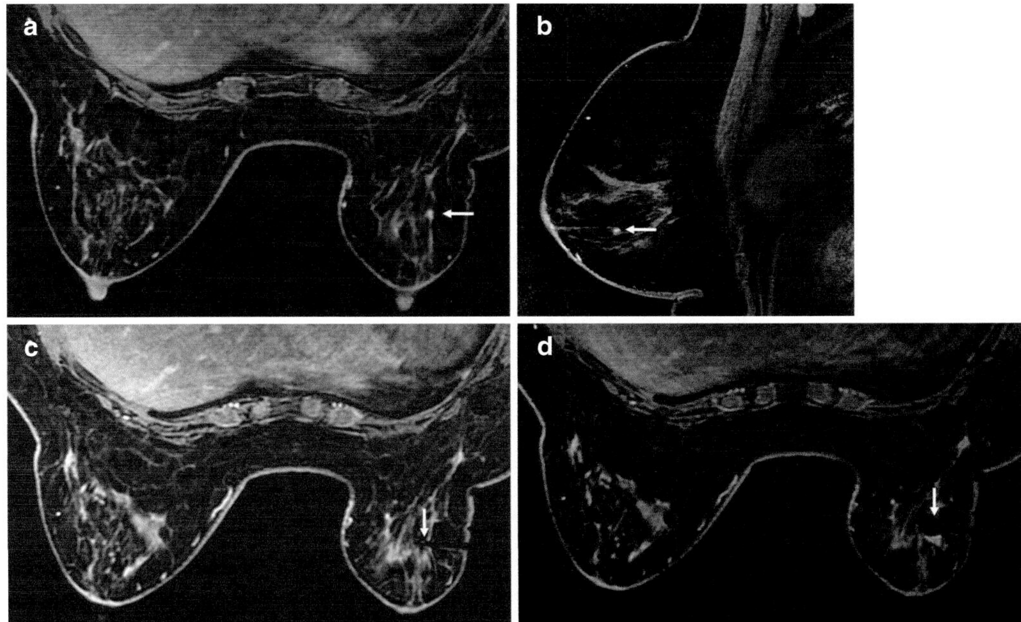

Fig. 19.12 43-year BRCA-positive woman with a new enhancing lesion in left lateral breast underwent MRI-guided biopsy. (**a**, **b**) Postcontrast images show a tiny focus of enhancement in the axial and sagittal planes (white arrows). (**c**) Pre-biopsy MRI shows the tip of the introducer (white arrow) at the level of the target confirming correct position. (**d**) Post-biopsy MRI shows a small hematoma/air (white arrow) at the site of the biopsy

biopsy needle through the introducer sheath. The MRI-compatible needles that are 7–12-gauge are used with commercially available vacuum devices.

Following generous sampling, an MRI-compatible tissue marker (clip) is placed in the biopsy cavity. The obturator is once again placed in the sheath carefully, ensuring the tip remains in the sheath. Pushing the obturator in completely and aggressively may inadvertently displace the biopsy clip distal to the biopsy site. A post-MRI biopsy check mammogram is then performed to document the position of the clip and subsequently guide further excision if required (Fig. 19.13).

In the rare event where there is nondeployment of the biopsy clip, an ultrasound can be used to find the biopsy cavity (hematoma) and a new clip can be placed under ultrasound guidance.

In situations of target nonvisualization, every effort must be made to look for surrounding landmarks which may assist in the biopsy, such as surrounding T2 bright lesions, distortion, or T1 masses.

Overcompression is generally difficult to compensate as releasing the compression would change all targeting coordinates. More so with passing time the contrast may wash out or the surrounding enhancing parenchyma may completely obscure the target lesion. In these cases, a repeat attempt or 6-month follow-up MRI are the only options.

Complications

1. Bruising and hematoma.
2. Infection.
3. Clip migration: The clip may sometimes move distal to the biopsy cavity due to hematoma or needle movement. If this occurs, a second clip may have to be placed in the biopsy cavity under ultrasound guidance.

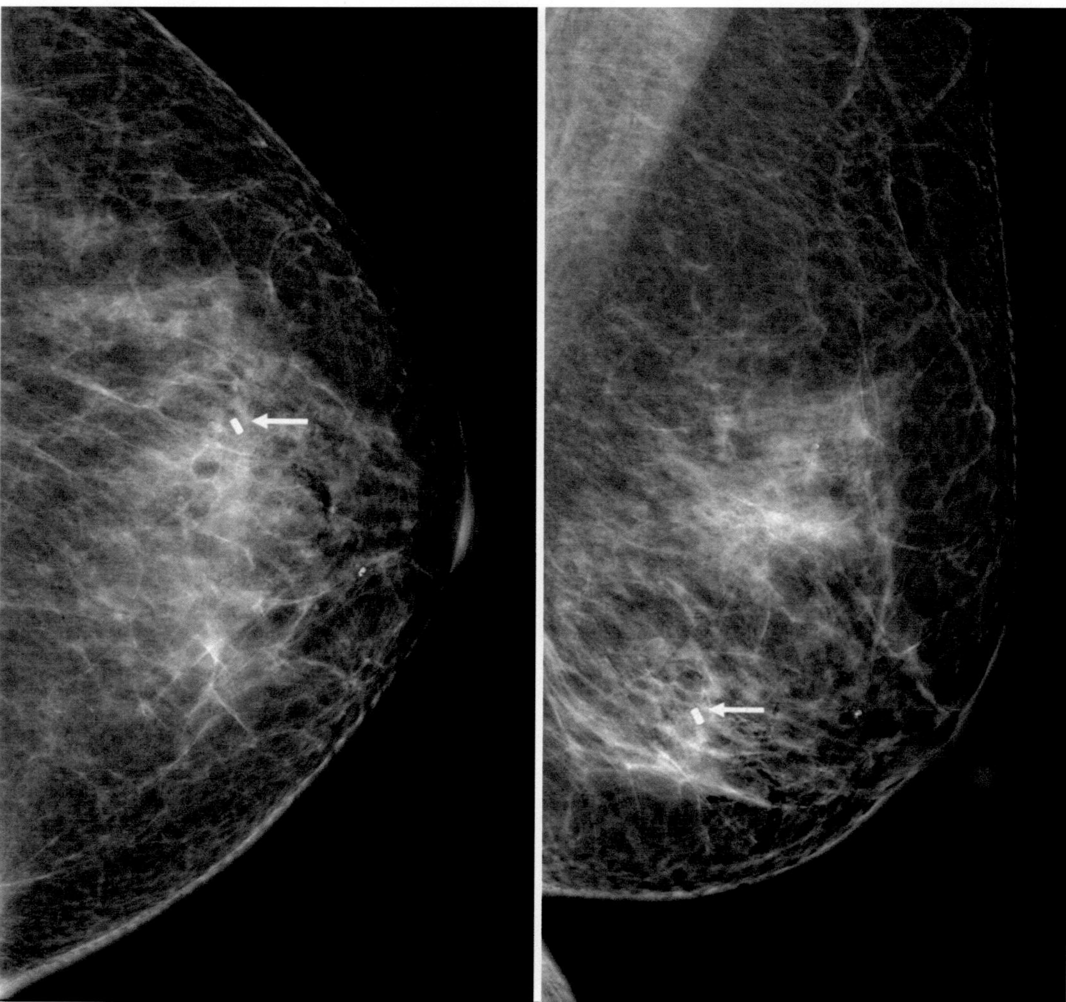

Fig. 19.13 Post-MRI biopsy left mammogram shows the marker clip in the expected location. Small hematoma and air tract are expected post-biopsy changes

19.9 MRI-Guided Needle Localization (Fig. 19.14)

MRI-guided needle localization is performed prior to surgical excision for lesions that are not visualized on conventional imaging and for various reason (including lack of MRI guided biopsy capability) did not undergo MRI-guided biopsy. The technique is similar to the biopsy procedure with some variations in the plastic needle guide, and commercially available MRI-compatible needle localizations wires should be used.

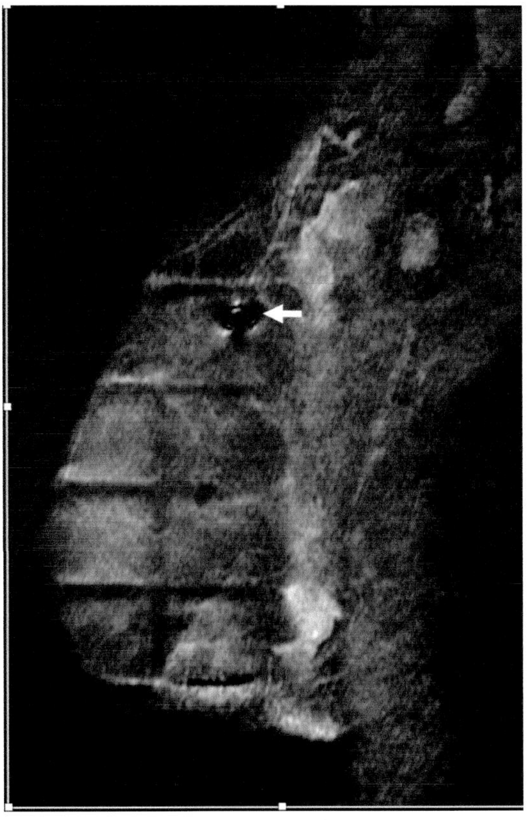

Fig. 19.14 Sagittal image of a right breast MRI positioned for a needle localization procedure shows the needle artifact (blooming) in the upper breast (thick white arrow). The compression grid is an alphanumeric grid which allows selection of site of biopsy based on lesion location

Suggested Readings

Helbich TH, Matzek W, Fuchsjäger MH. Stereotactic and ultrasound-guided breast biopsy. Eur Radiol. 2004;14(3):383–93.

Papalouka V, Kilburn-Toppin F, Gaskarth M, Gilbert F. MRI-guided breast biopsy: a review of technique, indications, and radiological–pathological correlations. Clin Radiol. 2018;73(10):908–e17.

20 Male Breast and Miscellaneous Cases

20.1 Case 20.1

History: 44-year-old male with left breast enlargement.

Questions

Q1. Describe the imaging findings (Fig. 20.1A–C).
Q2. What is the etiology of the above condition?
Q3. What are the radiological variations of the above diagnosis?

Answers

A1. Bilateral MLO (Fig. 20.1A) and CC (Fig. 20.1B) views reveal asymmetric subareolar mass on the left side with no suspicious features. There is a small volume of fibroglandular tissue seen on the right side. Findings are suggestive of bilateral gynecomastia, more prominent on left side. Ultrasound (Fig. 20.1C) shows comparative image from right and left subareolar region. A small amount of heterogeneous parenchyma is seen in right subareolar region(a), while large amount of parenchyma is seen in left subareolar region(b) (white arrows).

A2. There are many causes of gynecomastia.

1. Physiological:
   (a) Neonatal period due to circulating maternal hormones.
   (b) Puberty.
2. Drug induced:
   (a) Marijuana.
   (b) Anabolic steroids.
   (c) Estrogen.
   (d) Spironolactone.
   (e) Digitalis.
   (f) Thiazide diuretics, etc.
3. Hypogonadism.
   (a) Klinefelter's syndrome.
4. Neoplasms.
   (a) Testicular tumors.
   (b) Adrenocortical tumors, etc.
5. Systemic causes:
   (a) Cirrhosis.
   (b) Chronic renal failure.

A3. There are three different patterns of gynecomastia.

1. Nodular pattern: Fan-shaped subareolar density which blurs into surrounding fat. This type is reversible upon removal of the causative factor.
2. Dendritic pattern: Flame-shaped subareolar density with linear projections radiating out from it into the deep adipose tissue. This is a more advanced type of gynecomastia which is associated with fibrosis and therefore is clinically and radiologically irreversible.

N. Chotai, S. Kulkarni, *Breast Imaging Essentials*, https://doi.org/10.1007/978-981-15-1412-8_20

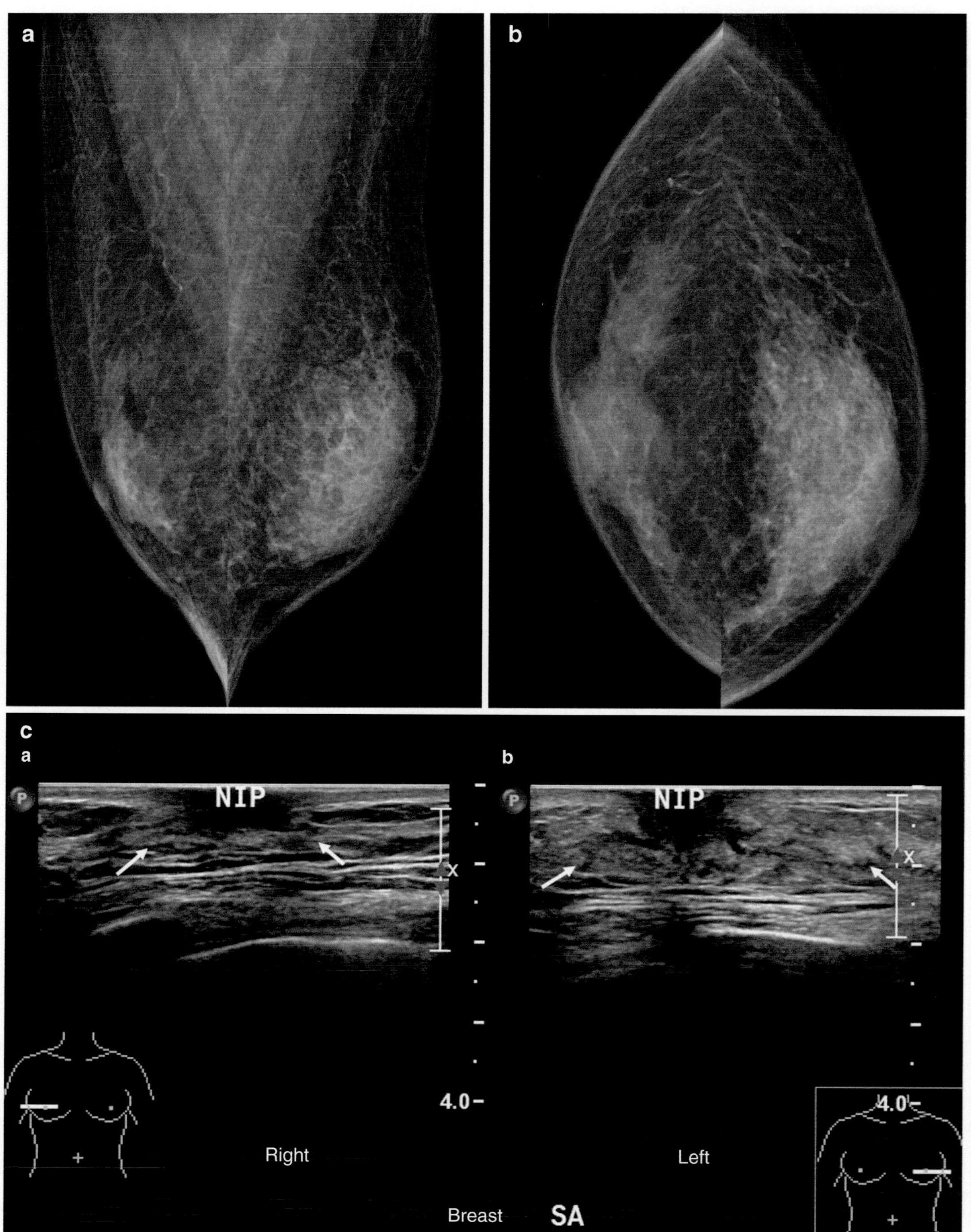

Fig. 20.1 (**a**) Bilateral MLO views. (**b**) Bilateral CC views. (**c**): Targeted ultrasound of bilateral subareolar region

3. Diffuse glandular pattern: This is usually seen in men receiving estrogen therapy. Heterogeneously dense breasts are seen bilaterally. They may contain patterns of nodular or dendritic gynecomastia and may resemble female breasts. Appearance

of ultrasound may mimic malignancy and therefore clinical history and lack of palpable finding can help differentiate benign from malignant.

Notes

Treatment of Gynecomastia

Physiologic causes such as hormonal imbalance during puberty usually regress spontaneously. In men with an identifiable cause, such as drug induced, gynecomastia can regress following discontinuation of the offending medication or treatment, unless the process has reached the irreversible fibrotic phase. Medical intervention in the form of androgens, selective estrogen-receptor modulators, and aromatase inhibitors may be helpful.

Cosmetic interventions such as reduction mammoplasty may be performed if the symptoms are unacceptable to the patients.

20.2 Case 20.2

History: 46-year-old male with right breast swelling.

Questions

Q1. Describe the imaging findings in Fig. 20.2a, b.

Q2. Provide possible differentials. What is the BI-RADS category?

Answers

A1. Right MLO and CC views (Fig. 20.2a) reveal a partially circumscribed mass in the upper outer quadrant of the breast (double white arrows), corresponding to the palpable mass marked with a radiopaque marker (thick white arrow). The mass shows irregular margins along its posterior aspect.

Corresponding ultrasound image (Fig. 20.2b) reveals a heterogeneous solid mass with microlobulated margins posteriorly, a few angular margins.

A2. Differential diagnosis includes:

1. Invasive mammary carcinoma.
2. Papillary carcinoma.
3. PASH.
4. Granular cell tumor.
5. Desmoid tumor.
6. Schwannoma.
7. Metastasis.

Category: BI-RADS 4.

Imaging features of the mass are suspicious and needs further assessment with an ultrasound-guided core biopsy.

Histopathology: Invasive ductal carcinoma.

Notes

Male Breast Cancer

Male breast cancer is rare and accounts for 1% of all breast cancers. It is usually unilateral and occurs bilaterally only in 1% of cases. BRCA gene mutations, family history, chest irradiation, Klinefelter's syndrome are the few causes which increase the likelihood of developing breast cancer in male patients. Male breast cancer presents at an older age than women and is likely to present at an advanced stage due to delay in diagnosis. Eighty percent of all male breast cancers are invasive ductal carcinoma followed by DCIS in 5%. They commonly present as a painless mass followed by other symptoms, including skin changes, nipple discharge, nipple changes, axillary lymph nodes, etc.

20.3 Case 20.3

History: 67-year-old male with left breast swelling. History of colorectal cancer.

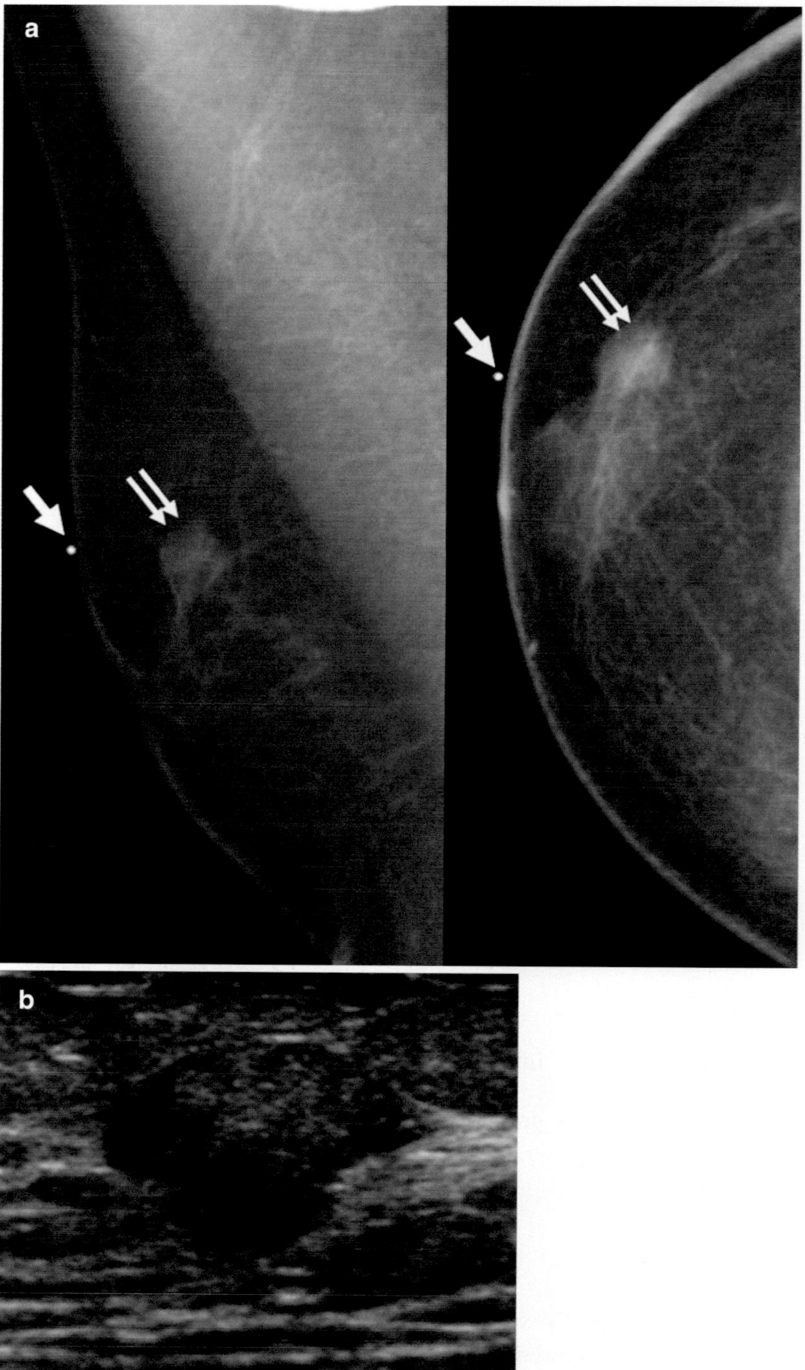

Fig. 20.2 (**a**) Right MLO and CC views. (**b**) Targeted ultrasound of right breast palpable lump

Questions

Q1. Describe imaging findings in Fig. 20.3a, b and give the BI-RADS category.
Q2. Provide possible differentials.

Answers

A1. Left MLO view (Fig. 20.3a) shows dense subareolar tissue with no discernable mass or calcifications. Corresponding ultrasound image (Fig. 20.3b) reveals a hypoechoic solid, slightly irregular mass which is indeterminate and requires further biopsy. Category: BI-RADS 4.
A2. Differential diagnosis will include:
1. Invasive mammary carcinoma.
2. Papillary carcinoma.
3. PASH.
4. Granular cell tumor.
5. Desmoid tumor.
6. Schwannoma.
7. Metastasis.

Given the personal history of colorectal cancer, the likely hood of metastasis is higher.

Histopathology: Colonic metastasis in the male breast.

Notes

Breast Metastasis

Metastatic lesions in the breast are rare, accounting of 0.5–3% of all malignant breast tumors in either gender. The common primary malignancies which can metastasize to the breast are melanomas, NHL, lung carcinoma, sarcomas, and gastric, renal, prostatic, or ovarian carcinomas. There is on average a 2-year interval between diagnosis of the primary nonmammary cancer and the detection of breast metastasis. Imaging appearances range from multiple well-circumscribed masses to palpable irregular masses with possible axillary lymph node involvement.

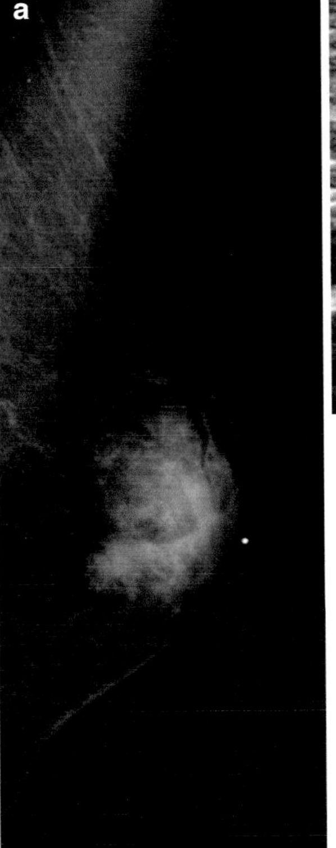

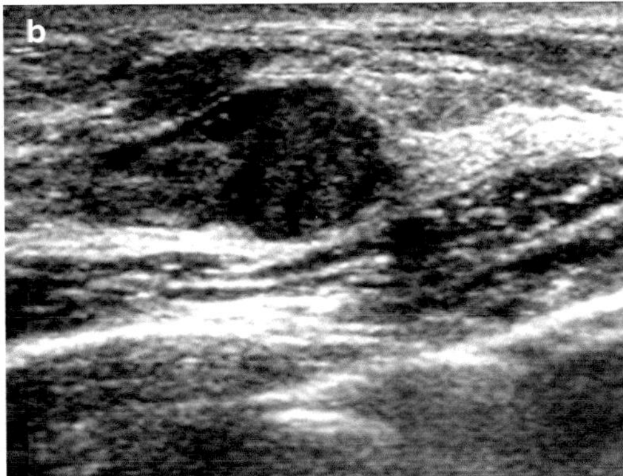

Fig. 20.3 (**a**) Left MLO view. (**b**) Targeted ultrasound of left breast palpable concern

20.4 Case 20.4

History: 43-year-old woman with left breast palpable lump over 3 months. History of fever and generalized weakness since a month.

Questions

Q1. Describe the findings on mammogram (Fig. 20.4a, b) and ultrasound (Fig. 20.4c). Give the appropriate BI-RADS.

Q2. What are the common differentials for multiple circumscribed breast lesions?

Q3. What is the definition of a primary breast lymphoma?

Answers

A1. Bilateral MLO (Fig. 20.4a) and CC views (Fig. 20.4b) show heterogeneously dense breast tissue. A metallic BB marker is placed over the upper outer quadrant of the left breast to annotate the site of clinically palpable lump. Two, partially circumscribed high-density masses are noted underlying the marker (double white arrows and thick white arrow). A few benign-appearing microcalcifications are seen in both breasts. Ultrasound images of left breast (Fig. 20.4c) show multiple iso- to hypoechoic masses in left breast at the 1, 2, 5, and 12 o'clock positions. Two dominant masses at the 1 o'clock and 2 o'clock positions likely correlate with the mammographic masses. The masses are generally circumscribed with some posterior enhancement, except for the dominant mass at 2 o'clock with some indistinct margin posteriorly. This lesion shows microlobulated margins. Findings are suggestive of multiple left breast masses, the dominant lesion being most suspicious on imaging. Ultrasound-guided biopsy is suggested. Category: BI-RADS 4.

A2. Common differentials to be considered for multiple circumscribed breast lesions include metastases, fibroadenomatas, multifocal-multicentric breast cancer, complicated cysts, breast lymphoma.

Histopathology: Histology report from the dominant mass was reported as lymphoma.

A3. The definition of primary breast lymphoma (PBL) includes the following four criteria:
1. Close anatomic proximity of mammary tissue and lymphoma.
2. No preceding diagnosis of extramammary lymphoma.
3. No evidence of disseminated disease, other than ipsilateral axillary lymphadenopathy.
4. Adequate quality of the histopathological specimen.

Notes

Primary Breast Lymphoma (PBL)

Incidence of primary breast lymphoma is <0.5% of all breast malignancies.

On imaging, no pathognomonic sign for breast lymphoma is described.

On mammogram, large circumscribed masses or asymmetry is the common imaging feature. Architectural distortion and microcalcifications are seldom seen in lymphoma.

On ultrasound, solitary or multiple, mixed echogenic to hypoechoic masses with regular or irregular outline are the commonest finding. Posterior acoustic shadowing that is frequently associated with breast carcinoma is generally not a feature in breast lymphoma.

MRI features are also not specific in breast lymphoma. Mass with restricted diffusion-weighted imaging, heterogeneous contrast enhancement are common features.

Some features on imaging that may favor lymphoma over carcinoma: (1) large size at presentation. Architectural distortion, microcalcifications, skin thickening and edema are less common in breast lymphoma than in breast carcinoma. (2) Multiplicity of lesions, specially circumscribed masses, should raise concern for lymphoma and metastasis in appropriate clinical settings.

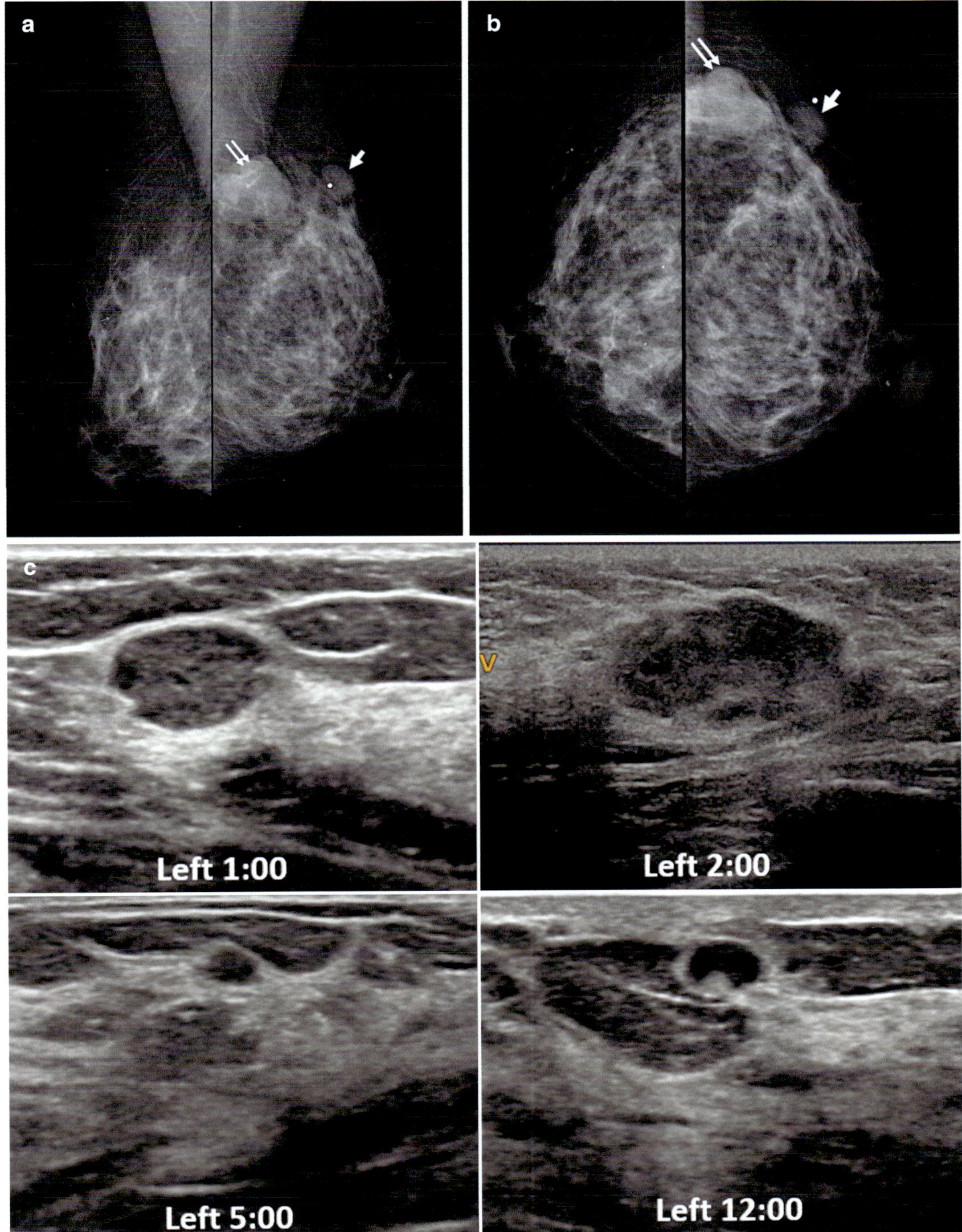

Fig. 20.4 (**a**) Bilateral MLO views. (**b**) Bilateral CC views. (**c**) Ultrasound of the left breast

Suggested Readings

Cuhaci N, Polat SB, Evranos B, Ersoy R, Cakir B. Gynecomastia: clinical evaluation and management. Ind J Endocrinol Metabol. 2014;18(2):150.

Lattin GE Jr, et al. Diseases of the male breast: radiologic pathologic correlation. Radiographics. 2013;33:461–89. https://doi.org/10.1148/rg.332125208.

Liberman L, Giess CS, Dershaw DD, Louie DC, Deutch BM. Non-Hodgkin lymphoma of the breast: imaging characteristics and correlation with histopathologic findings. Radiology. 1994;192(1):157–60.

Nguyen C, et al. Male Breast Disease: pictorial review with radiologic pathologic correlation. Radiographics. 2013;33:763–79. https://doi.org/10.1148/rg.333125137.

Sarıca Ö, Kahraman AN, Öztürk E, Teke M. Efficiency of imaging modalities in male breast disease can ultrasound give additional information for assessment of gynecomastia evolution? Eur J Breast Health. 2018;14(1):29.

Yang WT, Lane DL, Le-Petross HT, Abruzzo LV, Macapinlac HA. Breast lymphoma: imaging findings of 32 tumors in 27 patients. Radiology. 2007;245(3):692–702.

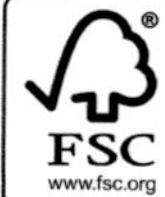

MIX
Papier aus verantwortungsvollen Quellen
Paper from responsible sources
FSC® C105338

If you have any concerns about our products,
you can contact us on
ProductSafety@springernature.com

In case Publisher is established outside the EU,
the EU authorized representative is:
Springer Nature Customer Service Center GmbH
Europaplatz 3, 69115 Heidelberg, Germany

Printed by Libri Plureos GmbH
in Hamburg, Germany